Public Health and Community Nursing
Frameworks for Practice

THIRD EDITION

Edited by

Dianne Watkins MSc EdD Cert Ed HV RM RN RNT
Director of External Relations, Learning and Teaching, Cardiff School of Nursing and Midwifery Studies, Cardiff University, Cardiff, UK

Judy Cousins MSc PGCE ONC RGN HV
Lecturer, Cardiff School of Nursing and Midwifery, Cardiff University, Cardiff, UK

Foreword by

Dean Whitehead BEd MSc PhD RN
Senior Lecturer, School of Health and Social Services, Massey University, Palmerston North, New Zealand

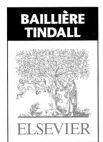
BAILLIÈRE TINDALL

ELSEVIER

Edinburgh London New York Oxford Philadelphia St Louis Sydney Toronto 2010

BAILLIÈRE
TINDALL
ELSEVIER

First edition published 1996
Second edition published 2003
Third edition © 2010, Elsevier Limited.

ISBN: 978 0 7020 2947 9

British Library Cataloguing in Publication Data
A catalogue record for this book is available from the British Library

Library of Congress Cataloging in Publication Data
A catalog record for this book is available from the Library of Congress

Notice

Knowledge and best practice in this field are constantly changing. As new research and experience broaden our knowledge, changes in practice, treatment and drug therapy may become necessary or appropriate. Readers are advised to check the most current information provided (i) on procedures featured or (ii) by the manufacturer of each product to be administered, to verify the recommended dose or formula, the method and duration of administration, and contraindications. It is the responsibility of the practitioner, relying on their own experience and knowledge of the patient, to make diagnoses, to determine dosages and the best treatment for each individual patient, and to take all appropriate safety precautions. To the fullest extent of the law, neither the Publisher nor the Authors assume any liability for any injury and/or damage to persons or property arising out of or related to any use of the material contained in this book.

The Publisher

ELSEVIER your source for books,
journals and multimedia
in the health sciences

www.elsevierhealth.com

Working together to grow
libraries in developing countries

www.elsevier.com | www.bookaid.org | www.sabre.org

ELSEVIER   BOOK AID
International   Sabre Foundation

The
publisher's
policy is to use
**paper manufactured
from sustainable forests**

Printed in China

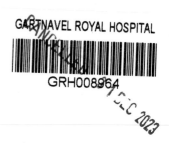
Public Health and Community Nursing

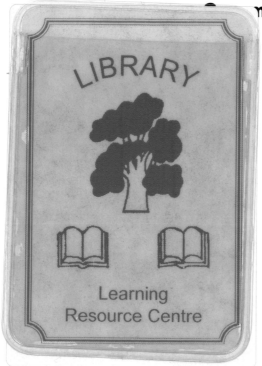

LIBRARY

Learning
Resource Centre

Commissioning Editor: Mairi McCubbin
Development Editor: Carole McMurray
Project Manager: Joannah Duncan
Designer: George Ajayi
Illustration Manager: Bruce Hogarth

Contents

Contributors

Graham Allan BA MA PhD
Professor of Sociology, University of Keele, Keele, UK

Carol Alstrom BSc MSc DipDN RN
Chief Nurse, NHS Isle of Wight, Primary Care Trust, UK

Bashyr Aziz PGCE PGDip RN OHNC SCPHN GradIOSH MIIRSM FHEA
Senior Lecturer in Primary Healthcare, University of Wolverhampton, Wolverhampton, UK

Helen Beswick MSc RGN
Community Matron, Bristol Primary Care Trust, Bristol, UK

Judith Carrier MSc PGCE DipPPSp RGN
Professional Head, Primary Care/Public Health Nursing, Cardiff School of Nursing and Midwifery, Cardiff University, Cardiff, UK

Joanne Chambers BSc BSc(DistrictNursing) PGcert RN
Emergency Nurse Practitioner, Bristol Primary Care Trust, Bristol, UK

Judy Cousins MSc PGCE ONC RGN HV
Lecturer, Cardiff School of Nursing and Midwifery, Cardiff University, Cardiff, UK

Sarah Cowley BA PhD PGDE RGN RCNT RHV HVT
Professor and Head of Public Health and Health Services Research Section, Florence Nightingale School of Nursing and Midwifery, King's College London, London, UK

David Stuart Coyle MEd CertEd RN
Senior Lecturer, University of Chester, Chester, UK

Graham Crow BSc MSc PhD
Professor of Sociology, University of Southampton, Southampton, UK; Deputy Director, ESRC National Centre for Research Methods

Denis D'Auria MA LLM MD DIH DipRCPath(Tox) CBiol MIBiol MFFLM FFOM FFOM(Lond)
Senior Lecturer in Toxicology and Occupational Medicine, Cardiff University; Honorary Consultant Occupational Physician, Cardiff and Vale NHS Trust, Cardiff, UK

Julie Davidson RGN
Nurse Independent/Supplementary Prescriber, Community Matron, Bristol Primary Care Trust, Bristol, UK

David L. Fone MD FFPH
Deputy Head: Department of Primary Care and Public Health Cardiff; Honorary Consultant in Public Heath Medicine, National Public Health Service for Wales, Cardiff, UK

Aileen Fraser MSc RGN NPD
Consultant Nurse for Older People/Safeguarding Adults, Bristol Community Health, North Bristol Primary Care Trust, Bristol, UK

Neil Frude MPhil PhD CPsychol FBPsS
Consultant Clinical Psychologist, Cardiff and Vale NHS Trust, Cardiff, UK

Ros Godson RGN
Professional Officer, Community Practitioners' and Health Visitors' Association, London, UK

Alison Hann BA(Hons) PhD
Lecturer, School of Health Science, Swansea University, Swansea, UK

Ben Hannigan BA(Hons) MA PhD PGCE RMN RGN DPSN
Senior Lecturer, Cardiff School of Nursing and Midwifery Studies, Cardiff University, Cardiff, UK

Lorraine Joomun MSc CHSdip PGCE RGN HV
Lecturer, Cardiff School of Nursing and Midwifery, Cardiff University, Cardiff, UK

Pat McCamley BSc SRN ONC DIP/DN
Clinical Lead, District Nursing, NHS, Primary Care Trust, Isle of Wight

Nigel Monaghan MSc BDS LLM FFPH FDS RCPS(Glasg)
Deputy Director of Health and Social Care Quality, National Public Health Service, Cardiff, UK

Shantini Paranjothy MB ChB MSc PhD
Lecturer in Public Health Medicine, Cardiff University, Cardiff, UK

Stephen Peckham BSc MA(Econ) HMFPH
Reader in Health Policy, Director NCCSDO, London
School of Hygiene and Tropical Medicine, London, UK

Celia Phipps BSc MSc RGN HV
Locality Manager (Adults), Bristol Primary Care Trust,
Bristol, UK

Kirsten Robson BSc PGC (AP) RN
Community Matron, Bristol Primary Care Trust, Bristol,
UK

Anna Sidey DNCert RSCN RGN
Independent Adviser in Community Children's Nursing,
Stretton, UK

Rhianwen Elen Stiff BSc MBBCh
Walport Academic Clinical Fellow in Public Health
Medicine, Cardiff University, Cardiff, UK

Janet Vokes BSc(Hons) RGN
ENT Leader, Bristol Community Health/North Bristol NHS
Trust, Bristol, UK

Dianne Watkins MSc EdD CertEd HV RM RN RNT
Director of External Relations, Learning and Teaching,
Cardiff School of Nursing and Midwifery Studies, Cardiff
University, Cardiff, UK

John Watkins BSc MB BCh MRCGP FFFPH
Clinical Senior Lecturer in Epidemiology/Consultant in
Public Health Medicine, Department of Primary Care and
Public Health, School of Medicine, Cardiff University,
Cardiff, UK

David Widdas RGN RSCN DN
Consultant Nurse for Children with Complex Care
Needs – Coventry and Warwickshire; Honorary Lecturer,
University of Coventry and the University of Birmingham

Ruth Wyn Williams BN(Hons) MSc PGDip RN(Adult) RNLD
PhD student, School of Healthcare Sciences, Bangor
University, Bangor, UK

Foreword

During my long and ongoing 'crusade' to champion all things health promotion for nurses and nursing – several things have remained a constant to me. One is a distinct lack of nursing-specific quality texts that encompass how, why and where health promotion should most distinctly occur. While I have espoused the validity of 'seamless services', where health promotion crosses the traditional divide of acute and community provision, most will acknowledge that the majority of health promotion activity occurs in the community setting – and within a public health context. With the advent of this new edition the above-mentioned issues are addressed. It is a quality text aimed primarily at nurses with an interest in public health. Although much of the book is aimed at nurses working in a community environment, it has relevance for all nurses wherever they work.

Another constant for me has been the ability (or lack of it) for most nurses to both understand and engage in the political landscape that underpins most health promotion practice (Whitehead 2003a, 2003b). Accompanying this, I have often been bemused by nursing's unwillingness to acknowledge and embrace the wider dimensions of health promotion that are more relevant for the practice of today's community-based health professionals (Whitehead 2004, 2005, 2006, 2007, 2008). This book directly faces up to those challenges. It espouses a much-needed awareness of the changing landscape of primary healthcare and public health. In doing so, it addresses the fundamental principles of a required wider agenda for health promotion through exploring dimensions such as population health, health and social policy and social capital – all correctly aligned to a socio-ecological model of practice. More importantly, this book does all this in such a way that it is accessible to both nurse practitioners and undergraduate and postgraduate students working in a variety of community-based specific disciplines. This book is also accessible through its sequential format. It begins with a section that explores the current landscape of public health and its frameworks (Sections 1 and 2) right through to a concluding section on 'challenges for the future' (Section 5).

Unique to this book, it extends its content to a framework where readers can appreciate the applicability of theoretical concepts to practice. In particular, this uniqueness extends to particular sections of the book that focus on both the importance of 'family-centredness' (Section 3) and discipline-specific roles (Section 4). While, for the most part, this book is located against the backdrop of UK-based policy and clinical examples this does not exclude it from a wider audience. Such is its range and diversity that most readers will benefit from its content in some way. It is with this in mind and the other above-mentioned strengths of this book that I wholeheartedly recommend this text to anyone who is interested in health promotion, community health and public health – and I hope that you enjoy it and gain from it as much as I have.

Dean Whitehead
MSc, PhD, BEd, RN
Senior Lecturer
Massey University
School of Health and Social Services
Palmerston North
New Zealand

References

Whitehead D 2003a Incorporating socio-political health promotion activities in nursing practice. Journal of Clinical Nursing 12(5): 668–677

Whitehead D 2003b The health-promoting nurse as a policy expert and entrepreneur. Nurse Education Today 23(8): 585–592

Whitehead D 2004 Health promotion and health education: advancing the concepts. Journal of Advanced Nursing 47(4): 311–320

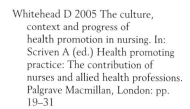

Whitehead D 2005 The culture, context and progress of health promotion in nursing. In: Scriven A (ed.) Health promoting practice: The contribution of nurses and allied health professions. Palgrave Macmillan, London: pp. 19–31

Whitehead D 2006 Health promotion in the practice setting: findings from a review of clinical issues. Worldviews on Evidence-Based Nursing 3(4): 165–184

Whitehead D 2007 Reviewing health promotion in nursing education. Nurse Education Today 27: 225–237

Whitehead D 2008 Arriving at a consensus for health promotion and health education in nursing practice, education and policy: an international Delphi study. Journal of Clinical Nursing 17(7): 891–900

The ever-changing political context continues to influence public and primary healthcare, hence the need for revising the content of this book, ensuring it offers as contemporary a view as any textbook can. The NHS is witnessing radical reforms in an attempt to redress the imbalance in health across social groups in society (Welsh Assembly Government (WAG) 2005, 2008, Scottish Executive Health Department 2005, Department of Health, Social Services and Public Safety (DHSSPS) 2005, Department of Health 2004, 2008). Inequalities in health influenced by structural and environmental issues, and beyond the control of the individual, are guiding public health practice, while the organization of public health and primary healthcare is again under review (Department of Health 2006, NHS Scotland 2005, WAG 2008). Different models of public health and primary care organizations are emerging across the four countries of the United Kingdom, with devolution playing a major part in determining differences between these. An increased emphasis on prevention, expedient transition of patients from acute to primary care, resource effectiveness, efficient commissioning of services and patient and public involvement, as well as protection of vulnerable groups, are major drivers for change.

This third edition of *Public Health and Community Nursing – Frameworks for Practice* brings these issues to the forefront and considers the implications for nurses in the delivery of public health and care in the community. It updates each chapter and responds to the changing landscape of working to improve health. This is evident from inclusion in this edition of chapters on: epidemiology and its application to practice, the influence of social capital on health, needs assessment and commissioning, promoting health: frameworks for practice, occupational health nursing, partnership working in health and social care, developments in promoting workforce health and advancing public health in nursing practice. These new chapters broaden the scope of the book and increase its public health focus.

The text remains broad based and is designed to support students undertaking graduate and postgraduate programmes, at a pre-registration and post-registration level. Students studying for first registration in the fields of mental health, learning disability and adult and children's nursing would benefit from using elements of this book as an accompaniment to their community modules and associated clinical placements. It would help them to understand the broad nature of public health and primary healthcare and the roles of various nursing professionals working within the field, as well as guiding them through those factors that adversely affect health and well-being.

Qualified nurses studying for either a specialist practice qualification in district nursing, community mental health nursing, community learning disability nursing, practice nursing, or community children's nursing, or nurses studying for a specialist community public health nurse qualification in health visiting, school nursing or occupational health nursing will find this book invaluable to their studies. Nurses undertaking study into public health at Masters level would also find useful material within this third edition. This new version has incorporated chapters specifically relating to occupational health nursing along with all the other disciplines, thereby increasing its acceptability to these groups of specialist community nurses. It aims to provide a stimulating resource for both public health and community nursing students and educators in clinical practice and higher education institutions. The book poses questions and issues for reflection, seminars and debate, as well as offering referenced and recommended reading to promote depth and breadth of study.

As editors we made a decision to continue with a 'framework' approach that links social and health policy with public health and community nursing practice. There is a deliberate overlap in some parts of the book to guide the reader through a multitude of subject areas that interlink, thus reinforcing important messages. Each chapter is cross-referenced with other chapters, which allows the reader to gain an in-depth knowledge of particular areas and assists with building the 'picture' of nursing in a public health, community, workplace and primary care environment.

Structure and organization of the book

The book is organized into five sections, each using a different perspective to explore the issues relevant to public health and community nursing practice. Section 1 focuses on the changing landscape of public health, highlighting relevant health and social policy developments and their consequent effects on the organization and management of public health and primary care.

Section 2 uses public health as a framework for practice, with chapters that explore the use of epidemiology as a method of gathering an evidence base for practice. The section continues with a vision of the modern public health movement and emphasizes the use of a social model of health. The emphasis in this section is on those factors that adversely affect health and the associated issues for preventative work. Needs assessment and the commissioning process are examined and a framework for undertaking a needs analysis is presented. The next chapter in this section outlines frameworks for promoting health, providing an overview of the theory of health promotion and how this fits into a public health framework. The final chapter in Section 2 outlines developments in promoting workplace health, and presents numerous frameworks for practice.

Section 3 reviews the family as a framework for public health and community nursing practice, outlining sociological and psychological perspectives. Society's view of what constitutes a family changes over time, and the perceived functions of a family all impact upon the way in which nurses deliver care in any environment. Violence and abuse in families is a major health-related problem and one which public health and community nurses need to be aware of when undertaking an assessment. Protecting children from abuse is of importance to all nurses, and an ecological framework for prevention of violence to children by their parents is presented in this chapter. In the final chapter in this section the family is discussed as a provider of healthcare, as well as the unit for nursing assessment. It presents a way of working with families that would suit all public health and community nurses, regardless of the specialism being studied.

Section 4 contains chapters pertaining to each of the specialist areas of community nursing previously mentioned. Each chapter outlines the historical development of that area of nursing, highlights issues relevant to current practice, and discusses the future development in relation to health and social policies. The section, read in its totality, will serve to provide an overview of nursing in a public health, workplace and primary healthcare setting, accurately describing how each diverse discipline contributes to the delivery of care through collaboration and team working.

The final section is concerned with partnership working in health and social care, alternative ways of working and advancing public health in nursing practice. New nursing roles associated with greater autonomy are rapidly developing in public health and primary care settings, leading to new issues associated with partnership working, accountability and promoting patient and public involvement. These concerns are addressed in the first chapter of this section. The next chapter illustrates the emergence of a diverse range of nursing roles in public health and community nursing practice. The editors present a final chapter in this section which brings together many of the issues discussed within the book and introduces a framework of engagement that outlines nurses' current involvement in public health. It debates ways in which nursing could further develop public health in practice and advocates for recognition of the nurse's contribution to the nation's health.

This book is by no means inclusive of all issues influencing public health in nursing practice. It does, however, provide an overview of the complexities influencing and shaping the current and future practice of public health and community nursing. An important message based on our personal beliefs is that, although we play a critical part in the lives of many people on their pathway to recovery or death, our role will only be valued if we value others. Each person's experience of illness or health is unique, shaped by personal life experience, and this must be respected. As public health and community nurses we are privileged to share people's homes and families and we must never abuse our position. This philosophy underpins each page of this new edition of *Public Health and Community Nursing – Frameworks for Practice*.

Dianne Watkins and Judy Cousins, Cardiff, 2010

References

Department of Health 2004 Choosing health. The Stationery Office, London

Department of Health 2006 Our health, our care, our say. The Stationery Office, London

Department of Health 2008 High quality care for all: NHS next stage review. Final report. The Stationery Office, London

Department of Health, Social Services and Public Safety 2005 Caring for people beyond tomorrow: a strategic framework for the development of primary health and social care. The Stationery Office, Belfast

NHS Scotland 2005 The national framework for service change in NHS Scotland: elective care action team – final report. Scottish Executive Health Department, Edinburgh

Scottish Executive Health Department 2005 Delivering for health. Scottish Executive Health Department, Edinburgh

Welsh Assembly Government 2005 Designed for life: creating world class health and social care for Wales in the 21st century. Wales Assembly Government, Cardiff

Welsh Assembly Government 2008 Proposals to change the structure of the NHS in Wales: Consultation paper. Wales Assembly Government, Cardiff

Section **One**

The changing landscape of public health

There are numerous issues that have and continue to influence the landscape of public health. These relate to the political agenda, developments in primary care, the emergence of the modern public health movement, changes in demography and disease patterns. New ways of identifying health and social needs are outlined in this section.

The first chapter opens with a review of recent health and social policy developments, their background, introduction and likely impact. It covers issues surrounding devolution, public health and primary care development and public involvement. Against this backdrop the second chapter examines definitions and growth of primary care in the United Kingdom, the impact of the General Medical Services contract and the changing patterns of work in primary care. The changing landscape of primary care will lead to greater diversification of roles. The chapter concludes by urging nurses to consider the impact of the changes outlined on primary health-care services, and on the development of public health and community nursing.

Chapter 3 follows with a discussion on innovation and change in public health. It commences with an overview of the function and historical development of public health practice and draws attention to the pressures for change. It explores the need to incorporate a social model of health in the drive to reduce the impact of poverty and key health issues are discussed from a public health perspective. The authors conclude with examples, drawn from a case study of health and social needs assessment carried out in the Caerphilly County Borough, South Wales, which illustrates a social model of health in action.

Recent health and social policy developments

Stephen Peckham and Alison Hann

KEY ISSUES

- The policy history of public health and primary care services
- The influence of devolution on UK health service delivery
- Quality, regulation and performance in UK healthcare
- The increasing emphasis on patient and public involvement in healthcare

Introduction

It is not surprising that health continues to dominate the political agenda in the UK. Like education it is a service that is open to all and used by the majority of the population at some point in their lives. It is possible to opt out by using private health services but this remains a minority group of people. Despite recent increases in National Health Service (NHS) funding, controversies over deficits, funding for new drugs and changes in hospital provision (especially relating to maternity and accident and emergency departments) have kept the NHS on the agenda. Despite national concerns, devolution has created some clear distinctions in rhetoric and health policy between England, Scotland, Wales and Northern Ireland. In England ideas of independence from the centre with more control given to clinicians and healthcare professionals to act in the interests of patients, forming an independent NHS board and creating an NHS constitution have dominated political discussion in 2006 and 2007. But this is at a time when both the Scottish Parliament and Welsh Assembly are taking a stronger, central role in health

policy. The NHS in England is also developing the role of the private and not-for-profit sectors in healthcare and further embedding a healthcare market while in Northern Ireland, Scotland and Wales the emphasis has been on partnerships, professional engagement and central planning – often to overcome fragmentation and improve integration.

Changes in healthcare are, however, driven by wider changes in society and substantial shifts in how social problems are addressed. While much of the map of healthcare in the last 20–30 years can be seen as a response to shifts in the types of health problems faced by people and to meet the demands of an ageing population, health is not something separate from the rest of the social context: it is inextricably bound up with income, housing, education and every other facet of public policy. There can be no lasting good health without income adequate to provide the required diet and clothing, or without adequate housing and the means to heat it. Health is improved and health inequalities diminished not just, or even primarily, by attention to health – housing, income and all the other aspects of welfare are just as likely to be in need of attention and to be capable of making a contribution to the health of the populace – a situation that has increasingly been realized by successive governments in relation to public health policy (Baggott 2004).

A central theme of New Labour's approach to social welfare has been termed the 'Third Way' highlighting the link between welfare and work with an emphasis on opportunity with responsibility, balancing state control with market approaches to deliver high quality, responsive services (Peckham and Meerabeau 2007). We can see how these ideas dominate debates about welfare services today with the emphasis on paid work, rights and responsibilities and the individual's relationship with welfare services encompassed in debates about self-care and proposals to increase choice in healthcare services. Choice currently dominates the public services agenda and how this, together with welfare pluralism and increasing privatization, impact on the type of welfare state in the UK is very important, particularly in relation to an analysis of inequalities within the UK. In health and social care choice has become a dominant paradigm with service users cast as consumers. In England, *Our Health, Our Care, Our Say* (Department of Health 2006) explicitly focuses on the role of the consumer as being responsible for managing their own health and choosing between different locations for treatment. How these approaches affect the current organization and delivery of health services is critical to an understanding of the NHS and healthcare. This chapter looks at some of these areas in more detail, exploring the impact of devolution, patient choice, public health and inequality and ensuring quality services. The chapter ends by highlighting some of the key challenges in healthcare and policy and how these are likely to impact on community health nurses.

Policy history

While this chapter focuses on more recent policy developments it is important to understand these policy changes within the overall context of health policy in the UK over the last 150 years. Much of the shape of the NHS and key problems to which policy is addressed are the result of professional and policy developments in the 19th century, at the birth of the NHS in 1947 and organizational changes in the 1970s, 1980s and 1990s. This history has been amply dealt with elsewhere (Klein 2006). In fact, many of the policy developments since 1947 have been to address key tensions which continue to haunt the delivery of healthcare in the UK today:

- the tension between central or local control and management
- the tension between medical and management power
- the tension between treating individuals and providing a population-based service within a capped budget
- the tension between treatment and prevention of ill health.

Furthermore, current policy developments can be seen as part of the continuing response to developments in health and welfare which have been termed the 'crisis in health' (Ham 2004). Many of the features of the 'crisis in health' were visible in all industrialized countries and had their roots in concerns about the rapidly escalating costs of healthcare, although the 'crisis' reflects concern about a range of issues of which those given in Box 1.1 are seen to be the most significant.

Part of the response to the 'crisis' was the recognition that changes in the epidemiology and demographics of disease required a different approach to health and healthcare from one that focused on the delivery of acute care. Thus in dealing with chronic illness and supporting older people, the role of general practice and community health services became more central. In the UK the response was to develop general practice and primary healthcare teams and led to an increasing engagement of government and the NHS in developing the quality and role of primary care (Peckham and Exworthy 2003). There was also a retrenchment with an initial focus

Box 1.1

Pressures for change: factors in the 'crisis in health'

- Demographic changes – the UK has an ageing population while at the same time a reduction in the proportion of the population of working age, leading to an increasing demand for healthcare at a time when health systems will be limited in their ability to respond to this demand.
- Epidemiological transition – a move from a major preoccupation with infectious diseases to one concerned with chronic conditions.
- Changing relationships between patients and healthcare professionals.
- Concern with social factors – the biomedical or curative approach to health is being questioned, with a search for a broader approach which takes into account social factors, recognizes the harmful effects of the environment and shifts the emphasis on to prevention of ill health.
- Continuing concerns about inequalities of health and the recognition that these are deep-seated.
- The ever-widening gap between demands made on healthcare services and the resources which the government is prepared to make available.

on high-spending hospitals but a recognition that control also needed to be exercised over the gate-keepers to the NHS. The last 20 years have also seen an increasing overlap between primary and community care services. The issue of collaboration between health and social care agencies is not a new one but there has been an increasing emphasis on health and social care partnerships during the 1990s and the Labour government placed partnership at the centre of its proposals and developments for the NHS and Social Services (Glendinning et al 2001). It is now widely recognized that while the pathologies of chronic disease are diverse, the needs of people with long-term conditions are broadly similar in that they have to learn to manage the disease, integrate it with their everyday life, engage in health maintenance activities, confront the progression of the disease and in many cases their death from the disease. For the health service to influence the overall prevalence of chronic illness and the morbidity of the population it needs to develop not only clinically effective interventions but also acceptable strategies to engage directly with the individual and the family. Some of these themes are clearly of continuing importance and approaches to developing community-based services and supporting people with chronic health problems are the subject of current developments in policies for self-care and service reorganization (Department of Health 2006, Kerr 2005).

Current contexts

However, while New Labour set out a UK-wide approach to health and healthcare in 1997 and 1998 that attempted to redress some of the problems it identified from the previous Conservative government's approach, the introduction of political devolution has introduced a new dynamic to health policy. Initial developments post-1997 suggested a more bureaucratic approach to ensuring national standards with national service frameworks (NSFs), national criteria for standards and quality of care, agreed approaches to clinical practice (through the National Institute for Health and Clinical Excellence (NICE) and the Commission for Health Improvement (CHI)) and a commitment to tackle inequalities in healthcare and health. Proposals included better access (such as the introduction of NHS Direct (NHS 24 in Scotland)), a commitment to driving up quality with a stronger emphasis on clinical governance, stronger professional regulation and improved education and training, a renewed focus on addressing public health problems and a recognition of the critical role of individuals in their own care with a shift, also, towards consumer or patient choice (Department of Health 1997, 2000, NHS Scotland 2000, NHS Wales 2001). The remainder of this chapter, therefore, examines the impact of devolution, the emphasis on performance and standards, public health and changing relationships with patients and the public.

Devolution

While initial responses in England, Wales, Scotland and Northern Ireland identified common issues in terms of moving away from the internal market and two-tierism of previous policy, devolution has gradually created substantive differences in the focus and direction of health policy with partnership more central to developments in Scotland and Wales whereas England has increasingly drawn on market-based approaches. Since the beginning of the NHS there have always been important differences in the organization and delivery of healthcare services between England, Northern Ireland, Scotland and Wales. Essentially England and Wales operated the same structure and organization, but Scotland had health boards rather than authorities, and Northern Ireland has combined health and social care departments. Many elements of the system were, however, the same including the general practitioner system, role and location of public health, and delivery of community services. Since the Labour government came to power in 1997 much has changed, following political devolution to the Scottish Parliament and Welsh Assembly and, although rather spasmodic, to the Northern Ireland Assembly.

Although the capacity for policy diversity post-devolution varies in each territory, the UK operates as a unitary state with a parliamentary system (based at Westminster) and there is some uniformity through new institutions such as NICE (England and Wales only) and the NHS Quality Improvement Scotland (although NICE guidelines are applicable to Scotland and the two organizations work together), the provision of national pay and conditions contracts such as the new contract for GPs (see Chapter 2) and similarities between some policies such as service frameworks. The important role of NICE is underlined by the high media profile it has – especially around the sanctioning of the use of new drugs (e.g. Herceptin in 2006) and on services (such as choice in maternity services and place of birth in 2006). NICE guidelines are sent to all NHS trusts and while not mandatory it is expected that trusts take the guidelines into account. Details of all guidelines and how they are developed are on the NICE website (http://www.nice.org.uk). Political devolution has continued to increase diversity as it has allowed greater policy experimentation but it may also facilitate uniformity. For example, comparisons are being made between health services performance in England where waiting lists are being reduced and Wales where performance has been criticized (Audit Commission in Wales 2004, Healthcare Commission 2005) and also in terms of public health policy where Scotland and Wales introduced a ban on smoking in enclosed public places before England.

Scotland already enjoyed considerable administrative devolution which is complemented by political devolution to the Scottish Parliament and measures adopted in Scotland (e.g. the introduction of free personal care and student grants) have demonstrated that the Scottish Parliament is determined to set its own political course. In many ways Scotland is becoming a distinctively different country. Since self-government came to Scotland in 1999 there has been a huge raft of legislation creating clear policy differences with the rest of the UK including free personal and nursing care, no student tuition fees, and a range of policies on health, social care and education. The Welsh Assembly is responsible for allocating NHS expenditure in Wales but as yet has no law-making powers although the provision for this is now available. Pressure for political change and the creation of a Welsh Parliament remains a very live debate particularly since elections in 2007 when to achieve a governing coalition in the Assembly the Welsh Labour Party agreed terms with Plaid Cymru to explore the establishment of a separate Parliament for Wales. In Wales the emphasis is on partnership and the coterminosity of local authorities and the local health boards (established April 2003), with their broad memberships, do provide opportunities for close cooperation and coordinated activity.

In contrast, in England, the Secretary of State is perhaps more politically remote from the delivery of healthcare than in Scotland and Wales, and the NHS has undergone successive reorganizations driven from the centre. Pressure from the centre for quick results is likely to continue to remain a key feature of the English NHS despite recent debates about increased autonomy, decentralization and independence for the NHS which have been associated with the new administration of Gordon Brown. Organizational change is a constant feature of English health policy and a review in 2005/06 led to a reduction in the number of strategic health authorities (SHAs) and primary care trusts (PCTs) (Department of Health 2005a). The reduction in the number of PCTs was also widely anticipated for a number of years, completing a consolidation of commissioning that started with the move from primary care groups (PCGs) to PCTs between 2000 and 2003. The key argument is that small commissioners were failing and lacked the skills and resources to commission effectively. Concerns about the quality and strength of PCT commissioning have also been highlighted given the accelerated expansion of foundation trust status to all NHS trusts in the next few years and the introduction of payment by results. The changes that these developments will bring to NHS contracts and financial flows (especially coupled with patient choice) present enormous challenges to healthcare commissioners. There are now half the number of PCTs (152) and there has been some rationalization of boundaries to bring greater coterminosity between social services departments and PCTs. However, it is hard to see any clear rationale for the changes across the country. The smallest PCT (Hartlepool) has a population of 90 000 while the largest (Hampshire) has a population of 1.2 million. One important impact of the focus on commissioning is the assessment being made about the provision of community health services by PCTs and encouragement to privatize these services or at least examine alternative models of provision such as independent social enterprise organizations or community interest companies (Department of Health 2006).

Size and capacity of primary care organizations have also been of concern in Wales and this has resulted in the amalgamation of the activities of the 22 local health boards into three regions (resembling the old health authority boundaries) in order to develop commissioning capacity in the wake of poor performance reports and financial problems (Audit Commission in Wales 2004, Healthcare Commission 2005, Welsh Assembly Government 2005). While the proposed regions are an attempt to create better service integration and avoid fragmentation in Wales, the response to similar concerns in Scotland has resulted in changes at a more local level. The NHS in Scotland has just completed development of a more formal localized structure with the establishment of community health partnerships – bringing together community healthcare service providers and coordinating a wide range of primary medical and community health resources – to provide the delivery and planning of health services at a local level (SEHD 2005). Greater integration and reduction of fragmentation are cornerstones of Welsh and Scottish health policy across both commissioning and provision. This is at odds with England where the need for larger commissioning organizations is developing alongside a greater fragmentation of healthcare provision with an emphasis on greater provider plurality and patient choice (Department of Health 2006).

Quality, regulation and performance

Since the late 1990s there has been a steady increase in healthcare regulation in the UK, but especially in England. Before this, regulation was mainly a matter of professional self-regulation underpinned by the state. However, a series of scandals since the mid 1990s (e.g. the Bristol Royal Infirmary and Alder Hay, as well as individual 'maverick' doctors such as Shipman, Leward and Ayling) led to an overhaul of the way in which hospital trusts and clinical practice were regulated, inspected and managed. Central to changes have been the reports on the Bristol, Alder Hay and Shipman cases where extensive inquiries made recommendations about making the NHS safer, more open and accountable and improving NHS performance in monitoring the performance of clinicians and other healthcare professionals (Department of Health 2001, Shipman Inquiry 2001, 2004). In the wake of these, and other, debacles, a number of bodies were created to set and monitor national standards and to assess NHS performance. For example, the Blair administration created a new healthcare professions regulatory council, and the CHI, renamed the Healthcare Commission in 2005, was responsible for investigating serious service failures, undertook independent reviews of complaints, regulated the registration of independent healthcare providers and undertook an annual 'health check' to assess the performance of healthcare organizations in England and Wales. It worked closely with the Commission for Social Care Inspection (itself an amalgamation of two previous regulatory agencies) to undertake joint inspections. The Commission also worked with the Care and Social Services Inspectorate in Wales and, in Scotland, the NHS Quality Improvement Scotland. In 2009, further changes occurred with Wales establishing its own inspection arrangements, and in England the Healthcare Commission and social care regulator merged to form the Care Quality Commission. The Commission is a statutory non-departmental public body which is accountable to Parliament as well as to health ministers. For foundation trusts there are additional regulatory structures. In England there are additional regulatory arrangements for foundation trusts through MONITOR which is predominantly concerned with financial and governance issues. Despite the strengthening of regulatory arrangements, major scandals have not been averted, and in 2009, a major clinical management issue leading to excess deaths was identified in a Staffordshire hospital.

Another important part of the government's regulatory approach was the setting of clinical standards through NSFs and NICE. NICE was established in 1999 to provide evidence on the cost-effectiveness of new and existing healthcare interventions, to develop clinical guidelines for various conditions and also to help the NHS with clinical audit, with Health Quality Scotland performing a similar function. NSFs are long-term strategies for improving specific areas of care; they set national standards and identify key interventions for a defined service or care group (such as older people) and are one of a range of measures which aim to raise quality and decrease service variations. Each NSF is developed with the assistance of an external reference group (ERG) which draws on the expertise of health professionals, service users and carers, health service managers, and partner agencies. NSFs currently cover coronary heart disease, cancer, paediatric intensive care, mental health, older people, diabetes, long-term conditions and renal services, children and chronic obstructive pulmonary disease. The NSFs also emphasize the importance of working across the health and social care boundary, particularly for people with complex needs such as the elderly or the mentally ill. (See Chapter 14 for further information relating to care of the elderly with complex needs and Chapter 18 for information on care of the mentally ill.)

Public health

In addition to the emphasis on primary and community care, the 'crisis in health' and renewed attention paid to health inequalities led to a renewed interest in public health (Baggott 2000). The NHS has predominantly been concerned with caring for the sick, and medicine has been primarily concerned with curing the sick rather than broader aims of promoting health and preventing disease. Despite increasing health expenditures in the post-war period there has been an increase in major chronic diseases such as cardiovascular diseases, as well as in cancer, accidents and alcohol-related conditions. Most importantly it became recognized that these are preventable and that the focus of health and healthcare should change, with an increasing emphasis on reducing morbidity and mortality rates through a broad range of public health measures (Baggott 2000). A new development, however, is that prevention may now entail medicalization and a great expenditure on medicines, if, for example, the recommendations for prescribing statins are put into practice.

One key theme of the government's approach to public health since 1997 has been the renewed emphasis on tackling health inequalities and the approach has broadly been within the context of the 'new public health' – an approach combining government and collective action with individual approaches to lifestyle change. Since 1997, the Labour government has taken various steps associated with tackling health inequalities. One of its first actions was to commission an independent inquiry into inequalities in health, chaired by Sir Donald Acheson, the former Chief Medical Officer. The inquiry reported in November 1998 and only three recommendations were directed to the NHS – underlining the relative contribution of healthcare services to tacking health inequality compared to poverty, education, employment, housing, transport and nutrition (Acheson 1998). However, while early public health policy did not specifically address health inequalities, the emphasis on addressing inequality was central to *Making a Difference* (Department of Health 1999), which promoted the importance of nurses, midwives and health visitors working with the wider community and across organizational boundaries undertaking health promotion activities. However, the lack of clarity and huge scope of the public health function, and the organizational diversity of public health practice has led to problems in defining public health roles and prioritizing public health activities by community health staff.

Similarly in Scotland and Wales there has been a focus on the need to address health inequalities which, in these countries, have been seen as key problem areas for many years (Baggott 2000). Both the Welsh Assembly and the Scottish Parliament have emphasized the development of public health measures and there are clear differences in the approach to public health in England, Scotland and Wales despite a similar emphasis on reducing health inequalities and tackling key public health problems. Distinct differences in the organization and shape of public health services are beginning to emerge in England, Northern Ireland, Scotland and Wales. In Scotland, the role of the Scottish Parliament is likely to become more significant and it may take a more multisectoral approach to public health. Moreover, the founding of the National Public Health Services in Wales, which brings the public health resources of the five former health authorities together under one national organization, promises strong national leadership in public health to support multidisciplinary action that cuts across policy and organizational boundaries. In Northern Ireland, future developments are less clear (Appleby 2005). Within the existing health and social care workforce, it is nurses who have received most attention, and their existing and potential contribution to the public health agenda has been both recognized and supported. In England, while inequalities and the need for government action are still seen as high priorities, there is a shifting emphasis towards self-care and individual responsibility for prevention and lifestyle choices (Department of Health 2004). The Treasury commissioned a further report on public health (Wanless 2004) and a further White Paper *Choosing Health* was published in 2004 setting public health policy. However, despite concerted government statements about developing public health approaches, financial constraints in 2005/06 tended to focus attention on the acute healthcare sector and limit resources for public health. So as we move further into this new century the role of public health and the commitment to eradicating health inequalities remain uncertain.

Perhaps the most important recent innovation affecting public health delivery in the UK has been the introduction of the new General Medical Services (GMS) contract and a financial incentive scheme – the Quality and Outcomes Framework (QOF) – rewarding specific areas of activity. The new contract introduced key changes to the incentive structures for public health activities in general practice (see Chapter 2). It is widely accepted that explicit financial incentives do encourage practices to maximize their potential income but it is not clear how this then affects wider public health activity. The concentration of incentives on financial payments rather than broader targets does create a problem for national and local public health policy makers. It is likely that until community development and community involvement in public health is positively and formally sanctioned at PCT level, such activity will remain marginal. Early evidence from studies on the new GMS contract suggests that there is substantial role substitution with nursing staff undertaking many of the new screening and health check roles prescribed by working to the QOF. This means that they will not be doing other activities with practice patients and it has traditionally been non-GP staff who have taken on wider public health roles in the practice. There is a danger that this activity will be lost due to an increasing inward orientation towards the clinical practices of the local general practice dominated by the medical model of care. Many professionals, then, confine their public health activity to a strictly clinical agenda. Those who do engage with the community on wider public health issues go beyond their formal role (Turton et al 2000).

Public involvement, the patient and choice

A key change in the last few years has been the way the relationship between patients and service users and the NHS and healthcare practitioners has shifted towards a more individualized one. Patient choice reflects an increasing emphasis on choice and consumerism in public services while the increasing policy emphasis on supporting self-care highlights individual responsibility and limits the role of public services in the maintenance of health and well-being. The choice and self-care agendas appear, in England, to be separate from changes to the structures and processes for patient and public engagement, while in Wales and Scotland the development of patient and public involvement

seems to be central to these areas (SEHD 2005, Welsh Assembly Government 2005). The self-care agenda focuses on the contribution of patients (and their carers) to their own health and well-being (Department of Health 2006). Essentially this means individuals taking responsibility for staying fit and maintaining good physical and mental health; meeting social, emotional and psychological needs; preventing illness or accidents; caring for minor ailments and long-term conditions; and maintaining health and well-being after an acute illness or discharge from hospital. This has key relevance to the development of primary and community health services and the roles of health professionals (see Chapter 2).

Choice is a common theme in UK health policy, reflecting a wider emphasis on choice in public services that aims to meet individual needs with more responsive services, challenge the power of professionals, drive quality improvements and improve equity, as well as being a good thing in its own right (Fotaki et al 2005). The rhetoric of choice is about giving patients more control and it raises important questions about the way healthcare is accessed, delivered and experienced and needs to be seen within a web of factors that influence access to and the use of healthcare services (Exworthy and Peckham 2006). However, policy differs between England, Northern Ireland, Scotland and Wales, reflecting differences in the ideological underpinning of how choices are constructed. For example, in England the emphasis is on consumerism and the use of choice as a driver for improving quality and efficiency alongside other supply side developments to create contestability, such as payment by results and private sector treatment. In England, patient choice is based on the belief that giving patients appropriate information on service providers will achieve greater responsiveness to patient needs, increase technical and allocative efficiency, enhance quality of services and, most contentious of all, improve equity (Fotaki et al 2005). Together with payment by results (where funding follows the patient) and practice-based commissioning (PbC), patient choice aims to introduce a market-type competitive environment in healthcare provision which will drive health service improvements. However, elements of choice already exist within the English NHS, with NHS Direct and walk-in centres providing alternative access points to primary care. A key danger of widening choice in healthcare through multiple providers will be a fragmentation of the healthcare system which may affect continuity of care if good information systems and methods for sharing information are not developed.

Governments in Northern Ireland, Wales and Scotland have not been so determined to widen choices of service providers and have tended not to be in favour of introducing a consumer market approach. In Wales, there is an emphasis on patient and public involvement (Audit Commission in Wales 2004, Fotaki et al 2005, Healthcare Commission 2005), although there is a Second Offer Scheme where patients can be offered a second choice of treatment and/or location if they have waited for more than the national waiting time targets. The Welsh Choice Scheme is centrally driven and is specifically aimed at reducing waiting times following criticism about the poor performance of the Welsh healthcare system (Audit Commission in Wales 2004, Wanless 2003). The main emphasis in the Welsh government's strategy is, though, to 'empower the community to have its voice heard and heeded, rather than simply being given a choice of treatment location' (Welsh Assembly Government 2005). The Assembly has created a public and patient involvement network with a central support service to develop patient and public engagement in service development and planning. In Scotland, *The NHS Plan* stressed the need to be responsive to patients' views – providing information on the quality of provider services (including the development of clinical performance indicators) so that clinical choices are made in consultation with patients (Department of Health 2000). Patient choice of secondary provider is now facilitated by the National Waiting Times Database which provides service users and their GPs with information to support GP referral decisions. In addition, the recent introduction of GP specialists and the establishment of the Referral Information Service have increased the availability of alternative routes to treatment and information aimed at increasing patient choice (NHS Scotland 2005). Finally in Northern Ireland the opportunity for choice is more limited given the size of the health system. The recent proposal to introduce a Second Offer Scheme (similar to Wales) has been welcomed and a recent review of health and social care services recommends further expansion of choice for specific treatments and specialties (Appleby 2005). The Northern Ireland scheme will, as in the Welsh scheme, be centrally driven, providing loca-

tion of treatment choice only for patients waiting 9 months or more for hip and knee operations and 6 months for cardiac and cataract operations.

Choice would seem to be supported by patients as studies of patient choice in the English and London choice pilots found that the majority of people opted for a different provider rather than wait (Exworthy and Peckham 2006). Operation of the Welsh Second Offer Scheme also suggests that patients are willing to choose different treatments and providers rather than wait for treatment (Audit Commission in Wales 2004). However, these studies also suggest that there are limitations to choice depending on socio-demographic characteristics and in relation to geographical location (Exworthy and Peckham 2006). The actual roll-out of choice has, however, been somewhat limited and a survey in May 2006 found that only 30% of patients recall being offered a choice of hospital for their first out-patient appointment (Department of Health 2006). The range of choices is also limited and does not include treatment choices, even though choice of treatment is something patients have called for and the evidence suggests that patients benefit from being involved in treatment decisions (Fotaki et al 2005).

While patient choice reflects an increasing emphasis on choice and consumerism in public services, self-care highlights individual responsibility and limits to the role of public services in the maintenance of health and well-being. In England *Our Health, Our Care, Our Say* (Department of Health 2006) stressed the importance of self-care and the support role of the NHS; this built on the earlier *Choosing Health*, which introduced health trainers and placed a greater emphasis on individual skills for preventing ill health (Department of Health 2004) while the Green Paper on adult social services, *Independence, Well-being and Choice*, highlighted the need to support people with long-term conditions to manage independently (Department of Health 2005b). In Scotland and Wales, current plans for service development also emphasize the need for NHS organizations to improve support for patients with long-term conditions as well as supporting their carers (Audit Commission in Wales 2004, NHS Scotland 2005).

In England, over 50% of the population have some form of chronic health problem. They are intensive users of health services and it is estimated that as many as 40% of general practice consultations and 70% of Accident and Emergency (A&E)

visits are for minor ailments that could be taken care of by people themselves, while 10% of inpatients account for 55% of inpatient days (Department of Health 2005c). The benefits of supporting self-care have been shown to be improved health outcomes, a better quality of life for those with long-term conditions, increased patient satisfaction and effective use of what is an enormous healthcare resource – patients and the public (Department of Health 2005c). However, to date the NHS has not been particularly good at supporting this process and it will be interesting to see whether a shift to self-care creates further problems for patients and their carers if responsibility for self-care is pursued by the NHS without providing appropriate support – especially for more vulnerable groups such as older people (Ellins and Coulter 2005, Coulter 2006). The wide and varied roles in nursing, midwifery and health visiting such as school nursing, practice nursing and community midwifery lend themselves to a variety of relationships with people living with long-term conditions, ranging from health promotion to caring for those with highly complex needs. Although it is recognized that a key role is helping people to manage long-term conditions, there has been limited proactive engagement with clients in trying to ascertain their needs (Peckham and Meerabeau 2007). Developing specialist nurse roles and enhancing the skills of generalist nurses to focus systematically on particular groups of patients (including the development of community matron type roles) have been shown to be effective approaches to supporting people with long-term conditions.

Conclusion

NHS policy is currently at a time of rapid development with a strong central drive towards a new, although not always clear, modernization programme. Two things would appear to be happening at the moment, which at first glance would seem to be diametrically opposed. The first is the emphasis on decentralization and devolution pushing responsibility for the NHS away from central government to the elected assemblies in Scotland and Wales and to front-line clinicians/managers within primary care organizations. At the same time central government and the Scottish and Welsh NHS are applying more central control on standards and quality. Thus we

may see increasing diversity in organizational structure in the future but clearer goals regarding standards and quality of care with nationally driven guidelines and national inspection, all emphasizing a national health service. This tension will become increasingly difficult as the government increases expenditure on the NHS over the next few years. The publication of the Wanless Report (2002) has led to an increasing Treasury presence in health policy and it is not clear to what extent this exercise of control will be increased in future years. How far such centralized control can sit alongside a more decentralized and fragmented service is not clear. Gordon Brown's move to being Prime Minister may have a significant impact given his association with increased funding, addressing health inequalities and high profile strategies relating to supporting children across the UK despite increasing political devolution.

As the Acheson Inquiry (1998) and the Wanless Reports (2002, 2004) demonstrate very well, many if not most of the causes of, and preventative actions for, health problems lie outside the remit of the Department of Health and the NHS. In addition, despite the recent recognition that healthcare (and social care) services need to support patients with long-term chronic conditions, patient views on the availability of support for long-term conditions suggest that the NHS is not providing appropriate or adequate services (Coulter 2006). The emphasis on self-care, while important, will require different sorts of services to ensure that there is not simply a shift of care from formal health and social care services to the informal sector, placing increased burdens on service users, their carers, families and communities.

Community health services are the centre of these shifts in approaches to health. The roles of community nurses will probably increasingly diverge across the UK as different organizational structures, regulatory frameworks and service emphases increase. The emphasis on collaboration and public health in Scotland and Wales will undoubtedly shape local roles. In the same way increasing service fragmentation, new non- or quasi-NHS organizations in England will place new challenges for nurses and nurse roles. However, changing expectations and the emphasis on self-care are likely to create common ground across the UK and more centrally challenge concepts about professional and lay roles in the provision of healthcare.

SUMMARY

- This chapter focuses on the UK National Health Service since 1997, with a summary of the period before then.
- Major organizational changes to the structure of the NHS since 1997, introduced by the Labour government, including legislation are covered.
- The introduction of the devolved electoral assemblies in Northern Ireland, Scotland and Wales and the impact on each other and on the NHS in England are discussed.
- The priority policy areas of the Labour government are political devolution, performance and quality, public health and developing and supporting the role of the patient with increased individual responsibility.

DISCUSSION POINTS

1. The extent to which devolution in Scotland, Wales and Northern Ireland will create new tensions within the NHS and health policy more generally.
2. The government is pursuing a more market style approach in England. What impact will this have on the organization and coordination of community health services?
3. In what ways could increased accreditation, regulation and patient/public scrutiny ensure higher quality care?
4. The importance of developing a public health role for community nursing.
5. How important is patient choice? How does self-care relate to issues of choice?

References

Acheson D (chair) 1998 Independent inquiry into inequalities in health. HMSO, London

Appleby J 2005 Independent review of health and social care services in Northern Ireland. Report to the NI Office

Audit Commission in Wales 2004 Transforming health and social care in Wales. Audit Commission in Wales, Cardiff

Baggott R 2000 Public health: policy and politics. Macmillan Press, Basingstoke

Baggott R 2004 Health and health care in Britain. Palgrave/Macmillan, Basingstoke

Coulter A 2006 Engaging patients in their healthcare. Picker Institute Europe, Oxford

Department of Health 1997 The new NHS. HMSO, London

Department of Health 1999 Making a difference. HMSO, London

Department of Health 2000 The NHS plan. HMSO, London

Department of Health 2001 Learning from Bristol: the report of the public inquiry into children's heart surgery at the Bristol Royal Infirmary 1984–1995, Cmnd paper 5207. HMSO, London

Department of Health 2004 Choosing health. TSO, London

Department of Health 2005a Commissioning a patient led NHS. DH, London

Department of Health 2005b Independence, well-being and choice. TSO, London

Department of Health 2005c Self care – a real choice, self care support – a real option. DH, London

Department of Health 2006 Our health, our care, our say. TSO, London

Ellins J, Coulter A 2005 How engaged are people in their health care? Findings of a national telephone survey. The Health Foundation, London

Exworthy M, Peckham S 2006 Access, choice and travel: implications for health policy. Social Policy and Administration 40(3): 267–287

Fotaki M, Boyd A, Smith L, McDonald R, et al 2005 Patient choice and the organisation and delivery of health services: scoping review. University of Manchester, Manchester

Glendinning C, Coleman A, Shipman C, Malbon G 2001 Primary care groups: progress in partnerships. British Medical Journal 323:28–31

Ham C 2004 Health policy in Britain. Macmillan, Basingstoke

Healthcare Commission 2005 State of healthcare 2005. Healthcare Commission, London

Kerr D 2005 Building a health service fit for the future. Scottish Executive, Edinburgh

Klein R 2006 The new politics of the NHS. Longman, London

NHS Scotland 2000 Our national health: a plan for action, a plan for change. SEHD, Edinburgh

NHS Scotland 2005 The national framework for service change in NHS Scotland: elective care action team – final report. SEHD, Edinburgh

NHS Wales 2001 Improving health in Wales – a plan for the NHS with its partners. National Assembly for Wales, Cardiff

Peckham S, Exworthy M 2003 Primary care in the UK: policy, organisation and management. Palgrave/Macmillan, Basingstoke

Peckham S, Meerabeau E 2007 Social policy for nurses and the helping professions. Open University Press, Maidenhead

Scottish Executive Health Department 2005 Delivering for health. SEHD, Edinburgh

Shipman Inquiry 2001 The 2001 first report. TSO, London

Shipman Inquiry 2004 The 2004 fifth report: safeguarding patients. Lessons from the past – proposals for the future. TSO, London

Turton P, Peckham S, Taylor P 2000
    Integrating primary care and public
    health. In: Lindsay J, Craig P Nursing
    for public health: population-
    based care. Churchill Livingstone,
    Edinburgh

Wanless D 2002 Securing our future
    health: taking a long-term view. HM
    Treasury, London

Wanless D 2003 Review of health and
    social care in Wales. Wales Assembly
    Government, Cardiff

Wanless D 2004 Securing good health
    for the whole population. HM
    Treasury, London

Welsh Assembly Government 2005
    Designed for life: creating world
    class health and social care for Wales
    in the 21st century. Wales Assembly
    Government, Cardiff

Recommended reading

Baggott R 2004 The politics of public
    health. Macmillan, Basingstoke

Klein R 2006 The new politics of the
    NHS. Longman, London

Peckham S, Meerabeau E 2007 Social
    policy for nurses and the helping
    professions. Open University Press,
    Maidenhead

2

Developments in primary care

Stephen Peckham

KEY ISSUES

- The centrality of primary care to developments in the NHS and health policy in the UK
- The lack of clarity over the exact definition of primary care
- The major challenges in primary care in terms of supporting self-care and people with long-term conditions
- The increasing emphasis on multidisciplinary and multiagency partnerships within primary care
- The increasing diversity of activity and ways of organizing primary care in the UK
- Primary care nursing as an increasingly important element of primary care

Introduction

Primary care plays a central role in the UK National Health Service (NHS) and has become a major focus of health policy since the 1990s. The changes introduced by the Labour government from 1997 have significantly shifted healthcare policy from an emphasis on secondary care – which has dominated health policy since before the Second World War – to placing primary care at the centre of healthcare development, commissioning and public health. These changes to the healthcare system resulted from a sustained period of healthcare reform in the 1990s and early 21st century - not only in the UK but also in many other developed countries. This chapter examines the implications of these changes in the UK and highlights how these changes have impacted on the delivery of healthcare services.

The 20th century saw the emergence of primary care as a specific area of healthcare, albeit dominated for the most part by general practice. However, this process was accompanied by a separation of the generalist model of primary care from the specialist approach of secondary care services. This separation was evident for the first third of the century and was formalized by the creation of GPs as independent contractors within the NHS, even though GPs' gatekeeping role was considered vital to the functioning of the NHS. In many ways, other primary care professions (especially community nursing) experienced a similar separation from the rest of the healthcare system by virtue of their distinctive professional developments in local authorities. The integration of GPs and community nursing became most apparent with the effective development of primary care teams from the 1960s onwards.

While the managerialism of the 1980s, and the internal market in the 1990s, has been seen as inimical to primary care teamwork, these two developments were instrumental in placing primary care at the centre of health policy and in a pivotal role in the organization and management of healthcare. It is no surprise therefore that the 1990s witnessed the most concerted attempt to shape primary care through policy reform, in part because of the pressures and needs elsewhere in the NHS. Though autonomy has been valued by all professions throughout, and the legacy of the generalist/specialist separation and of the 1948 settlement persist, the government has become less deferential to the professions. For much of the century, the government was wary about upsetting the professions (primarily medicine) given their status within society and the power which they wielded. However, with the rise of managerialism, policies have made fundamental advances in shaping the organization and management of primary care. This is resulting in a wider and more inclusive definition of primary care, a greater managerial role in what had been a professional enclave, and a more central role for primary care in meeting NHS objectives. For example, in England the recent proposals by Lord Darzi emphasize the need for stronger primary care. However, while issues such as access, quality, education and professional regulation, and developing premises and facilities remain important, recent changes in commissioning and contractual arrangements (discussed later in this chapter) have shifted attention to how national and local policy makers can stimulate these changes. There are also changes in the organization of primary care and in the roles of healthcare practitioners such as GPs and nurses, and though an increasingly inquisitive and sceptical public is placing more demands on practitioners, primary care has thus moved from the margins to the mainstream of health policy in the UK. As discussed in Chapter 1, any discussion of healthcare organization must consider the effect of political devolution in the UK and the development of not one, but four NHSs. As in other areas of healthcare, this has had a significant impact on primary care services, and while on the whole unchallenged by much reform, the enduring nature of general practice may fundamentally alter in the future in England and certainly the shape of community health services will change, forging clearer divisions between England and the rest of the UK.

The growth of primary care in the UK

Central to the organization of primary care services in the UK are general practice and community health services and since the Second World War there has been an enormous expansion of these services. From the 1960s there has been a steady increase in the workload and, consequently, the numbers of staff. Today primary care is a major employer with, in England, Scotland and Wales, over 120 000 people now working in general practice with over 40 000 additional members of the primary healthcare team (PHCT) who also work in, or with, practices (Table 2.1).

Table 2.1 Change in the numbers of practice staff in England[a], Scotland[b] and Wales[c]

Number of GP practice staff	1990s	Current
General practitioners[d]	35 494	42 876
Practice nurse	11 301	16 646
Admin/clerical	56 158	65 079
Direct patient care[e]	1 688	5 446
Community nurse[f]	0	268
Other	589	1 673

Source: RCGP General practice statistics July 2006, ISD(M)8 Scottish Health Statistics.
[a]Full-time equivalent (FTE) figures for England 1995 and 2005.
[b]Figures for Scotland 1990 and 2003 – practices do not have to return figures since April 2004.
[c]FTE figures for Wales 1994 and 2005.
[d]GP data is for 1995 and 2005 (FTE = 31 475 in 1995 and 35 020 in 2005).
[e]Other clinicians/therapists and practitioners employed by the practice (e.g. dispensers, physiotherapists, counsellors, complementary therapists, phlebotomists).
[f]England only.

A simple review of the history of UK health policy demonstrates little interest in general practice and community health services until the mid 1980s. As Moon and North (2000) argue:

… the current status that general practice enjoys as a speciality within medicine and the influence that GPs wield are in sharp contrast with its origins and much of its history, during which general practice was overshadowed by the more prestigious branches of medicine. (p. 13)

Traditionally, the sidelining of general practice and community health in the UK is seen as a by-product of the establishment of the NHS in 1948. The settlement achieved ensured that the focus of government was on the secondary and tertiary sectors given the dominance of hospital-based services (Klein 2006). Two consequences of the establishment of the NHS were the independent practice status of general practice, outside of the mainstream NHS administration, and the retention of community and public health services within local authorities (Klein 2006, Ottewill and Wall 1992,

Timmins 1995). For the UK this tended to push policy interest in these areas to the sidelines. This is not to say that these areas were ignored as there has been a continuing debate within the UK about the relationship between community health and hospital services (Ottewill and Wall 1992) and since the 1950s an interest in the development, quality and role of the general practitioner services (Moon and North 2000). However, the interest of government in primary care services rapidly escalated from the mid 1980s. This interest grew for a number of reasons but can be seen as arising from the coincidence of a number of trends as shown in Box 2.1 (Peckham and Exworthy 2003).

While identified as separate contributors to policy and organizational changes, there are clear interrelationships between these areas. In the UK, general practitioners have traditionally adopted a managed care approach, being both first point of contact for healthcare for the majority of the population, pro-

viding immediate healthcare to individuals and families and making referrals to secondary care (Fry and Hodder 1994, Starfield 1998). As Starfield notes, the UK system of general practice is the most universal and comprehensive in the world. Thus they have a critical role to play in dealing with long-term chronic illness. Similarly, the UK has one of the most comprehensively developed community health services which has increasingly become integrated with general practice. Interestingly this integration combines both primary *medical* care and, to a certain extent, primary *healthcare*. Thus the need to address changes in disease management from mainly acute episodes to the management of chronic disease places a greater burden on primary care and has perhaps led to the 'rediscovery' of the GP's role. At the same time there have been significant changes in demand by patients leading to pressure on consultation times, length of time waiting for an appointment and particularly out-of-hours work. It is not clear, however, what the varying contributions of providers and patients are in this upturn in demand, nor is there any simple answer to dealing with these problems (Rogers et al 1999). All these issues are explored in more depth by Peckham and Exworthy (2003) but it is important to recognize the complex background that lies behind current developments in policy and practice.

This discovery of the important role of primary care within the UK NHS has occurred at a time when there has also been a re-examination of the role of the GP and developments in primary care nursing. It is perhaps the convergence of these factors which has provided an impetus to the exploration of new models of primary care organization. These developments have also led to a re-evaluation of the nature of primary care. Certainly recent debates about who should deliver primary care and the potential opening up of a community health services market with a greater role for private and non-profit organizations (in the form of social enterprises of community interest companies) in England may bring substantial changes to the traditional model of general practice. At the same time, the increasing use of performance and incentive systems and flexibilities around service payments introduced in the new General Medical Services (GMS) contract in 2004 have substantially changed the way practices are run (Guthrie et al 2006, Wang et al 2006). Before examining this and key issues relevant to primary care it is worth spending some time thinking about what we mean by primary care and recent developments in the UK.

Box 2.1

Trends affecting the development of primary care

- Broader changes in the delivery of healthcare services associated with the 'crisis in healthcare' and the 'crisis of the welfare state'.
- An interest in the organizational relationship of general practice to the NHS as the key to managing activity.
- A desire to extend managerial control over primary care and, following the failure of earlier cost-control measures, to engage general practitioners in financial management.
- The growth of the 'new public management' and consequent changes in approaches to the management and organization of public services particularly to curb expenditure, contain demands and increase efficiency and effectiveness.
- Changes in patients' expectations about being treated more promptly and closer to home.
- A fragmenting medical profession with changing professional expectations – especially for GPs – towards more flexibility in their working arrangements and career choices.
- The rise of professionals as managers and a desire to control the gatekeepers to the NHS as general practice was seen as the last untouched bastion of clinical and medical autonomy.
- An increasing emphasis on localization and community-based services.

Re-evaluating primary care

Primary care has long been acknowledged as one of the major strengths of British health and social care arrangements, with its focus on universality of access, emphasis on continuity of family and individual care, and its role as a gateway to other services (Starfield 1998). However, the theory and practice of primary care has been undergoing re-evaluation and change (Macdonald 1992, Starfield 1998, WHO/UNICEF 1978), a situation reflected in the re-examination of primary care in the UK (Peckham and Exworthy 2003).

This re-evaluation from within primary care services has been accompanied by impetus for change coming from national policy and growing concerns about how well practices are supporting people with long-term conditions and supporting self-care and public health (DHSS 1986, 1987, Department of Health 1996, 1997, 2000a, 2006). Initially, the main thrust for change was on quality and then, with the introduction of the internal market and fundholding, on the purchasing role of primary care, which was intended to lead to greater efficiency and responsiveness (Le Grand et al 1998). At the same time, there has been a reassessment of the role of general practice, and latterly, more radical solutions have been sought, with a range of new developments, from the mid 1990s onwards. These included primary care act pilots (PCAPs) which are exploring new organizational arrangements for general practice, total purchasing – where groups of practices held the whole purchasing budget for their population, and GP commissioning which brought together GPs and health authorities on commissioning. These latter two were the forerunners of, primary care trusts (PCTs) and care trusts – in England, Scottish local community health partnerships, local health and social care groups in Northern Ireland and local health boards (LHBs) in Wales.

One central feature of this new focus on primary care is the increasing tension over what we mean by primary care itself. In particular current policy developments and responses to the challenges of increasing technological advances and increasing specialization, public health, self-care and supporting people with chronic conditions highlight a tension between traditional approaches to general practice as primary medical care and wider understanding of primary care as community-based care and support (Peckham and Exworthy 2003). Current government policy across the UK emphasizes the promotion of primary and community care, with the intention of ensuring a more efficient response to the needs of vulnerable groups, by managing the care of these groups as much as possible in the community and by developing interagency work and focusing on long-term care. In a sense this recognizes the need for general practice to change although at present general practitioners remain the central figures, and general practice the pre-eminent organizational structure in UK primary care.

The current context of primary care in the UK

Primary care became seen as both an issue ('problem') to be tackled and also as a solution to 'difficulties' elsewhere in the NHS during the 1980s and especially the 1990s. As the contribution of primary care to the wider NHS became increasingly recognized, there was a greater need to incorporate it into the NHS's organization and management. Perhaps the most significant trigger for this was a process of managerialization which took place right across the public sector – the rise of new public management (NPM). It established new patterns of policy, organization and management. Although it initially had a marginal effect on primary care, NPM began to permeate primary care through the introduction of managerialism in community health services and other providers, the shift in focus from family practitioner committees to family health service authorities and the more managerial approaches (often associated with information technology) within individual general practices.

This process of incorporation continued into the 1990s with a series of reforms which were an attempt both to reorganize primary care and to act as an additional lever upon secondary care. This was most clearly evident in the GP fundholding scheme and Trust status but also through a series of policy statements. Although the internal market had profound inter- and intraprofessional consequences, the policy direction continued to move towards further integration with the introduction of primary care organizations (PCOs – primary care trusts in England, local health boards in Wales and community partnerships in Scotland), not least because these were not voluntary schemes. Once community health services had been reorganized into PCOs, primary care was effectively incorporated into the NHS. A process which had begun some 30 years earlier had finally been realized.

However, such incorporation has not been absolute and nor is it complete. Primary care has always been noted for its diversity, in terms of service provision and quality. Despite many initiatives oriented around quality improvement (often associated with NPM) in the 1980s and 1990s, the linkage between management and quality only formally became established with the introduction of clinical governance in 1997 and now somewhat enshrined in the new GMS contract. As mentioned previously, primary care is also becoming increasingly characterized by diversity in its organizational form. Incorporation has not been, and is unlikely to be, a uniform process, applying to all areas and to all services, equally. Devolution has created further complexities and diversity in primary care (Exworthy 2001, Peckham 2007) but there are common themes in policy across the UK such as the new GMS contract introduced in 2004 (discussed below) which demonstrate a new emphasis on developing primary care services with the potential to change the traditional general practice model of organization. In addition, recent developments in England point to increasing divergence with a greater role envisaged for new forms of organization to deliver primary and community healthcare services including private companies and social enterprise and community investment organizational models, while in Scotland and Wales the emphasis has been on service planning, partnership and collaboration and developing organizational and clinical networks. These changes, while focusing on organizational models, reflect a growing interest and recognition of the need to support self-care and informal care (Department of Health 2006, Kerr 2005) with a growing recognition that long-term and chronic health problems are not satisfactorily addressed within the UK NHS (Coulter 2006). Self-care is increasingly perceived as central to developments in health and social care and various English policy documents such as *Our Health, Our Care, Our Say* (Department of Health 2006) have stressed the importance of self-care and the role of the NHS in supporting it; the public health White Paper *Choosing Health* introduced health trainers and placed a greater emphasis on building skills of people for preventing ill health (Department of Health 2004) and the Green Paper on adult social services *Independence, Well-being and Choice* high-

lights the need to support people with long-term conditions to manage independently (Department of Health 2005a).

Over 50% of the population have some form of chronic health problem and people with chronic disease are more likely to be users of the health system, accounting for some 80% of all GP consultations, while 10% of inpatients account for 55% of inpatient days (British household panel survey, Office for National Statistics 2001). Older people are more likely to have multiple chronic problems and be intensive users of healthcare services and '15% of under 5s and 20% of the 5–15 age group are reported to have a long-term condition' (Wilson et al 2005: 658). In addition, it is also estimated that as many as 40% of general practice consultations and 70% of A&E visits are for minor ailments that could be taken care of by people themselves (Department of Health 2005b). The benefits of supporting self-care have been shown to be improved health outcomes, a better quality of life for those with long-term conditions, increased patient satisfaction and effective use of a huge resource to the NHS – patients and the public (Department of Health 2005c).

While there is widespread public support for self-care, recent surveys suggest that the UK NHS is poor at providing support for self-care and individuals require the confidence and knowledge to successfully embark on self-care, with some demographic groups such as older people requiring more support than others (Department of Health 2004, 2005c, Ellins and Coulter 2005, Coulter 2006). To date there is little evidence to show that PCTs have utilized the flexibilities offered by primary care contracts to develop greater support for people with long-term conditions or developed strategic approaches to support self-care (Wilson et al 2005).

The new GMS contract

In 2004 the new GMS contract was introduced in the UK. The contract marked a major change in the way GPs are contracted with the NHS. Under the old contract individual GP principals held an individual contract that, despite changes in substance, remained based on the original contract established in 1948. GP incomes were made up from a mixture of funding for registered patients, undertaking specific activities and support for practice development such as nursing and administration staff (Moon and North 2000). The introduction of salaried GPs and nurse practitioners were, for example, identified as new approaches but there has been little encroachment on the organization of practices, and nurse-led practices or nurse practitioners remain scarce. Of the first wave of pilots only two were nurse-led and in total only nine nurse-led practices have been developed (seven of which were developed by the local PCT). Structural barriers to non-GP-provided practice remain ingrained in professional guidelines and statutory responsibilities for prescribing and patient care (Houghton 2002). While salaried GPs were not a primary aim of the Primary Medical Services (PMS) scheme, about half of the first wave of practices employed salaried GPs – particularly in deprived, inner city areas – although adoption of salaried GPs in non-PMS practices grew at a similar rate (Sibbald et al 2000). While these services have been innovative in the extent to which greater emphasis is placed on multi-professional models with less GP involvement, they have not, as yet, significantly challenged the dominant general practice model of a small team of GPs supported by other staff.

The new GMS contract has been developed from pilots of new contractual forms introduced in the late 1990s under PMSs designed to stimulate innovation in practice (Meads et al 2004, Riley et al 2003, Smith et al 2005). The main principles of the new contract are:

• a shift from individual GP to practice-based contracts
• contracts based around workload management with core and enhanced service levels
• a reward structure based on a new Quality and Outcomes Framework and annual assessments
• an expansion of primary care services
• modernization of practice infrastructure (especially IT systems).

The new contract also provides two important variations for alternative and specialist provider medical services (APMS and SPMS). These provide opportunities to widen private sector involvement in primary care and for the development of more specialist services in the community. While wider private sector interest has been steadily growing and in some cases larger healthcare companies (such as UK Care and United Healthcare) have bid for general practice contracts, to date GP-led private companies have

been most successful. The reasons for this are complex but the dominant GP model of independent GP contractors and continuing British Medical Association hostility to private provision means that developing private sector services with GPs remains easier to establish in local health systems.

One important aspect of the new GP contract introduced in April 2005 has been the Quality and Outcomes Framework (QOF). This has received relatively little general media coverage, although its operation has caused headlines in medical circles and a high degree of congratulatory medical press coverage. QOF has been described as offering a unique experiment in the use of incentives to reward quality, providing financial rewards to general practices based on a points system of over 150 quality indicators covering clinical, organizational and patient-focused aspects of practice (Smith and York 2004). A key aspect of QOF is the use of financial targets to change GPs' clinical behaviour. Previous research examining the relationship between financial incentives and public health, following the introduction of the new GP contract in 1990, found that financial reward for practices bore no relation to local need (Langham et al 1995).

There have been major successes in areas where targets have been set or additional resources have been provided but there are already concerns about the processes being developed to manage QOF and evidence suggests some skewing of clinical focus and some non-targeted areas of practice are being ignored (Campbell et al 2005, Fleetcroft and Cookson 2006). There is emerging evidence, though, that the use of the QOF is changing relationships in practices, with responses to the QOF being seen by those professionals affected as primarily a technical problem requiring attention to the design of information systems in order to rationalize practice and collect the relevant data, rather than being seen as the basis for guiding clinical practice (Checkland 2006). Research examining the effect of QOF in the first 2 years of operation has found that there are small inequalities between practices in the provision of simple monitoring interventions (e.g. blood pressure, asthma checks), but larger inequalities for diagnostic, outcome and treatment measures with poorer areas being more disadvantaged – a situation further exacerbated by exclusion reporting, where practices can exclude patients with complex clinical problems or 'non-compliance' and thus improve QOF scores (McClean et al 2006, Sigfrid et al 2006). What impact this will have on the quality of care is not clear at the present time but despite these concerns the QOF process should lead to improvements in clinical care as it provides targets associated with additional funding.

Other changes include the recent introduction of access targets in England, which has led to increasing numbers of practitioners dealing with the care of an individual patient as a result of meeting the 24/48 hour targets for GP appointments; this raises questions about continuity of care and clinical quality, since the risk of error increases as more practitioners are involved in a patient's care (Blendon et al 2002). As with many performance systems, the evidence of 2 years' data suggests that practices will prioritize maximizing their performance against targets. These continue to be centrally negotiated and include an expanded range of clinical areas and more emphasis on health promotion activities. Discussions are underway between the British Medical Association (negotiating on behalf of GPs) and the Department of Health on focusing QOF more on self-care support and interventions to reduce demand in primary care.

The other major innovation – again restricted to England – is the introduction of practice-based commissioning (PbC). The purpose of PbC is to achieve better patient care, make financial savings and to reconfigure services by shifting investment to primary care. Since April 2005, all practices in England have been able to hold an indicative budget that covers their commissioning activity and, progressively, practices are allowed to take control over the commissioning of services starting with elective surgery and outpatient appointments but eventually covering a large element of all commissioned healthcare. With a close resemblance to fundholding introduced in the 1990s, the success of PbC will similarly be dependent on practices being appropriately resourced, having the right level and mix of skills in practices (technical and clinical), having good healthcare professional support and engaging clinicians in the commissioning process (Smith et al 2004). Certainly the fact that PbC is in reality a mandatory approach (although technically voluntary) means that practices must have a different attitude to PbC and the government expected all practices to engage in PbC at some level by the end of 2006, but take-up has been slow and very limited in activity (Checkland et al 2008). How far PbC will deliver practice autonomy is also in doubt as it is likely that PbC will operate within practice networks as well as within the overall strategic frame-

work of the PCT and the NHS, introducing new tensions between the different levels of the NHS but also introducing a key distinction between England and the rest of the UK.

General practice in the UK also faces a number of other challenges and changes resulting from changes in the workforce, greater pressure to apply evidence-based medicine and treatment protocols and meet centrally set targets. It is into this complex context that the new contract has been introduced. These challenges are not unrecognized by the profession and the need for general practice to respond to social change was the topic of a Royal College of General Practitioners working group on the future of general practice (Wilson et al 2006).

Changing pattern of professional work in primary care

Current changes in organization and practice in primary care will provide challenges and new opportunities for professional practice. However, the pattern of professional work in primary care has rarely been static, reflecting fluctuations in the balance between and within professions as well as the myriad changes in the organization and management of primary care. Nevertheless, the medical profession has remained largely dominant in various incarnations of interprofessional working. Nonetheless, the degree of interprofessional working grew in the latter part of the 20th century such that it is now a well-established feature of primary care in the UK (see Chapter 21 for further information on partnership working in health and social care).

The 1990s was a period of huge change for primary care nursing/community nursing as a result of the rise in the number of practice nurses and the development of nurse practitioners. The growth in the number of practice nurses was aided by subsidies to practices who employed practice nurses. Their numbers rose spectacularly from 1920 in 1984 to 9100 in 1994 (Green and Thorogood 1998: 100). Though working with the practice population and for the practice, practice nurses also experienced a huge rise in, and expansion of, their workload (associated with the 1990 GP contract), and with practice nurse roles now extended especially into chronic disease management (e.g. asthma), health promotion, smoking cessation, family planning and treatment of minor illnesses, numbers have risen to over 15 000. In addition, the number of therapy staff such as osteopaths, counsellors and physiotherapists has also risen.

The increase in practice nurses and the wider primary healthcare team has occurred alongside developments in community services with an increase in both professional roles and also professionals such as care assistants and healthcare assistants. The extension of nurse prescribing and nurse consultant roles are key developments which, coupled with changes in the organization of primary care (such as walk-in centres, telephone support and new models of service delivery), are likely to see substantial changes in work patterns and relationships in community and primary care nursing in the immediate future. Certainly in relation to the new contract there has been concern that nurses are in fact picking up much of the new activity for monitoring patients to meet QOF targets but that it is the GPs who have received the financial reward (Amicus/CPHVA 2006).

But the role of the GP is also changing – although it would be wrong to say that their role will be substantially different in the short term as a result of current policy developments. One key change over the last 10 years has been the feminization of general practice. More women than men now enter general practice training. This has led to pressures on working patterns and has particularly fed pressures to change out-of-hours support. Working practice has also been changed through the Primary Care Act pilot schemes which have introduced changes to the GMS contracts, with an increase in the number of salaried GPs. Clearly the context of practice will change. Increased accreditation, changes in organization and increases in medical knowledge will directly affect practice. However, it is likely that the daily routine of general medical practice will change little – the frontline is where continuity will be retained. The central role of general practice is to manage patient care and make appropriate referrals for further care or investigation. This is central to both medical practice and the way the NHS operates. However, the increasing use of GPs with a special interest to manage common conditions in primary care, undertake investigations or triage patients prior to secondary referral is changing the way primary care works. This is likely to be extended as group and network based approaches to primary care – with practices linked through primary care organizations or through purchasing arrangements in England – change the nature of relationships between practices.

One area of major change has been in out-of-hours services and emergency care – particularly since the introduction of the new GMS contract, which provided for practices to withdraw from out-of-hours care shifting responsibility to primary care organizations. Out-of-hours services have been the focus of considerable and rapid workforce change, as local NHS organizations work to ensure that patients are provided with a service that meets quality standards such as those set out in the independent review of out-of-hours care (Department of Health 2000b). The House of Commons Select Committee (2004) report on *GP Out-of-Hours Services* identified several areas with innovative developments in skill mix (p. 10), but it supported calls for 'better use of skill mix to deliver out-of-hours care' (p. 35) in order to deliver a better quality of service to patients, noting that the service is complex to provide and that there will be training needs associated with the changing workforce. Examples of workforce change have already included employing salaried GPs, increasing role substitution by nurses and paramedics, establishing community interest companies, and forging integration of GP cooperatives with NHS Direct (NHS 24 in Scotland) and local ambulance services for initial call handling. Out-of-hours services are also providing new roles for nursing staff and innovative approaches to role substitution between healthcare professionals.

Conclusion

The landscape of primary care is changing fast. While general practice will remain the cornerstone for the immediate future, policies across the UK will lead to a greater diversification of primary care organization. In particular, we can expect community and primary care nurses to take on additional responsibilities both in terms of clinical practice and organizational management. There is though an increasing level of technicality in the provision of primary care, creating a challenge to the notion of primary care as being holistic with the practitioner dealing with the whole person. At the same time the routinization of much care through QOF is also structuring both the type of work undertaken by practice staff but also subtly shifting the relationship between the practice and the patient. The changing nature of professional, patient and lay-carer roles with the emphasis on choice and self-care also challenges the notion of practitioner as expert. Thus, in the future we can expect to see an increasing blurring of roles such as that which is already happening in nursing and social care for people with learning difficulties, where integrated professional training already exists. This may in future lead to a blurring of roles between carers and nursing professionals in particular.

Nurses provide much of the new developing agenda within primary care such as NHS Direct, out-of-hours care, walk-in centres, routine health checks and screening services. Primary care in the future may also offer greater diversity for nurses with the range and level of roles expanding, providing new career paths. In England proposals for developing polyclinics may also provide new opportunities

for nursing roles, and the development of new forms of community health services as PCTs divest themselves of provider functions could open up new models of working within the primary care sector alongside traditional general practice (Department of Health 2006, 2008). While the general shift within nursing is towards expanding professional roles there is a danger in primary care that greater standardization of activity through the use of protocols (e.g. in NHS Direct or for QOF) will downgrade nursing responsibilities and tasks and open up the development of low-grade nursing auxiliary functions instead of more developed and central roles for primary care nurses. There may also be a push for greater generalization in nursing (from medics) with their main role as continuing to support primary medical practice.

SUMMARY

- Primary care is now recognized as playing a central role in the NHS.
- There has been a huge growth in the number of primary care workers since the 1960s and the trends which have affected this are discussed.
- The re-evaluation of primary care over the past 20 years and the current context within the UK NHS, particularly since the coming to power of the Labour government, are aimed at access, informing patients, extending high-quality care, providing modern primary care settings and the training and education of staff.
- Public health has become an important aspect of primary care and is incorporated

within the performance framework of the new GMS contract but focuses on clinical and individual interventions rather than wider community-based approaches.
- The latter part of the 20th century saw a 'professionalization' of the UK NHS workers in primary care, which has had an impact on the roles of all involved with, in particular, the lines between medical and nursing staff becoming blurred.
- The need to ensure that health and social care services address the needs of people with long-term conditions and also to support self-care are central to current debates about the future development of primary and community care services.

DISCUSSION POINTS

1. How important are organizational changes in primary care to shaping clinical practice and patient care?
2. To what extent will local practitioners be able to shape local healthcare services?
3. How will developments such as walk-in centres, NHS Direct and different organizational forms affect nurse roles in the future and traditional general practice?

4. How will nurse roles expand in the future? To what extent will specialisms in nursing remain, or will there be a move towards more generalist nurses?
5. How will multidisciplinary working and increasing carer and patient self-care affect nurses' roles?

References

Amicus/CPHVA 2006 Press release: Practice nurses get '10 per cent of top GPs pay' but do 50% of the work, says Amicus/CPHVA. Amicus/CPHVA, London

Blendon RJ, DesRoches CM, Brodie M, et al 2002 Views of practicing physicians and the public on medical errors. New England Journal of Medicine 347: 1933–1939

Campbell S, Roland M, Middleton E, Reeves D 2005 Improvements in quality of clinical care in English general practice 1998–2003: longitudinal observational study. British Medical Journal 331: 1121–1125

Checkland K 2006 Collecting data or shaping practice? Evidence from case studies in general practice about the impact of technology associated with the new GMS contract. PSA Annual Health Group Conference, Oxford, September 2006

Checkland K, Coleman A, Harrison S, Hiroeh U 2008 Practice based commissioning in the National Health Service: interim report of a qualitative study. National Primary Care Research and Development Centre, University of Manchester

Coulter A 2006 Engaging patients in their healthcare. Picker Institute Europe, Oxford

Department of Health 1996 Primary care: delivering the future. HMSO, London

Department of Health 1997 The new NHS: modern, dependable. HMSO, London

Department of Health 2000a The NHS plan. HMSO, London

Department of Health 2000b Raising standards for patients: new partnerships in out-of-hours care. An independent review of GP out-of-hours services in England. London, HMSO

Department of Health 2004 Choosing health. TSO, London

Department of Health 2005a Independence, well-being and choice. TSO, London

Department of Health 2005b Creating a patient-led NHS: delivering the NHS improvement plan. Department of Health, London

Department of Health 2005c Self care – a real choice, self care support – a real option. Department of Health, London

Department of Health 2006 Our health, our care, our say. TSO, London

Department of Health 2008 High quality care for all: NHS next stage review. Final report. TSO, London

DHSS 1986 Primary health care: an agenda for discussion. Cmnd 9771. HMSO, London

DHSS 1987 Promoting better health: the government's programme for improving primary health care. Cmnd 249. HMSO, London

Ellins J, Coulter A 2005 How engaged are people in their health care? Findings of a national telephone survey. The Health Foundation, London

Exworthy M 2001 Primary care in the UK: understanding the dynamics of devolution. Health and Social Care in the Community 9(5): 266–278

Fleetcroft R, Cookson R 2006 Do incentive payments in the new NHS contract for primary care reflect likely population health gains? Journal of Health Services Research and Policy 11(1): 27–31

Fry J, Hodder JP 1994 Primary health care in an international context. Nuffield Provincial Hospitals Trust, London

Green J, Thorogood N 1998 Analysing health policy: a sociological approach. Longman, London

Guthrie B, McLean G, Sutton M 2006 Workload and reward in the Quality and Outcomes Framework of the 2004 general practice contract. British Journal of General Practice 56 (Nov): 836–841

Houghton M 2002 We bought our own GP. Nursing Times Mar 28–Apr 1; 98(13): 28–29

House of Commons Select Committee 2004 GP out-of-hours services (6 August 2004). TSO, London

Kerr D 2005 Building a health service fit for the future. Scottish Executive, Edinburgh

Klein R 2006 The new politics of the NHS. Longman, London

Langham S, Gillam S, Thorogood M 1995 The carrot, the stick and

the general practitioner: how have changes in financial incentives affected health promotion activity in general practice? British Journal of General Practice 45: 665–668

Le Grand J, Mays N, Mulligan J-A (eds) 1998 Learning from the NHS internal market: a review of evidence. King's Fund, London

Macdonald J 1992 Primary health care: medicine in its place. Earthscan, London

McClean G, Sutton M, Guthrie B 2006 Deprivation and quality of primary care services: evidence for persistence of the inverse care law from the UK Quality and Outcomes Framework. Journal of Epidemiology and Community Health 60(11): 917–922

Meads G, Riley AJ, Harding G, Carter YH 2004 Personal medical services: local organisational developments. Primary Health Care Research Development 3: 193–201

Moon G, North N 2000 Policy and place: general medical practice in the UK. Macmillan, Basingstoke

Office for National Statistics 2001 General household survey. The Stationery Office, London

Ottewill R, Wall A 1992 The growth and development of the Community Health Services. Business Education Publishers, Sunderland

Peckham S 2007 Not one but four: the NHS in 2007? Social Policy Review 19. Policy Press, Bristol

Peckham S, Exworthy M 2003 Primary care in the UK: policy, organisation and management. Palgrave/Macmillan, Basingstoke

Riley AJ, Harding G, Meads G, Underwood AR, Carter YH 2003 An evaluation of personal medical services pilots: the times they are a changin. Journal of Interprofessional Care 17(2): 127–139

Rogers A, Hassell K, Nicolaas G 1999 Demanding patients? Analysing the use of primary care. Open University Press, Buckingham

Sibbald B, Petchey R, Gosden T, Leese B, Williams J 2000 Salaried GPs in PMS pilots: impact on recruitment, retention, workload, quality of care and cost. In: National evaluation of first wave NHS Personal Medical

Services pilots: integrated interim report from four research projects. NPCRDC, Manchester

Sigfrid LA, Turner C, Crook D, Ray S 2006. Using the UK primary care Quality and Outcomes Framework to audit health care equity: preliminary data on diabetes management. Journal of Public Health 28(3): 221–225

Smith J, Mays N, Dixon J, et al 2004 A review of the effectiveness of primary care-led commissioning and its place in the NHS. The Health Foundation, London

Smith J, Dixon J, Mays N, et al 2005 Practice based commissioning: applying the research evidence.

British Medical Journal 331(7529): 1397–1399

Smith P, York N 2004 Quality incentives: the case of UK general practitioners. Health Affairs 23(3): 112–118

Starfield B 1998 Primary care: balancing health needs, services and technology. Oxford University Press, New York

Timmins N 1995 The five giants. Penguin, Harmondsworth

Wang Y, O'Donnell CA, Mackay DF, Watt GCM 2006 Practice size and quality attainment under the new GMS contract. British Journal of General Practice 56(Nov): 830–835

WHO/UNICEF 1978 Primary health care: the Alma Ata conference. WHO, Geneva

Wilson T, Buck D, Ham C 2005 Rising to the challenge: will the NHS support people with long term conditions? British Medical Journal 330: 657–661

Wilson T, Roland M, Ham C 2006 The contribution of general practice and the general practitioner to NHS patients. Journal of the Royal Society of Medicine 99: 24–28

Recommended reading

Moon G, North N 2000 Policy and place: general medical practice in the UK. Macmillan, Basingstoke

Ottewill R, Wall A 1992 The growth and development of the Community

Health Services. Business Education Publishers, Sunderland

Peckham S, Exworthy M 2003 Primary care in the UK: policy, organisation and management. Palgrave/Macmillan, Basingstoke

Starfield B 1998 Primary care: Balancing health needs, services and technology. Oxford University Press, New York

Innovation and change in public health

David Fone, Shantini Paranjothy and Rhianwen Elen Stiff

KEY ISSUES

- Public health and public health functions
- Practitioners of public health
- Pressures for change
- Innovations and changes
- A case study of modern public health practice in Caerphilly County Borough

Introduction

This chapter provides a framework for understanding recent innovations and change in public health practice. It explores the history of public health from the pioneering days in Victorian times to the pressures for change that have led to the redefinition of the functions of public health and the development of modern public health practice.

A case study of innovation in local collaborative public health practice highlights how modern public health can work to improve community health and reduce health inequality.

What is public health?

Public health is about understanding and improving the health of populations or communities, rather than the health of individuals. The key feature is of a geographically defined population, such as a country or region, or at smaller levels, the local authority or the electoral ward. Within these, public health practitioners may focus on people with a particular illness, such as coronary heart disease, or a client group such as children or the elderly.

Population measures for health improvement include population screening programmes for breast and cervical cancer to identify disease at an early stage for treatment, health promotion activities aimed at the underlying determinants of poor health, such as smoking cessation programmes, and health protection which may include, for example, preparation for and managing outbreaks of infectious disease, non-infectious hazards such as threats to the health of the public from chemical spills, and measures to improve environmental safety, such as reducing danger from unfenced ponds or measures to improve traffic-calming.

The scientific basis of public health practice is the discipline of epidemiology, which is often described as the study of the distribution of diseases in populations. In fact, the science of epidemiology is broad ranging and of fundamental importance to everybody who is working towards improving the health of the population. Epidemiological methods can help us understand the aetiology and natural history of disease, measure the size of health problems to inform planning for action and evaluate the effectiveness and cost-effectiveness of interventions to improve health.

One of the fundamental principles of epidemiology and public health is that the subject of interest must be defined. The most commonly used definition of public health was suggested in the Acheson Report (1988), which reviewed the public health function: 'the science and art of preventing disease, prolonging life, and promoting health through the organised efforts of society'.

This definition makes it clear that public health is not the responsibility of one professional group or organization, but is a process which involves the whole of society. In a report on strengthening the public health function, the Chief Medical Officer for England (Department of Health 2001a) considered that 'this definition is still widely used because it reflects the essential elements of modern public health' (Beaglehole and Bonita 2004). The UK Faculty of Public Health recognizes the public health approach as:

- population based
- emphasizing collective responsibility for health, its protection and disease prevention
- recognizing the key role of the state, linked to a concern for the underlying socio-economic determinants of health as well as disease
- having a multidisciplinary basis, which incorporates quantitative, as well as qualitative, methods
- emphasizing partnerships with all those who contribute to the health of the population.

(See http://www.fphm.org.uk/about_faculty/what_public_health/default.asp.)

What are the public health functions?

Much consideration has been given to defining the public health functions required to move towards a better understanding of how to improve population health through public health practice. Ten public health core activities have been defined by the US Health and Human Services Public Health Service (1995). They are shown in Box 3.1.

The UK Faculty of Public Health defines three overlapping domains in which public health specialists practise. These are health improvement, improving services and health protection (see: http://www.fphm.org.uk/about_faculty/what_public_health/3key_areas_health_practice.asp). The range of activity within each domain is given in Box 3.2.

The UK Faculty of Public Health core values are that public health practice should be equitable, empowering, effective, evidence based, fair and inclusive. Together with the three domains, these inform the Faculty's nine key areas for public health practice:

- surveillance and assessment of the population's health and well-being

---

Box 3.1

The ten public health functions

1. Preventing epidemics
2. Protecting the environment, workplaces, food and water
3. Promoting healthy behaviours
4. Monitoring the health status of the population
5. Mobilizing community action
6. Responding to disasters
7. Assuring the quality, accessibility and accountability of medical care
8. Reaching out to link high-risk and hard-to-reach people to needed services
9. Researching to develop new insights and innovative solutions
10. Leading the development of sound health policy and planning

---

- assessing the evidence of effectiveness of health and healthcare interventions, programmes and services
- policy and strategy development and implementation
- strategic leadership and collaborative working for health
- health improvement
- health protection
- health and social service quality
- public health intelligence
- academic public health

(See: http://www.fphm.org.uk/about_faculty/what_public_health/9key_areas.asp.)

The functions of public health show that everyone, both public and professionals, has responsibilities for improving public health. Public health is clearly not just one activity but requires a broad multidisciplinary team to implement the defined public health functions. The functions will be discharged by many people working for a variety of different organizations in different settings, but all with the same aim of improving the health of the population.

Who practises public health?

It became increasingly apparent that in order to respond to the health inequalities agenda, new

Box 3.2

Public health domains (UK Faculty of Public Health)

Health improvement

- Inequalities
- Education
- Housing
- Employment
- Family/community
- Lifestyles
- Surveillance and monitoring of specific diseases and risk factors

Improving services

- Clinical effectiveness
- Efficiency
- Service planning
- Audit and evaluation
- Clinical governance
- Equity

Health protection

- Infectious diseases
- Chemicals and poisons
- Radiation
- Emergency response
- Environmental health hazards

The UK Faculty of Public Health core values are that public health practice should be equitable, empowering, effective, evidence based, fair and inclusive. Together with the three domains, these inform the Faculty's nine key areas for public health practice:

1. Surveillance and assessment of the population's health and well-being
2. Assessing the evidence of effectiveness of health and healthcare interventions, programmes and services
3. Policy and strategy development and implementation
4. Strategic leadership and collaborative working for health
5. Health improvement
6. Health protection
7. Health and social service quality
8. Public health intelligence
9. Academic public health

See: http://www.fphm.org.uk/about_faculty/what_public_health/9key_areas.asp.

modes of multidisciplinary collaborative teamwork were required. A broader view of the different roles and scope of public health practitioners necessitated a careful consideration of training and professional standards of public health practice. An important debate on the need for appropriately trained and accredited public health specialists who are not medically qualified developed and the question of leadership in public health was aired in the *British Medical Journal* (McPherson et al 2001).

A national tripartite project between the Faculty of Public Health, the Multidisciplinary Public Health Forum and the Royal Institute of Public Health and Hygiene redefined the three levels of public health practice as generalists, practitioners and specialists. This was reflected in the report of the Chief Medical Officer for England on strengthening the public health function (Department of Health 2001a), where he identified three broad categories of people who work to improve public health:

1. *Specialists*: those whose primary role is maintaining and improving the public's health. They come from a variety of professional backgrounds and experience including social science, public health science, environmental health, public health medicine, pharmacy, nursing, health promotion and dentistry. They will have completed specialist training in public health. Specialists will lead public health programmes across organizational boundaries to manage change at strategic and operational levels.

2. *Practitioners*: those for whom public health is part of their role. Public health practitioners include people whose role includes (but not exclusively) furthering health by working with communities or groups. They include health visitors, health promotion specialists, community development workers and environmental health officers. As well as their core professional training and qualification, public health practitioners may have had more specific training in the public health sciences and practice, for example taking a Masters in Public Health degree.

3. *Generalists*: those whose roles have an influence on the wider socio-economic and environmental determinants of health and whose role would benefit from an awareness of public health issues. This may be either at a strategic or

policy level, such as government officials or managers in the NHS or those working with communities or individuals, such as voluntary workers, teachers or housing officers.

The Faculty of Public Health has outlined the nine key areas as the basis for standards of specialist practice (see above). Training schemes, to the standards required to achieve the core competencies as defined by the Faculty and to become a 'specialist', are now available to both doctors in specialist training and to graduates from non-medical backgrounds. In addition, trainees are required to become Members of the Faculty of Public Health by examination. Having achieved membership and satisfactorily shown that they have gained all the skills required by the curriculum, a trainee is eligible for specialist registration, either with the General Medical Council Specialist Register, or the UK Voluntary Register for Public Health Specialists for non-medical graduates. At this point all are eligible for consultant in public health or equivalent posts within the NHS.

An alternative route to 'specialist' status is available to people with experience of working within the field but who have not participated in a dedicated training scheme via a process of 'retrospective recognition'. Those applying are required to demonstrate their experience and capabilities through completion of a portfolio of work. Currently, this allows people to be granted specialist status only in the defined area of public health in which their experience lies, for example pharmaceutical public health or health promotion.

The UK Voluntary Register for Public Health Specialists is currently working on establishing a framework for public health practitioners. Further information may be obtained from the Faculty of Public Health career guidance website: http://www.publichealthconferences.org.uk/careers/ and the UK Voluntary Register for Public Health Specialists website: http://www.publichealthregister.org.uk/.

Local job descriptions will vary, but the key principle of the role of public health specialists is to take a local leadership role, facilitating and leading partnership working between the statutory organizations with a public health remit, such as primary care organizations and the local authority, with links into wider public health networks. A new cadre of well-trained and enthusiastic public health specialists is the key with which the door to modern public health practice is being opened.

History of public health

As medical science developed in the 19th century, a growing awareness that the major causes of epidemic infectious diseases, such as cholera, were preventable through ensuring a clean water supply and safe disposal of sewage led to growth of the public health movement. Edwin Chadwick, a lawyer and engineer and secretary to the Poor Law Commission, was one of the pioneers of the day and the architect of the first Public Health Act of 1848. This was a defining moment in the history of public health. It established a General Board of Health and local boards were set up which became the forerunners of local government. The 1848 Act gave the boards of health permissive powers to monitor and enforce control of the environment, through activities such as inspecting drains. It recommended the appointment of Medical Officers of Health to advise on matters relating to the health of the community. These appointments were not obligatory until the next major Public Health Act of 1875, which obliged local health boards to improve a range of sanitary and environmental provisions.

But what was the role of the Medical Officer of Health? One of the most perceptive comments on this subject was made by P.H. Holland Esq., the General Board of Health inspector sent to assess the condition of Merthyr in 1853. In a letter to C. Macauley Esq, the secretary of the General Board of Health, dated 15 December 1853, he recommended the appointment of a Medical Officer of Health and believed that:

> *the labour of such officer will do much to* **remove the ignorance** *which has permitted such evils to arise, to* **arouse the apathy** *which allows their continuance, and to overcome the opposition which impedes their removal. Such officers would* **show** *the fearful amount of suffering disease and death produced for want of means for bringing pure water into the town, and for taking foul water out of it. They would* **prove** *that the losses occasioned by avoidable sickness and its consequences reduce a well paid population to poverty.*

A sequence of four public health activities was envisaged to carry out these duties. These are shown in Box 3.3.

Box 3.3

Four public health activities for the Medical Officer of Health, 1853

1. Epidemiological investigation of disease prevalence and incidence (**to show**).
2. Evidence-based assessment of the socio-economic impact of the disease burden (**to prove**).
3. Dissemination of knowledge about disease and their causes (**to remove ignorance**).
4. Advocacy for changing environmental conditions (**arouse the apathy**).

As a result of the Public Health Acts of the 19th century, public health practice was based in local authorities. Environmental health departments employed environmental health officers whose role was to investigate and control outbreaks of communicable disease, and be responsible for enforcing standards relating to food, water supplies and sewage disposal, housing and air quality. The responsibilities of the Medical Officer of Health widened to include responsibility for community health services, such as maternity and child welfare, and responsibility for the new municipal hospitals.

Local authorities continued to provide these public health services until the 1974 NHS reorganization. After 1974, the Medical Officer for Health role became the responsibility of health authorities and the medical specialty was renamed community medicine. This fragmented the public health service and removed the focus for public health doctors away from public health and their colleagues in nursing and environmental health to a more medical administrative role. This 'new' specialty of community medicine further lost its way in successive NHS reorganizations and in 1988 the Acheson Report (1988), taking stock of the 'crisis' in public health, suggested renaming the specialty back to public health medicine. He recommended the appointment of Directors of Public Health as an executive director and member of the health authority board. The professional role of the Director of Public Health was to assess the health needs of the health authority resident population, to publish an annual independent report on the health of the population and play a key role in organizing the necessary multisectoral and multidisciplinary links to implement change to improve the health of the population.

However, despite this role, the specialty of public health medicine in health authorities became increasingly isolated in the 1990s from the wider practice of public health. Public health physicians were increasingly drawn into the commissioning of secondary and tertiary hospital services within the NHS purchaser/provider split. The health service reforms of 1990 brought in by the NHS and Community Care Act 1990 established an 'internal market' healthcare system in which health authorities and some GP fundholding practices acted as *purchasers* of healthcare, setting up contracts for provision of services with hospitals, the *providers* of healthcare. Despite the rhetoric that services should be commissioned on the basis of healthcare need and interesting theoretical frameworks for healthcare needs assessment (Stevens and Raftery 1994, see: http://hcna.radcliffe-oxford.com/introframe.htm), there was little evidence that assessment of health need actually drove the process; contracting for healthcare within the internal market was essentially a financial accounting process, with small marginal shifts in provision over time.

This was the situation up until as recently as 1997. Since then, modern multidisciplinary public health practice has continued to evolve in response to the pressures for change that are described in the following section.

Pressures for change

The fundamental pressure for change has been the refocusing of the public health agenda back to its core purpose of improving the health of the population and reducing health inequalities through action on the wider societal determinants of health. An understanding of social exclusion, which refers to individuals living in communities on the margins of society as a result of a cycle of problems such as low educational achievement, unemployment, poor health and crumbling community infrastructure, was made possible through societal change which included an increasing awareness of these issues and a greater individual and community involvement in solutions. All those practising public health realized the need to move away from the traditional medical model of public health practice to a multiprofessional approach in order to rise to the challenges posed by health inequalities. The newly elected Labour government in 1997 provided the necessary policy frameworks for change.

Inequalities in health

The fundamental pressure for change has been the awareness of increasing evidence for health inequalities within the UK and the need for action to address them. Although absolute levels of health have improved in the UK over the last 20 years, the effect has been simultaneously to widen the health divide between affluent and deprived populations (Shaw et al 1999).

In the late 1970s, the Labour government established the Black Committee on Inequalities in Health, chaired by Sir Douglas Black. Their report published in 1980, the Black Report, has since become a landmark in the history of understanding inequalities in health (Department of Health and Social Security 1980, Townsend and Davidson 1988). The report highlighted the substantial variations in health that existed in the UK, arguing that these inequalities were caused by inequality in material well-being and poverty. However, the report was rejected by the Conservative government of the day on the grounds that implementation of the recommendations was financially unrealistic. The report was effectively suppressed as the government restricted the number of copies published to a few hundred and there was no official publicity.

Although increasing evidence on health inequalities was published during the 1980s (Whitehead 1987), it was not government policy to explicitly address them. Eventually the overwhelming research evidence that was being published did lead the Conservative government to establish a Health Variations Group in 1994 (the word 'inequalities' was never used), chaired by the Chief Medical Officer for England. Their comprehensive and enlightened report (Department of Health 1995) identified that although some activity within the NHS was addressing the so-called 'variations' in health, it was taking place at the margins of health authority business. The report reinforced the need for 'alliances' with local government, voluntary and community organizations to make progress, and made a series of recommendations that paved the way for change later in the decade.

Following the election of the new Labour government in 1997, an independent inquiry into inequalities in health was commissioned, chaired by Sir Donald Acheson. Their report (Department of Health 1998a) made 39 recommendations for action. A detailed examination of the evidence presented to the inquiry was published a year later (Gordon et al 1999), summarizing the evidence base for each recommendation.

The three areas considered by the independent inquiry to be crucial to reducing inequalities in health are shown in Box 3.4.

> **Box 3.4**
>
> **Three areas crucial to reducing inequalities in health**
>
> 1. All policies likely to have an impact on health should be evaluated in terms of their impact on health inequalities.
> 2. A high priority should be given to the health of families with children.
> 3. Further steps should be taken to reduce income inequalities and improve the living standards of poor households.
>
> Source: Department of Health (1998a).

What innovations and change are happening?

Innovation and change will be considered under the three domains of health improvement, improving services and health protection.

Health improvement

Surveillance and assessment of the population's health and well-being

Growing acknowledgement of the need for a greater understanding of inequalities in health at a local level, for local planning, has given a new focus to public health practitioners in the surveillance and assessment of the population's health and well-being. This focus has moved away from large population areas to geographically defined small areas (such as administrative local government units of the electoral ward, population of around 5000 people). At this small area level, information on disease and health status is usefully displayed in maps. Maps of disease will highlight areas of greatest risk and reveal patterns of local geographical variation that may not be suspected from inspection of the same data as numbers in tables. Maps are an important source of information for local planners, as well as generating hypotheses on causal mechanisms that can be tested in further research studies.

There is a long history of geographical public health and the use of maps of disease to highlight health inequality. The first example is that of John Snow and the Broad Street pump in Soho, London in 1854 (Donaldson and Donaldson 2003). The increasing availability of information at a small spatial level, coupled with the growth in computer technology and geographical information systems (GIS), small area statistical methods and advances in disease-mapping techniques, has led to a much wider use of geographical information in health needs assessment. These techniques have greatly enhanced the presentation and analysis of information as a basis for strategic planning to address health inequality.

New Internet-based interactive GIS technology has resulted in the wider availability of small area data for planning. For example, the Office for National Statistics Neighbourhood Statistics website (see online: http://www.statistics.gov.uk) has a wide range of multiagency data at electoral ward and unitary authority for England and Wales that can be downloaded and used to calculate local rates for presentation in tables and maps.

There are some important epidemiological pitfalls that should be avoided in converting these data into disease maps. First, to convert Neighbourhood Statistics data, which are presented as number of events, into a rate requires the choice and availability of an appropriate denominator. Second, if the numbers of events, or population size of an electoral division is small (commonly the case in rural areas of the UK), then the differences between small areas are likely to be due to random variation rather than differences in true underlying risk. Third, the appearance and interpretation of a map can vary with choice of data ranges and colour scales used to present the data. An excellent introduction to the subject including discussion of these pitfalls is given in Lawson and Williams (2001).

An example of innovation in the surveillance and assessment of population health using geographical multiagency social, economic, environmental and health data at the small area level is shown in Case study 3.1 (see pp. 39–43).

Policy and strategy development and implementation – collaborative working for health

The whole thrust of the new Labour government's policy response to reducing health inequalities lies through multisectoral partnership working between the NHS, corporate local government and other organizations to address the social, economic and environmental determinants of health. A series of measures has been implemented to work towards this aim. In this section we will focus on measures taken in England, but the NHS in Wales and Scotland has published similar policy documents. A useful discussion of the similarities and differences between the White Papers from the three countries is given in an NHS Confederation Briefing Paper (see online: http://www.nhsconfed.net).

First, the government took the traditional step of reorganizing the NHS, this time with the aim of enhancing the role of primary care to play a leading role in health improvement and reducing inequalities. Government White Papers were published (Department of Health 1997) which ended the internal market and established primary care groups in England. These were based on groups of GP practices and where possible coterminous local authority areas of population size around 100 000 to 200 000 people. The boards of primary care groups are multiprofessional, and include GPs, community nurses, pharmacists, optometrists, dentists, local authority representatives and voluntary sector representatives. In addition to responsibilities for local health services, they were given new population health responsibilities to 'improve the health of, and address health inequality in, the local community' (Department of Health 1999). This was an important step towards integrating the expertise and local knowledge on health and social well-being held by primary care practitioners, such as community nurses, into the local planning arrangements to improve health (see Chapter 4 for further discussion of how community nurses can use baseline data as a starting point for planning health improvement strategies).

The government responded to the recommendations of the independent inquiry on inequalities in health with a White Paper on public health entitled *Saving Lives: Our Healthier Nation* (Department of Health 1999). This document was presented as an action plan to tackle poor health. Its emphasis was clearly to improve the overall health of the population, through partnership working between all sectors with an influence on health, to be monitored nationally through a series of targets to reduce deaths from coronary heart disease and stroke, cancer, accidents and suicide (Box 3.5), with the expectation that local targets will be set locally.

Box 3.5

Saving Lives: Our Healthier Nation: national targets

By the year 2010:

- cancer: to reduce the death rate in people under 75 **by at least a fifth**
- coronary heart disease and stroke: to reduce the death rate in people under 75 **by at least two fifths**
- accidents: to reduce the death rate **by at least a fifth** and serious injury **by at least a tenth**
- mental illness: to reduce the death rate from suicide and undetermined injury **by at least a fifth**.

Source: *Saving Lives: Our Healthier Nation* (Department of Health 1999).

However, no explicit national targets were set at the time to reduce health inequality.

Saving Lives: Our Healthier Nation acknowledged the crucial role that nurses have to play in promoting health and preventing illness. Emphasis was given to the role of health visitors, school nurses, midwives and occupational health nurses as public health practitioners. The government's view was summarized as 'to develop a family-centred public health role, working with individuals, families and communities to improve health and tackle health inequality'.

In 2001, the government published a consultation document in England on a set of core national health inequalities targets (Department of Health 2001b). The report reinforces the broader societal and partnership approach required to tackle health inequalities, including the NHS, academic institutions, local government departments, community and voluntary sector organizations, employers, the business community and trade unions. Following the consultation process, national health inequality targets were published in 2002 and progress can be found in 'Tackling health inequalities: status report on the Programme for Action' (see online: http://www.dh.gov.uk/en/Publicationsandstatistics/Publications/PublicationsPolicyAndGuidance/DH_4117696).

More recently, the public health White Paper *Choosing Health: Making Healthy Choices Easier* (Department of Health 2004, see online: http://www.dh.gov.uk/en/Publicationsandstatistics/Publications/PublicationsPolicyAndGuidance/

DH_4094550) aims to continue with efforts to reduce health inequalities and improve health through providing practical solutions to a number of public health concerns identified through extensive consultation with the public in England. Three core principles of a new public health approach underpin this strategy:

1. *Informed choice*: provision of credible and trustworthy information to help people make their own decisions about choices that impact on health, and achieved in part through developing the work of the Public Health Observatories. However, it was felt that there are special governmental responsibilities for children and in cases where one person's choices may cause harm or nuisance to another, e.g. exposure to second-hand smoke.

2. *Personalization*: tailoring support to the 'realities of individual lives, with services and support personalized sensitively and provided flexibly and conveniently' in order to be effective in tackling health inequalities.

3. *Working together*: government should lead, coordinate and promote effective collaborative partnerships across communities with local government, the NHS, business, advertisers, retailers, the voluntary sector, the media, faith organizations and many others.

The consultation process established a shared set of priorities for action:

- reducing the numbers of people who smoke
- reducing obesity and improving diet and nutrition
- increasing exercise
- encouraging and supporting sensible drinking
- improving sexual health
- improving mental health.

This strategy has produced many examples of collaborative approaches to improving the health of the public and providing the means by which the public can make decisions to improve their own individual health. Examples range from working with the food industry to develop better information on the nutritional content of packaged food to commissioning Health Direct as an online information service providing advice and links to existing services such as support for parents, provided by Sure Start (see online: http://www.healthdirect.co.uk/index.html).

The first Sure Start local programmes were established in 1999 as the result of the 1998 Comprehensive Spending Review. Sure Start local programmes were an area-based initiative, initially targeted at deprived communities, which worked by bringing together early education, childcare, health and family support for the benefit of families and young children from before birth to 4 years of age. The aim was to provide the best opportunities for children to flourish once they attended school.

Since its inception, the programme has extended considerably. The Sure Start, Extended Schools and Families Group now supports families from pregnancy right through until children are 14, or 16 for children with disabilities.

Sure Start, Extended Schools and Childcare Group forms part of the Children, Young People and Families Directorate of the Department for Children, Schools and Families. Through collaborative working with local authorities, primary care trusts, Jobcentre Plus, local communities, public agencies and voluntary and private sector organizations, Sure Start aims to achieve better outcomes for children, parents and communities by: ensuring delivery of free early education for all 3- and 4-year-olds; providing affordable, quality childcare and after-school activities in every area; and providing children's centres and health and family support, particularly in disadvantaged areas where they are most needed. It works with parents to build aspirations for employment and for their children's education.

The government's 10-year childcare strategy, *Choice for Parents, the Best Start for Children*, was published alongside the pre-budget report on 2 December 2004. The aims are to ensure provision of choice and flexibility for parents in obtaining and maintaining work and family life balance, e.g. through extended parental leave, increasing availability of Sure Start Children's Centres and high-quality affordable childcare for all. The strategy was formalized in the Childcare Act of 2006, placing duties on local authorities and reforming early years' regulation and inspection arrangements.

Further information about Sure Start initiatives can be obtained at: http://www.surestart.gov.uk/.

Skilled for Health (see: http://www.continyou. org.uk/content.php?CategoryID=292) provides practical support for people who lack basic skills to help them use health information. Sure Start itself is planned to further develop and roll out programmes to improve support for parents in understanding issues that impact on their children's social, emotional and physical development. Expansion of the home volunteer visiting programme through Home Start for families under stress is also envisaged. Healthy Start is a new initiative since 2005 which provides disadvantaged pregnant women and mothers of young children with vouchers for fresh food and vegetables, milk and infant formula. The National Healthy Schools programme encourages schools to foster better health in all aspects – healthy environment, smoking, healthy food and physical activity. All schools should be aiming for healthy school status by 2009.

The consultation process to produce *Choosing Health* identified establishing smoke-free workplace and public environments as a contentious issue. Subsequent legislation has seen all enclosed public spaces and workplaces become smoke free. Both *Choosing Health* and *Health, Work and Well-being; Caring for our Future* (see: http://www.dh. gov.uk/en/Publicationsandstatistics/Publications/ PublicationsPolicyAndGuidance/DH_4121756) acknowledge the importance of work in offering self-esteem, companionship, structure and status as well as income. Both strategies outline ways to improve the health of the working population through endeavours such as reducing barriers to work to improve health and reduce inequalities, improving working conditions to limit work-related ill health and injury, encouraging a healthy workplace and providing occupational health services.

Perhaps five innovations embodied the wider collaborative approach to tackling health inequalities and improving health. These are Public Health Observatories, health improvement programmes, health impact assessment, Health Action Zones and Healthy Living Centres.

Health Improvement Programme

The government White Paper *Saving Lives: Our Healthier Nation* introduced the Health Authority Health Improvement Programme as the strategic planning mechanism to bring the necessary partnerships together to tackle local health inequality and bring about health improvement (Department of Health 1999). Health improvement programmes included a comprehensive local health needs assessment to identify health inequalities and set out a range of local priorities for evidence-based action to address them, improve the health of the local population and improve local healthcare services.

Health improvement programmes aimed to address policy areas that have a major impact on social exclusion, such as drugs and alcohol, crime and disorder, community care, asylum seekers and the health of prisoners. Local priorities also focused on the major groups of diseases, such as coronary heart disease, cancers and respiratory disease and other areas of concern, such as sexual health and injury prevention. Health promotion strategies, such as tobacco control, and health protection strategies, such as communicable disease control, non-infectious environmental hazards, healthy transport and housing, are an important output of partnership planning. As with any strategy, a detailed consideration of resource requirements was needed, as well as plans for monitoring and evaluation of the impact of the Health Improvement Programme.

The Health Improvement Programme has continued to develop within the policy frameworks of the four nations. In England, for example, they have been brought in under the umbrella of *Choosing Health: Making Healthy Choices Easier* (Department of Health 2004, see: http://www. dh.gov.uk/en/Publicationsandstatistics/Publica tions/PublicationsPolicyAndGuidance/DH_ 4094550). In Wales a different approach has been taken and new 'Health, social care and well being strategies' (see: http://new.wales.gov.uk/topics/ health/publications/health/strategies/hscwbs trategies?lang=en) replaced the Health Improvement Programme in 2003. Further information for Scotland can be found on the website of the Scottish Executive (http://www.improvementservice.org.uk/ health-improvement/health/programme-activities/ or http://www.scotland.gov.uk/Resource/Doc/47034 /0013854.pdf); for Northern Ireland see: http:// www.dhsspsni.gov.uk/eq-antipoverty.

Health Action Zones

Health Action Zones (Department of Health 1997) were introduced to develop local innovative strategies to tackle health inequalities, deliver measurable improvements in public health and health outcomes and modernize local treatment and care services. They were an innovative approach to public health collaborative action, 'Linking health, regeneration, employment, education, housing and anti-poverty initiatives to the needs of vulnerable groups and deprived communities'. Twenty-six Health Action Zones were established in England, representing areas of England with some of the highest levels of

---

Box 3.6

Health Action Zones: five levels of collaborative action

1. Strategic – to establish the vision and key themes pertaining to its achievement.
2. Governance – to secure the accountability of HAS activity, and to establish means of monitoring performance and the agreed framework within which the HAS partners will work.
3. Operational – the activities that will help deliver the vision.
4. Practice – the ability of professionals and others to work with users and communities in new ways.
5. Community – the development of confidence, skills and infrastructure to engage in multisector partnership working.

Source: Barnes et al (2001). Further details are available on the Health Action Zones website at http://www.investingforhealthni. gov.uk/zones.asp.

---

social deprivation and poor health. They range in population size from 180000 to 1.4 million people, covering over 13 million people in total. Health Action Zones are coordinated by a local partnership board, representing the NHS, local authorities, the voluntary and private sectors and community groups.

A national evaluation of Health Action Zones report (Barnes et al 2004; see: http://stage.library. nhs.uk/ppi/ViewResource.aspx?resID=143475) and the interim report of initial findings from a strategic level analysis (Barnes et al 2001) highlighted the successes and difficulties faced in making Health Action Zones work. Of interest is the detailed analysis of what collaboration actually means in practice. Five levels are considered necessary (Box 3.6). In England, Health Action Zone activities have now been incorporated into the development of sustainable mainstream practice within primary care trusts.

Healthy Living Centres

The Healthy Living Centre initiative was set up in January 1999 by the New Opportunities Fund (now known as the Big Lottery Fund), the lottery body established under the National Lottery Act. Healthy Living Centres were provided with 5-year funding and aimed to support national and local health strategies to tackle inequalities in health, including

Saving Lives: Our Healthier Nation and local health improvement programmes.

Healthy Living Centres aimed to promote a social model of health through interventions focused in disadvantaged areas and population groups, for example from Health Action Zones. They were locally based, and relevant to people of all ages. Their development was seen as an opportunity to develop multisectoral and multiprofessional partnerships across many different organizations to create a valued community resource to provide facilities and services in new ways to people who may not be accessing existing services. This might include, for example, parenting classes or smoking cessation schemes.

The funding deadline for new Healthy Living Centre closed in January 2002, and therefore most Healthy Living Centres have now completed their 5-year Big Lottery grants. Opportunities exist for maintaining the work of Healthy Living Centres through application for funding via other Big Lottery initiatives such as 'Reaching Communities' in England or 'Healthy Families: Way of Life' in Wales. Alternatively, in some locations, local public health teams are supporting the perpetuation of Healthy Living Centres work.

Health impact assessment

Health impact assessment acknowledges the important effects that a wide range of policies across a wide range of sectors may have on health and may be applied to a policy, a programme or a single project. These might include, for example, the siting of a new airport runway, road building schemes, new factory developments or a local planning application.

Health impact assessment has been defined in a number of ways. One definition given by Ratner et al (1997) is:

Any combination of procedures or methods by which a proposed policy or program may be judged as to the effects it may have on the health of a population.

The overall aim of health impact assessment is to provide a means of ensuring that the potential impact on health is taken into account as part of the decision-making process for policies, programmes and other developments. Health impact assessment may be prospective, in which prediction of the likely health effects is made, concurrent, in which the consequences are assessed as the policy or programme is being implemented, or retrospective, in which the health effects are assessed after policy implementation. Most health impact assessments undertaken to date have been retrospective, but as methodologies become tested, many more prospective studies will be undertaken. An interesting example of health impact assessment is that of the New Home Energy Efficiency Scheme (Kemm et al 2001).

The Welsh Impact Assessment Support Unit (WIASU) provides a valuable resource for those currently participating in, or wishing to undertake, a health impact assessment. The unit provides advice, guidance and support through the provision of awareness-raising presentations, training sessions, facilitation of rapid appraisals and support for other ongoing health impact assessments. The unit is currently involved in a World Health Organization/ European Commission Project entitled: 'The effectiveness of health impact assessment'. The project aims to map the use of health impact assessment, evaluate its effectiveness and develop the determinants for its successful use. The results of Task One of the European study can be found on the 'Project Results' page of the European Observatory website (http://www.euro.who.int/observatory/Studies/ 20040310_1).

Further information on WHIASU may be found at: http://www.wales.nhs.uk/sites3/home.cfm?orgid =522 and further examples of health impact assessment case studies may be found at: http://www. wales.nhs.uk/sites3/page.cfm?orgid=522& pid=10108.

Public Health Observatories

The fundamental importance of high-quality public health information required for health and social needs assessment, surveillance and monitoring of disease, monitoring and evaluation, and setting of meaningful targets to reduce health inequality has been recognized by the government. Eight Public Health Observatories were initially established in England (Department of Health 1999), with the following remit:

- monitoring health and disease trends and highlighting areas for action
- identifying gaps in health information
- advising on methods for health and health inequality impact assessments
- drawing together information from different sources in new ways to improve health
- carrying out projects to highlight particular health issues

- evaluating progress by local agencies in improving health and cutting inequality
- looking ahead to give early warning of future public health problems.

The Association of Public Health Observatories (APHO) now represents and coordinates a network of 12 Public Health Observatories working across the five nations of England, Scotland, Wales, Northern Ireland and the Republic of Ireland.

A key output has been the production of the health profiles for England, (a deliverable of the *Choosing Health* White Paper). Each health profile is local authority specific and provides an overview of the local population's health. Profiles can be utilized to inform local needs assessment, policy, planning, performance management, surveillance and practice. They provide a means of comparison locally, regionally and nationally as well as over time, and are a means of suggesting areas for targeted resource allocation.

The APHO is contributing to the delivery of the government's Public Health Intelligence and Information (I&I) Strategy *Informing Healthier Choices: Information and Intelligence for Healthy Populations* (see: http://www.dh.gov.uk/en/ Publicationsandstatistics/Publications/Publications PolicyAndGuidance/DH_075488) through four areas: improved data and information provision; stronger, more focused organizations; workforce training and support; and the development of a national health information and intelligence system. It is envisaged that collaborative working with regional cancer registries, health protection agencies and others will produce a more integrated health intelligence function for their area. The recent *Strong and Prosperous Communities – The Local Government White Paper in England* (see: http:// www.communities.gov.uk/publications/localgov ernment/strongprosperous) will provide fresh impetus to developing public health work with local government colleagues, e.g. building on health profiles.

Further information on the wide-ranging work of the Public Health Observatories can be accessed online at: http://www.apho.org.uk/apho/index.htm.

Improving services

In 1998, the UK government set out its strategy for reorganization of the NHS, with the aim of creating a modern health service that delivers high-quality services for all (Department of Health, 1998b, also see the NHS Plan 2000 at: http://www.dh.gov.uk/

en/Publicationsandstatistics/Publications/ PublicationsPolicyAndGuidance/DH_4002960). The need for clear national standards for healthcare was acknowledged in these documents and structures within the NHS for setting standards and monitoring performance were outlined, such as the National Institute for Health and Clinical Excellence (NICE, see: http://www.nice.org.uk/), the national service frameworks (NSFs, see: http://www. dh.gov.uk/en/Sitemap/DH_A-Z_AZSI?index Char=N) and the Commission for Health Improvement (now known as the Healthcare Commission, see: http://www.healthcarecommission.org.uk).

NICE is an independent organization responsible for providing national guidance on the promotion of good health and the prevention and treatment of ill health. They provide evidence-based guidance for public health practice, the use of health technologies and in clinical practice.

Since April 1998, NSFs have been developed for a number of clinical disease areas such as coronary heart disease and chronic obstructive pulmonary disease, and for services such as paediatric intensive care and care groups such as older people and children. NSFs were developed to address variations in standards of care and to achieve greater consistency in the availability and quality of health services, thus providing a systematic approach towards improving standards and quality across healthcare sectors. NSFs were developed by multidisciplinary groups, bringing together health professionals, service users and carers, health service managers, partner agencies, and other advocates. The groups consider the available evidence to set national standards and define service models for a service or care group, and establish performance measures against which progress within agreed timescales can be assessed.

The Healthcare Commission has been set up to promote improvements in the quality of healthcare and public health in England and Wales. In England, they are responsible for assessing and reporting on the performance of both NHS and independent healthcare organizations, to ensure that a high standard of care is provided. In Wales, they work closely with the Health Inspectorate Wales, who are responsible for the NHS in Wales.

Health protection

Traditionally, health protection activity by public health specialists in the UK was largely centred around the control of communicable diseases such as tuberculosis, *E. coli* and meningococcal disease. More recent challenges in health protection include emerging infections such as sudden acute respiratory syndrome (SARS) and avian influenza, and active surveillance is ongoing to address these issues. These emerging threats to public health have also renewed the focus for ensuring that an appropriate public health response can be initiated and coordinated at a local, national or international level depending on the situation. Therefore emergency preparedness has become a key area of work for public health specialists working in health protection. Today health protection has a much broader remit, covering not only infectious diseases, but also chemicals and poisons, radiation and environmental health hazards. Examples of recent major incidents in the UK that required public health protection response include the Buncefield oil depot fire (Palmer et al

2006). Understanding and managing the public's perception of risk following such events is an important area of work within this domain.

The Health Protection Agency was set up in the UK in 2001 as an arm's length body to provide an integrated approach to protecting UK public health through the provision of support and advice to the NHS, local authorities, emergency services, the Department of Health and the devolved administrations. In 2003, the Agency became a special health authority (SpHA), and in 2005 it was established as a non-departmental public body, incorporating the functions of the National Radiological Protection Board (NRPB). The key function of the Agency is 'to protect the community (or any part of the community) against infectious diseases and other dangers to health'. More information on the Health Protection Agency and the services they provide can be obtained from their website (http://www.hpa.org.uk/).

Case study 3.1 The Caerphilly Health and Social Needs Study – information for action

This case study aims to show how a modern collaborative and multidisciplinary public health approach across organizational boundaries can integrate all ten public health functions within local work to achieve positive benefits to the health and social well-being of a local geographically defined population.

The study is based in the county borough of Caerphilly, situated within the former Gwent Health Authority area (Figure 3.1), one of the 22 unitary authorities in Wales.

The county borough of Caerphilly was formerly dominated by the mining industry. However, the past 20 years has seen a dramatic decline in the traditional heavy industries of coal and, whereas in 1950 there were 29 pits employing 24 000 people, the last of the borough's pits closed in 1990. Throughout this period of pit closure, the borough, and indeed much of south-east Wales, suffered major changes in its social and economic structure and high levels of unemployment. Many families are seeing a second generation grow up in unemployment and poverty.

This social and economic decline has resulted in the county borough of Caerphilly containing some of the most deprived electoral wards in Wales and England. Two census wards situated in the Upper Rhymney Valley in the north of the borough are in the highest ranking 5% of wards in England and Wales on both the Breadline Britain and the Work Poverty Indices (Glennerster et al 1999).

In order to take forward the new public health agenda set out in the Welsh Public Health Strategy Green Papers *Better Health Better Wales* (Welsh Office 1998a) and the *Strategic Framework* (Welsh Office 1998b), Gwent Health Authority and Caerphilly County Borough Council made commitments to partnership working. Both authorities had started the process of developing local plans to improve health: Gwent Health Authority was leading on the development of the Health Improvement Programme (HIP) and Caerphilly County Borough Council had developed a comprehensive public health strategy for the Corporate Plan 1998–2001 (Caerphilly County Borough Council 1998) which included action on community regeneration strategies to address inequalities within the most deprived Upper Rhymney Valley area of the borough.

Planning local initiatives for local targeting of resources to reduce health inequalities requires analysis of epidemiological data on social, economic and environmental determinants of health and health outcomes at the small area level. In order to gain a greater understanding of the health and social needs of the Caerphilly County Borough, the collaboration between the Directors of Environmental Services and Housing (local authority) and Public Health (health authority) proposed a four-stage study, the Caerphilly Health and Social Needs Study (Box 3.7).

A study steering group was established, with representatives from the health authority, the local

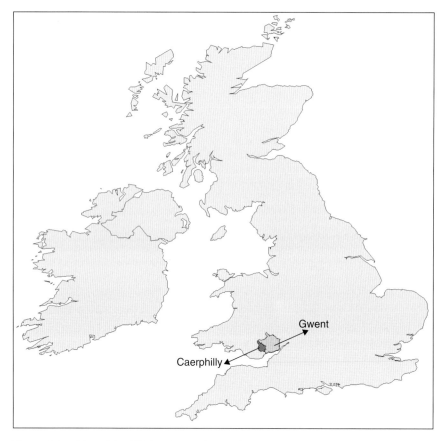

Figure 3.1 • Map of the UK showing the former Gwent Health Authority area and Caerphilly County Borough.

health group (equivalent to a primary care group in England) and the local authority. The steering group therefore had links into general medical practice, community nursing and the Local Health Alliance, which has a wide membership including the Community Health Council, local voluntary groups and local organizations.

The work of the study was undertaken through a working group. This included public health specialists and practitioners, including consultants and senior lecturers in public health medicine, research officers in information, epidemiology and GIS, social scientists, and officers from the Directorates of Environmental Health and Housing, Education, and Social Services within the local authority.

Methods

We chose the 1998 electoral division as the area level for analysis, defined by the April 1998 boundary changes to

the original 1991 census wards. The total population of the borough is 170 000, living within 33 electoral divisions.

The working group identified new sources of data from the local authority in the Chief Executive's, Education, Environmental Services and Housing and Social Services directorates. Data from the Chief Executive's directorate included Department of Social Security (DSS) claimant count data on means-tested and non-means-tested benefits and unemployment counts requested from the National Online Manpower Information Service (NOMIS) database. The Council Tax and Benefits division of the local authority supplied data on the proportion of houses in each council tax band A to H. The Education Department supplied data on educational achievement at GCSE (Key Stage 4), together with data on free school meal uptake and children with special educational needs. From a five-stage classification on the identification and assessment of special educational needs, data were aggregated for

Box 3.7

Caerphilly Health and Social Needs Study

Aims

- To achieve a greater understanding of the relationship between social, environmental and economic deprivation and health in Caerphilly County Borough, in comparison to the other boroughs in the Gwent Health Authority area, and to inform the development of local community regeneration strategies for health improvement and better targeting of resources.
- To establish a robust methodology for sharing and joint analysis of information between Gwent Health Authority and Caerphilly County Borough Council, and to inform the development of the health needs assessment information required by the Local Health Group and Local Health Alliance for developing the Health Improvement Programme.

Objectives

- To report the descriptive and comparative epidemiology of social, environmental and economic deprivation at the small area level in Caerphilly County Borough and the Gwent Health Authority area, sharing and integrating data from the following health and local authority data sets:
  - census data – local base statistics; local authority data, e.g. free school meals, unemployment
  - vital statistics (population, births and deaths); Welsh Public Health Common Data set
  - To use geographical information software to present profiles of Gwent and the county borough of Caerphilly, to highlight areas of greatest social, economic and environmental need and health outcomes.
- Further analysis of the data sets to identify gaps in knowledge, highlight areas for special study and generate hypotheses on the relationship between social, environmental and economic deprivation and health within Caerphilly County Borough which may be tested by further research.

---

stages 3, 4 and 5, where, as a minimum, teachers and the special educational needs coordinator are supported by specialists from outside the school.

Sharing of data between the health and local authorities was facilitated by the Gwent Information Exchange Protocol, which takes into account the requirements of the Data Protection Act legislation.

The education and social services data were shared as an anonymous postcoded data set. These postcodes were linked to the electoral division of residence using *Map Info* GIS software. In order to convert the data into electoral division-based rates, population denominators were extracted from the health authority general practice administrative age–sex register and, where required, household denominators were taken from the 1991 census. Denominators for the education data were based on school roll data supplied by the National Assembly for Wales Schools Census (Stats 1) return.

A wide range of health data that are routinely obtained and analysed by the Directorate of Public Health in the health authority were used in the study. Among these were mortality data from the Office for National Statistics (ONS) for many different causes of death, including all-causes, coronary heart disease, cerebrovascular disease, respiratory disease, all malignant neoplasms, lung cancer, breast cancer and all accidents and adverse effects. The Welsh Cancer Intelligence and Surveillance Unit supplied data on the incidence of all malignant neoplasms, lung cancer, female breast cancer, colorectal and prostate cancer.

We classified each of the data sets identified by the study into one of six domains: income, unemployment, housing, health, education and Social Services. For local planning purposes, thematic maps of all variables were prepared to highlight variation between electoral divisions within the borough. In the maps, each electoral division is assigned to one of five colour scales, based on dividing the range of the distribution of the variable into equal fifths. This enables easy identification of the lowest ranking electoral divisions for any particular variable.

Examples are shown in Figure 3.2. Four maps (council tax bands A and B, children in families on income support, referrals of children to social services and GCSE (Key Stage 4) educational achievement) are shown to illustrate their value in highlighting areas of greatest need and inequality.

How were the study data used?

A Health and Social Needs Profile Report (see: http://www.wales.nhs.uk/sites3/documents/368/ACF25EA.pdf) was written and local ownership of the data and the interpretation of the disease maps were obtained through presentations to meetings of the executive directors of the health and local authorities and of the full council. The use of the profile in population-based health and

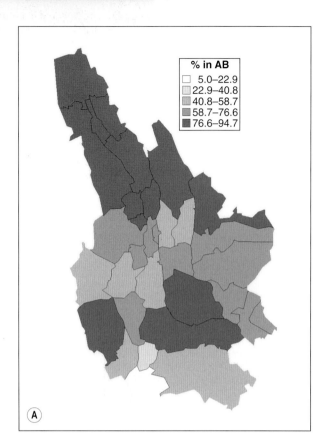

(A)

% in AB
- 5.0–22.9
- 22.9–40.8
- 40.8–58.7
- 58.7–76.6
- 76.6–94.7

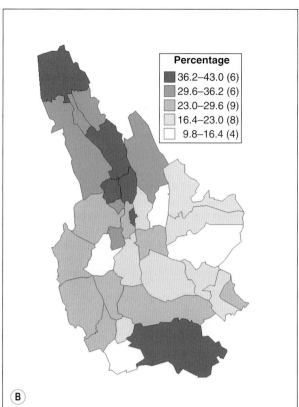

(B)

Percentage
- 36.2–43.0 (6)
- 29.6–36.2 (6)
- 23.0–29.6 (9)
- 16.4–23.0 (8)
- 9.8–16.4 (4)

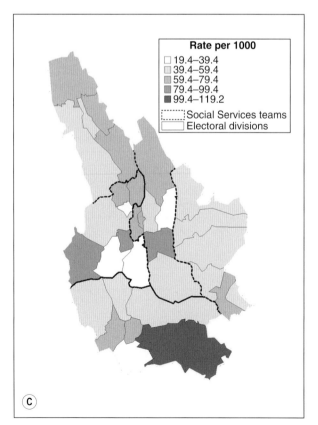

(C)

Rate per 1000
- 19.4–39.4
- 39.4–59.4
- 59.4–79.4
- 79.4–99.4
- 99.4–119.2

Social Services teams
Electoral divisions

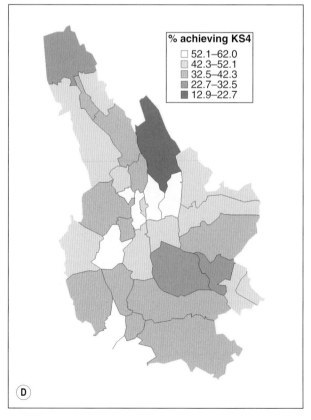

(D)

% achieving KS4
- 52.1–62.0
- 42.3–52.1
- 32.5–42.3
- 22.7–32.5
- 12.9–22.7

social needs assessment and a variety of local strategic planning processes has provided the local health group with the means to fulfil its population-based duties of improving health and reducing health inequality in the local community. The profile is a policy tool for advocating change, enabling local agencies to move forward on the local partnership agenda to improve health and reduce health inequality.

The first use of the profile was in the Caerphilly LHG Local Action Plan of the Health Improvement Programme. The local authority also has statutory service planning responsibilities and the profile enhanced the information used to formulate the Children's Services Plan (Caerphilly County Borough Council Directorate of Social Services 2000a), Social Care Plan (Caerphilly County Borough Council Directorate of Social Services 2000b) and the Housing Strategy and Operational Plan (Caerphilly County Borough Council 2000).

The profile has also been used by the partnerships in the borough to inform bids to a range of additional funding opportunities including a successful bid to the New Opportunities Fund Healthy Living Centre Initiative and a portfolio of primary care bids to the new Health Inequality fund for the prevention of coronary heart disease. These have been linked to a local community regeneration strategy aimed at addressing the wider socio-economic factors in one of the most deprived wards in the borough (Caerphilly County Borough Council and Partners 2000). This strategy forms close links between a new primary care centre and the development of proposals for a new community school, community resource centre and transport links.

The Local Government Act 2000 placed a new duty on Caerphilly County Borough Council to coordinate the production of an overarching 'Community Strategy' for their area. The duty comes with new powers to promote the social, economic and environmental well-being of local residents. Community planning is well advanced in the borough and has been agreed by a Standing Conference of over 50 partner organizations. To ensure effective community involvement, seven local area forums have been established. The first forums have agreed a local plan of action, informed by the data from the study and consistent with county borough-wide strategic priorities. These plans have been used as a major building block for the Local Partnership's Objective 1 Action Plan (Wales European Task Force 1999). Objective 1 funds are available to the poorest areas within Europe, providing considerable potential to improve health and reduce health inequalities within Caerphilly County Borough.

Conclusion

Public health has a long history of action on the wider determinants of health to improve health and reduce health inequality. In the 19th century this focused on improving sanitation and communicable disease control. After a long period of fragmentation of the public health functions and practitioners, public health has been revitalized by government policy initiatives on health inequalities and refocusing of its role and functions in a modern concept of public health – this involves multiprofessional and multiagency working to bring about social change and improvement in population health and reduction of inequality.

This is highlighted in the case study of health and social inequality in Caerphilly County Borough, which integrates public health action across all the defined functions of public health to bring about worthwhile change.

Figure 3.2 • Thematic maps of selected variables. (A) Council tax bands A and B (source: CCBC 1999). (B) Percentage of children aged 0–15 living in families claiming income support (source DSS 1998). (C) Social Services referrals of children aged 0–14, rate per 1000 (source: CCBC 1999). (D) Percentage of pupils achieving at least five GCSEs at grades A–C (KS4) (source: CCBC 1999).

SUMMARY

- Public health is about understanding and improving the health of populations or communities.
- The most commonly used definition of public health is 'the science and art of preventing disease, prolonging life, and promoting health through the organized efforts of society'.
- The Faculty of Public Health has defined nine key standards for modern public health practice.
- Public health is now a modern multiprofessional concept, practised by specialists, generalists and members of society.
- The major pressure for the change and innovation leading to the modern practice of public health has been the policy drive to tackle inequalities in health.
- There has been a renewed focus on protecting the health of the public from emerging infectious diseases and strengthening emergency preparedness and response to a wide range of threats to health.

DISCUSSION POINTS

1. How can community nurses make a contribution to reducing inequalities in health in their local area? What constraints are there on this public health role?
2. What are the elements of specialist training for community nurses who wish to practise as public health specialists?
3. How can community nurses provide leadership in national and local public health practice?

Acknowledgements

We are grateful to colleagues Professor Stephen Palmer, Dr Edward Coyle, Mr Andrew Jones and Dr John Watkins for interesting discussions on the development of modern public health practice.

References

Acheson D 1988 Report of the Committee of Inquiry into the Future Development of the Public Health Function. Public health in England. HMSO (Cm 289), London

Barnes M, Sullivan H, Matka E 2001 Building capacity for collaboration: the national evaluation of Health Action Zones. Birmingham, University of Birmingham

Barnes M, Sullivan H, Matka E 2004 The development of collaborative capacity in Health Action Zones. A final report from the national evaluation. Birmingham, University of Birmingham

Beaglehole R, Bonita R 2004 Public health at the crossroads, 2nd edn. Cambridge University Press, Cambridge

Caerphilly County Borough Council 1998 Corporate plan of priorities 1998–2001. Caerphilly County Borough Council, Caerphilly

Caerphilly County Borough Council 2000 Housing strategy and operational plan 2000–2003. Caerphilly County Borough Council, Caerphilly

Caerphilly County Borough Council Directorate of Social Services 2000a Review Plan 2000–2001 of the Children's Services Plan 1998–2001. Caerphilly County Borough Council, Caerphilly

Caerphilly County Borough Council Directorate of Social Services 2000b Review Plan of the Social Care Plan 1998–2001. Caerphilly County Borough Council, Caerphilly

Caerphilly County Borough Council and Partners 2000 New Tredegar Economic and Community Regeneration Strategy. Support Document for Local Regeneration Fund (LRF) submission. Caerphilly County Borough Council, Caerphilly

Department of Health 1995 Variations in health. What can the Department of Health and the NHS do? HMSO, London

Department of Health 1997 The new NHS: modern, dependable. Cmd 3807. HMSO, London

Department of Health 1998a Independent inquiry into inequalities in health. HMSO, London

Department of Health 1998b A first class service: quality in the new NHS. HSC 1998/113

Department of Health 1999 Saving lives: our healthier nation. Cmd 4386. The Stationery Office, London

Department of Health 2001a The report of the Chief Medical Officer's project to strengthen the public health function. Department of Health, London

Department of Health 2001b Tackling health inequalities. The Stationery Office, London

Department of Health 2004 Choosing health: making healthy choices easier. Cmd 6374. The Stationery Office, London

Department of Health and Social Security 1980 Inequalities in health: report of a research working group (the Black Report). HMSO, London

Donaldson LJ, Donaldson RJ 2003 Essential public health, 2nd rev. edn, Petroc Books, Newbury

Glennerster H, Lupton R, Noden P, Power A 1999 Poverty, social exclusion and neighbourhood: studying the area bases of social exclusion. CASE paper 22. Centre for Analysis of Social Exclusion, London School of Economics, London

Gordon D, Shaw M, Dorling D, et al (eds) 1999 Inequalities in health. The evidence presented to the independent inquiry into inequalities in health, chaired by Sir Donald Acheson. The Policy Press, University of Bristol

Kemm J, Ballard S, Harmer M 2001 Health impact assessment of the new Home Energy Efficiency Scheme. National Assembly for Wales, Cardiff

Lawson AB, Williams FLR 2001 An introductory guide to disease mapping. Wiley, Chichester

McPherson K, Taylor S, Coyle E 2001 Public health does not need to be led by doctors. British Medical Journal 322: 1593–1596

Palmer S, Gallacher J, O'Connell S 2006 The public health impact of the Buncefield oil depot fire. Health Protection Agency, July 2006. Online: http://www.hpa.org.uk/publications/2006/buncefield/default.htm

Ratner PA, Green LW, Frankish CJ, et al 1997 Setting the stage for health impact assessment. Journal of Public Health Policy 18: 67–69

Shaw M, Dorling D, Gordon D, Davey Smith G 1999 The widening gap: health inequalities and policy in Britain. Policy Press, Bristol

Stevens A, Raftery J (eds) 1994 Health care needs assessment, the epidemiology based needs assessment reviews. Radcliffe Medical Press, Oxford

Townsend P, Davidson N 1988 Inequalities in health: the Black Report, 2nd edn. Penguin Books, London

US Health and Human Services Public Health Service 1995. For a healthy nation: returns on investment in public health. US Government Printing Office, Washington DC

Wales European Task Force 1999 West Wales and the Valleys Objective 1. Single Programming Document for the period 2000–2006. NAfW, Cardiff

Welsh Office 1998a Better health better Wales. Welsh Office, Cardiff

Welsh Office 1998b Strategic framework: Better health better Wales. Welsh Office, Cardiff

Whitehead M 1987 The health divide: inequalities in health in the 1980s. Health Education Council, London

Recommended reading

Donaldson LJ, Donaldson RJ 2003 Essential public health, 2nd rev. edn. Petroc Press, Newbury
This is perhaps the standard introductory text to the principles and practice of public health and *offers a comprehensive overview of the subject.*

Marmot M, Wilkinson RG (eds) 2006 Social determinants of health, 2nd edn. Oxford University Press, Oxford

A comprehensive summary of the research evidence on the wider determinants of health.

Section **Two**

Public health frameworks

This section outlines frameworks for practice that can be utilized to take forward public health in nursing practice. It explores in more detail the knowledge base of epidemiology, the influence of social capital on health, needs assessment and commissioning of services, provides a framework for promoting health in all spheres of practice and updates the reader on developments in taking forward workplace health.

The first chapter in this section provides an overview of epidemiology and its utility in practice. It describes how the study of epidemiology is used to monitor disease, investigate causation and disease distribution, and evaluate the effectiveness of preventative programmes and treatments. The advantages and disadvantages of different kinds of research studies are discussed and subsequently linked to their relevance for public health practice, with reference to particular examples. The chapter provides the reader with the knowledge required to understand the scientific basis of epidemiology and how it can be used in needs assessment.

The second chapter explores social capital and highlights how this is a highly contested concept within the field of social theory. The chapter illustrates how its importance for public health is not well understood. A detailed analysis of social capital and its impact on health and inequalities is provided. The theory underpinning social capital and its attributes is analysed and a tripartite definition discussed.

The third chapter in this section discusses needs assessment and the commissioning process and provides a framework for undertaking a needs analysis. The strengths and weaknesses of using types of evidence to identify need and to prioritize resources accordingly are discussed, together with the use of this information to inform the commissioning cycle.

The next chapter in this section outlines frameworks for promoting health. It provides an overview of the theory of health promotion and how it fits into a public health framework. Health promotion approaches and models that can be utilized to underpin practice are explored. Concepts outlined in this chapter are further explored in the final chapter of the book.

The final chapter in this section is of particular use to those who practise in workplace settings. Differences between the concepts of risk and hazard are examined and the management of these is outlined within the current UK legislative framework.

Epidemiology and its application to practice

John Watkins

KEY ISSUES

- The past decade has seen an increase in emphasis on evidence-based practice
- The rapid expansion of the published literature on health and healthcare
- Increasing professional accountability and explicit quality standards
- The challenge of keeping up-to-date and being able to critically appraise the literature

Introduction

From primitive times man has sought to elucidate the causation of human disease. There is evidence that even in prehistoric communities, elders were selected as 'medicine men' and practised a primitive form of medicine based on tribal belief and folk law, much of which developed into a symbiotic relationship between man and his environment. Even today the aboriginal tribes that persist across the world demonstrate this deep understanding of the living world and their place within it. For example, the indigenous peoples of Australasia survived for thousands of years, before the invasion of modern man, with no written language yet passed down from one generation to the next the beneficial and medicinal properties of the foliage and fauna in their environment. One can only speculate that the origin of what was later to become modern therapeutics was arrived at by much trial and error, with some successes but a considerable amount of failure and death. In parallel to the discovery of effective agents, much disease and treatment benefit over time has been ascribed to either divine intervention or false claims of effectiveness, due to the lack of understanding of the natural course of diseases.

For much of history, man has had to be content with observing and monitoring disease with little understanding of either the aetiology or biological processes afoot and no understanding of the best course of treatment, other than the empirical knowledge handed down from one generation to the next.

Outlined in this chapter are the basic principles and broad areas of endeavour that represent the science of epidemiology, by which light can be shone on the darkness of folklore and misunderstanding. During the last 100 years the methodological tools of epidemiology have been developed and have become a powerful way of elucidating the aetiology and causation of disease, its early detection and a means by which treatment effectiveness can be evaluated.

In this chapter we will briefly look at the origins of the modern science that is epidemiology, how it is used to monitor disease, investigate causation and evaluate treatment effectiveness. Along the way we will illustrate this process by highlighting success and indicate how epidemiology should be embraced as a basic and necessary science for the practice of healthcare.

Causation of disease

The greatest minds of history have contemplated the aetiology, causation and treatment of disease. Hippocrates writing in 400 BC accepted that 'the science of medicine makes use of principles which can be of real assistance … but it would not be fair to expect medicine to attempt cures that are all but impossible nor be unfailing in its remedies' (Chadwick and Mann 1950). Implicit in this statement is that even 2500 years ago there was the realization that there was a limit to one's knowledge of disease, not all treatments were effective in all people at all times, and those that were to be used needed to undergo some scientific process of evaluation.

It is true today, as it was in the time of Hippocrates, that the overwhelming cause of death is infectious disease, and it is only in the developed world that diseases of degeneration and ageing have become dominant. This led Robert Koch and Friedrich Loeffler to develop in 1884 a set of criteria, later known as Koch's postulates (Box 4.1) for infectious disease aetiology (Grimes 2006).

Epidemiology is a science that is interested in the cause, occurrence, distribution, natural history and treatment of disease. Some 30 years before Koch produced his seminal work, John Snow in 1854 demonstrated these principles. During August and September 1854 London experienced a severe epidemic of cholera resulting in nearly 100 deaths. Snow found that by mapping the place of residence of the deaths that had occurred during this period, he was able to identify that the hand water pump in Broad Street was at the epicentre of the deaths and likely to be related in a causal way. His action in getting the local authorities to remove the handle on the water pump resulted in a curtailment of the epidemic and saved many lives. This event is often hailed as one of the first triumphs of modern epidemiology with its impact on public health policy (Johnson 2007).

Then, as now, Koch's postulates were never seen as absolutes in that many infectious agents can be present in humans without causing disease, e.g. polio and HIV viruses, in violation of Koch's first postulate. Similarly his third postulate recognizes the fact that many organisms experimentally inoculated with an infectious agent do not necessarily develop disease; the lack of disease in many of the residents of Broad Street in 1854 would support this, as not all residents exposed to infected water succumbed to cholera.

One of the founding fathers of modern medical statistics, Sir Austin Bradford Hill, in his Presidential address to the Royal Society of Medicine in 1965 addressed the issue of causation of disease from the perspective of occupational exposure; however, the tenet of his talk is just as relevant for wider discussions of causality (Hill 1965). Starting from the point of view that cause must precede effect if there is in fact a causal relationship between an agent and a disease, Bradford Hill suggested a number of factors that need to be taken into account in order to judge whether any such association was likely to be causal (Box 4.2).

Using the example of cigarette smoking and its association with lung cancer, which will be discussed in more detail later in this chapter, it is well known today that this association is causal. If we apply the criteria in Box 4.2 to this agent/disease combination we are able to see how we might gain confidence in the conclusion that there does in fact exist a causal chain at work.

The *strength of an association* between factors and a disease manifests itself if the disease occurs much more frequently, or exclusively, in those exposed. For example, in this case, heavy smokers have a significantly higher rate of lung cancer deaths than non-smokers.

Box 4.1

Koch's postulates

1. The suspected causal organism must be constantly associated with the disease.
2. The suspected causal organism must be isolated from an infected organism and grown in pure culture.
3. When a healthy susceptible host is inoculated with the pathogen from pure culture, symptoms of the original disease should develop.
4. The same pathogen must be re-isolated from organisms infected under experimental conditions.

Box 4.2

Aspects of an association between an agent and a disease that help in deciding if the association is in fact causal

1. Strength of the association
2. Consistency
3. Specificity
4. Temporality
5. Biological gradient
6. Plausibility
7. Coherence
8. Experiment
9. Analogy

Consistency refers to the finding being seen repeatedly over and over again, e.g. that a disease is related to exposure to a particular agent. Again turning to cigarette smoking, lung cancer is seen universally in all cultures and all societies where smoking has taken hold.

Specificity relates to the relationship between the agent and the disease in question. Cigarette smoking is known to be associated with a number of serious common diseases, for example coronary heart disease which is also common, though less so, in non-smokers; however, carcinoma of the lung is by comparison almost exclusively related to exposure to tobacco smoke and this is more so for particular pathological types of the disease.

Temporality means that cause must proceed effect; in this case one must be exposed to cigarette smoke over many years before one develops the disease and similarly one's risk diminishes over time after stopping smoking.

Biological gradient can be interpreted as an agent and disease displaying a dose–response relationship, i.e. those exposed the greatest develop the disease more commonly. This is true for smoking and lung cancer, where there is a steady gradation in the risks of developing the disease from non-smokers, through mild to moderate consumption, with heavy smokers, on average, having the greatest risk.

Coherence with known facts about the disease, its putative agent and evidence from other sources: Bradford Hill used the example of the temporal relationship between smoking rates in the population over time and the rise in deaths from lung cancer during the 20th century, reinforced by the differential rates of adoption of smoking by women in Britain, which was very much a post-war phenomenon, to illustrate this point. As women took up smoking in the second half of the 20th century, we saw a concomitant rise in deaths from lung cancer that mirrored the effects observed in males.

Experiment poses the question as to whether the effects can be replicated experimentally or in some quasi-experimental way. For cancer of the lung and cigarette smoking there is now enough accumulated evidence from the developed and developing world to show that as cigarette smoking increases in populations so does its health consequences, particularly lung cancer.

Analogy: one can ask is an association causal, from a *plausibility* point of view, i.e. does it make sense and are there analogies to be drawn with other agents and this disease? For example, cigarette smoke is inhaled and the organs that are most exposed to the agent are the air passages of the nasopharynx, bronchi and lungs; cancer of these tissues is strongly associated with cigarette smoking. We also know that inhalation of the radioactive gas radon during coal mining results in an increased rate of carcinoma of the lung; by analogy therefore it makes it easier to accept the biological plausibility that an inhaled carcinogen can cause lung disease.

Resting on the shoulders of giants, the modern edifice we call evidence-based practice can be broken down into a series of careful steps: disease surveillance, as epitomized initially by John Snow, hypothesis generation, again turning to Snow whose hypothesis was that an agent, cholera, was waterborne and related to the Broad Street pump, experimental intervention, removal of the pump handle, or as in Koch's case, isolation of an organism and experimental infection of another to prove causality. In addition, Bradford Hill has given us the intellectual instruments by which to decipher the evidence gathered. In the next section we will look at the surveillance role of epidemiology before moving on to the methods by which epidemiological investigation is carried out.

Surveillance

Webster's New World Medical Dictionary (2001) describes surveillance as 'the ongoing systematic collection and analysis of data and the provision of information which leads to action being taken to prevent and control a disease, usually one of an infectious nature'. Worldwide, a considerable amount of time and effort goes into the collection, collation and interpretation of data on disease occurrence, by which healthcare organizations and nations can plan healthcare services and their response to emerging threats.

In most westernized democracies, surveillance systems exist to monitor infectious disease, particularly those that can be prevented by vaccination. For example, both the United Kingdom and the United States monitor the common diseases of childhood, measles, mumps and rubella, which are notifiable to public health bodies, the data from which are used to monitor disease control and vaccine effectiveness. In addition the World Health Organization (WHO) has a network of sentinel centres around the world for specific diseases. Influenza, a disease which has the potential to kill millions of people worldwide, as it did in 1918, is one example of international collaboration between states and institutions to monitor, collect, collate, identify and characterize disease in order to detect any emergent threat immediately.

Severe acute respiratory syndrome (SARS) is a respiratory disease in humans which is caused by the SARS coronavirus; between November 2002 and July 2003, 8096 individuals in 29 countries were infected with this virus and 774 deaths occurred (Vijayanand et al 2004). The initial disease, from a smouldering start in mainland China, where it had probably spread to humans from bats who are asymptomatic to the disease, either directly, or through civet cats, then spread first to Hong Kong and then across the developed world. After China, Canada and Singapore were the countries worst affected, and because of the nature of the disease, healthcare workers, in particular, in the early stages of the epidemic were very badly affected. This single event was a wake-up call to the developed world that new and emergent diseases still pose a significant threat to humankind and that eternal vigilance is required to quickly identify and contain disease. In the years following the SARS epidemic, there has been a realization that a greater threat to humankind may emerge from the highly pathogenic strain of avian influenza, H5N1, that has, since it first appeared in 1997, devastated the world's bird populations and has infected over 300 people up to 2008, with a mortality rate of over 50%. Worldwide surveillance systems are now in place across the world linked into major laboratories in countries such as the UK, USA and Australia so that influenza and severe respiratory illness can be quickly identified and preventative measures, such as antiviral drugs in the case of influenza, can be rapidly deployed.

In the developing world the old killers of malaria, TB and the newer and more deadly, threat, HIV, are devastating the populations of sub-Saharan Africa. In these countries disease surveillance is less well developed, or even non-existent as in countries such as Zimbabwe, Iraq and Afghanistan.

Quantifying threats to public health

In the previous section we looked at the role of surveillance in the ongoing monitoring and detection of infectious disease; in addition to this, national governments also collect vital statistics on births, deaths and disease occurrence within their borders. Surveillance information is often combined with population data, obtained from national census, in the case of the UK once every 10 years, to create a powerful epidemiological database. Census data provide information on the health, wealth and well-being of a nation's citizens and also demonstrates ongoing trends in births and deaths, areas of increased mortality to be identified and the general slow change in disease importance to be monitored. It is beyond the scope of this chapter to cover, in detail, the use of routine data for epidemiological purposes; however, in order for the reader to gain some knowledge for further self-directed learning, a number of terms will be defined.

The health of the people is really the foundation upon which all their happiness and all their powers as a state depend. (Benjamin Disraeli)

The health of a nation can be measured in a number of ways, which broadly fall into two distinct categories. One relates to deaths in the population, i.e. mortality, and the other to the amount of illness present, morbidity, and these in turn give rise to more complex measures such as, life expectancy at birth and quality-adjusted life years (QALYs), respectively, which will not be covered here.

Mortality

While knowing the number of deaths that occur is in itself useful, additional details such as cause of death, age, sex, date and place of death, place of residence and occupation (or last employed position) all add much more to our ability to turn routine data into information with which to plan and target services.

Box 4.3 presents an example of how data on the number of deaths occurring in a population can be combined with data on age and population demographics to produce much more meaningful measures that may be used to compare the health of a population of interest with another, for example the health of one region of the UK with the health of the UK as a whole, as measured by deaths occurring.

Box 4.3

Measures of mortality

- Number of deaths – simple count of deaths occurring
- Crude mortality rate occurring in a defined population – all deaths during a calendar year/population at mid year
- Mortality by age – simple count of deaths by age
- Age-specific mortality rates
- Disease-specific mortality rates
- Standardized mortality ratio

Crude mortality rate

By taking the number of deaths that occur in a particular calendar year, in a defined population of interest, and dividing this by the mid-year estimate of the number of individuals within that population, we arrive at the crude mortality rate; this may be specified as a rate per unit of population, e.g. per 1000. This term is useful and gives some crude indication as to the relative rates of death between a population of interest and another, e.g. between states in the USA or between nations in Europe. The problem with this type of measure is that it makes no use of demographic data on the age distribution within populations. It would therefore only be useful in comparing populations where the population age structure was identical.

Age-specific and disease-specific mortality rate

To overcome problems with interpretation of mortality data related to age, it is often convenient to calculate age-specific mortality rates, i.e. the number of deaths occurring in, say, a 5-year age band per unit of the population in that age band. This will give rise to age-specific mortality rates for a population. By this method the mortality experiences of age-band-specific tiers of the population can be compared with others.

If we wish to look at the impact of a specific disease on a population it is sometimes useful to use the count of the number of deaths from that disease in a population, divided by an estimate of the population size. Again, just like age-specific mortality,

this may be useful in comparing the impact of a disease within, or between, nations. For example, if we carry out this analysis on regions within the UK, we will find that, for ischaemic heart disease, more deaths occur per unit of the population in Scotland, Wales and the northern regions of England than occur in the Home Counties around London, or the West Country. These regional differences, highlighted by disease-specific mortality rates, are the start of an epidemiological enquiry into disease aetiology and prevention.

Standardized mortality ratio

The standardized mortality ratio or SMR is a means by which the mortality experience of two disparate populations can be compared. For example, let's consider two populations represented by the population pyramids shown in Figure 4.1.

The structures of the two populations represented by Figure 4.1A and 4.1B are very different, in that population A represents a population dominated by the young, as often seen in developing countries, while population B, has a much more evenly distributed population often seen in the developed world where infectious disease has been defeated, population birth control has been introduced and one has a right to expect to live into old age. If we wish to compare the health of these two populations, crude mortality, or even mortality rates, would give an erroneous picture due to the imbalance created by the differences in demographic structure. In order to calculate the SMR for population A compared to population B, we carry out the following steps.

Step 1

For each of populations A and B, we calculate the age-band-specific mortality rate for males and females in each population.

Step 2

For population A, we then calculate, for each age band, the number of deaths we would have expected to occur if the population of community A had the same age structure as population B.

That is, if in the age band 45–49 years in males from population A, which represents 1.7% (from Figure 4.1A) of the total population, we saw 110 deaths in a specific year, we now can pose the

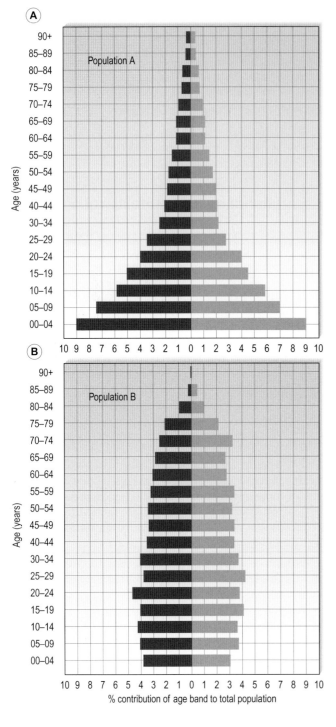

Figure 4.1 • (A) Population A – population pyramid typical of a developing economy. (B) Population B – population pyramid typical of a developed world economy.

% contribution of age band to total population

question, how many deaths would we see if population A had an age structure such that the 45–49 age group represented the same proportion of the population as it does in population B, i.e. 3.3% (Figure 4.1B)?

We now pose the question, how many deaths would we see if population A had an age structure such that the 45–49 age group represented the same proportion of the population as it does in population B, i.e. 3.3% (from Figure 4.1B)?

To answer this question we carry out the following computation:

$$\text{Death rate in age band 45–49 in population A} \times \frac{\text{\% of total population B in 45–49 age band}}{\text{\% of total population A in 45–49 age band}}$$

$$= 110 \times \frac{3.3}{1.7} = 214.5$$

So if population A had the same age structure as population B we would expect to see 214 deaths in the age band 45–49 during the year in question.

If, however, during this time period, in population B, the number of deaths in the age band 45–49 is less than 213 this signifies that there were fewer deaths in B than A than one would expect. If there were greater than 214 deaths the converse would be true, i.e. people were dying at a greater rate, in this age band, in population B.

Step 3

Repeat step 2 for all age bands, then sum the total number of deaths for population A one would expect if it had the same population age band structure as B.

Step 4

$$\text{The SMR} = \frac{\text{Population death rate in population A} \times 100 \text{ (with reference to B's pop.)}}{\text{Total population death rate for population B}}$$

By convention the ratio of death rates is multiplied by 100. We have now derived a methodology that allows us to compare deaths in two populations.

If the SMR value for a given population compared to another is greater than 100 then it means that overall the mortality is greater in the population under consideration than the comparator area and

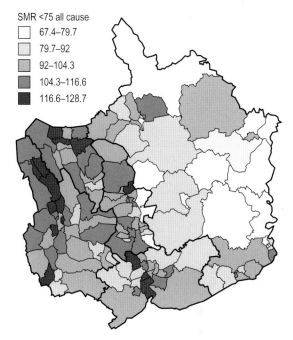

Figure 4.2 • Standardized mortality ratio in south-east Wales by electoral ward compared to the England and Wales population as a whole. (Source: Fone, Jones, Watkins, et al 2002 Caerphilly Health and Social Needs Study.)

hence, more unhealthy, while SMRs less than 100 mean the converse.

Figure 4.2 is a map of the communities of southeast Wales in the United Kingdom. This map displays the SMRs for premature, all-cause mortality under the age of 75 years, for each community; from this map we can see that some areas have an SMR greater than 100 compared to the reference population, which is England and Wales as a whole, while other areas have SMRs less than 80. This map represents real differences in the life chances of individuals who live out their lives not 20 miles apart. Differences of SMR of this magnitude, 120 compared with 80, represent differences in life expectancy of about 5 to 10 years for every man, woman and child living in the high SMR areas compared to the areas with lower ratios (see Chapter 3 for further information).

Disease-specific SMRs for populations can be calculated in a similar way to that described above using disease-specific deaths by age and sex rather than overall death rates; this represents a powerful tool in monitoring the impact of acquired human disease on populations, e.g. cigarette smoking and lung cancer.

Case fatality rate

Particularly for infectious disease, an often used measure of lethality of a disease agent is the case fatality rate. This quite simply put is the ratio of the number of deaths from a particular condition in those who have contracted the condition. For example, as of 18 March 2008 there have been 373 cases of avian influenza due to H5N1 virus and 236 deaths; this gives a case fatality rate of 63%, which puts avian influenza almost to the top of human lethal infectious diseases.

Mortality in childhood

As countries move from developing to developed world structures, the distribution of health, disease and deaths moves from infectious to chronic disease and the deaths seen before the age of 5 years decrease. This decrease is mainly due to improved maternal and child health, reduction in overcrowding and improved sanitation, water supplies, nutrition and social reform, changes seen in most developed countries for over 100 years but still a long awaited dream in many of the emerging nations around the world. Healthcare with immunization and vaccination programmes and improved prenatal care have been the final steps in giving every child born in a westernized home the greatest chance of survival. In order to capture this changing pattern of survival in early childhood and to allow us to compare nations and regions within nations, a number of specific measures of mortality in early childhood have been developed (Box 4.4).

Each of the parameters in Box 4.4, with regard to child health, provides an insight into the impact different aspects of the care have prior to birth and in the first year of life. For example, stillbirth rate

is directly related to the quality of maternal health and well-being and the care given during pregnancy; it can be severely affected by disease and malnutrition leading to fetal death. Perinatal mortality adds an extra dimension to this, in that it includes deaths that also occur in the first week of life. Hence it is a measure of the quality of intrapartum care and the early postnatal period, as much as it is of maternal health and well-being. Neonatal mortality in the first 28 days of life reflects on the quality of care in the postpartum period, while infant mortality extends this out to cover the first year of life. Low infant mortality rates are intimately related to the quality of infant nutrition and the uptake of effective vaccine programmes in the first year of life.

Figure 4.3 shows some selected infant mortality rates using data available from the WHO (see: http://www.who.int/healthinfo/morttables/en/index.html). From this it can be seen that in war-torn countries, such as Afghanistan, one in six children born will die before their first birthday. On the other hand, Cuba, with its socialized medicine, has much better health outcomes, as measured by infant mortality, at levels comparable with many western countries, yet has a gross domestic product similar to many African nations.

Box 4.4

Mortality in early childhood

- Infant mortality rate = number of deaths of infants <1 year/number of live births in year
- Neonatal mortality rate relates to deaths in first 28 days of life (rate/unit of population)
- Stillbirth rate is 'stillborn' after 28 weeks' gestation who never breathed (rate/unit of population)
- Perinatal mortality rate relates to stillborn plus deaths in the first week of life (rate/unit of population)

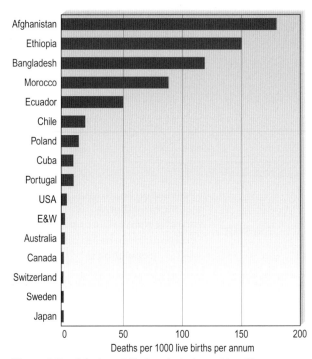

Figure 4.3 • Infant mortality in selected countries. (Source: World Health Organization.)

Morbidity

Morbidity is less straightforward a concept to understand than mortality; it is a measure of ill health or disease in a population and as such can be specified in a number of ways. Like mortality, we can carry out a simple count of the number of cases of a particular condition that occurs; however, this simple count will tell us nothing about the extent of the disease in a population. It is therefore more meaningful and useful to specify disease occurrence as a rate, i.e. number of cases per unit of time in a particular population, or as a proportion, i.e. proportion of the population affected by a condition. This time-dependent rate is often called an incidence rate, while the proportion of cases in a population is known as prevalence. Prevalence can be further divided into point and period prevalence, point prevalence being the proportion of cases in the population at an instant in time, while period prevalence would be a proportion of the population with the disease measured over the course of a period of time, e.g. 12 months.

For infectious disease, another often quoted measure of morbidity would be attack rate, which will be the number of people at risk of developing a condition who fall ill.

Figure 4.4 is a diagrammatical representation of a 'pot' of human disease; using this analogy we can get some idea of the meaning and application of the various measures of morbidity and how these may be used to quantify disease. In this analogy, the contents of the pot are analogous to the amount of disease present in the population at any one time, i.e. prevalence. The contents of the pot are added to by new cases appearing over time, incidence; the contents of the pot diminish by evaporation and in this case, the analogous events to this will be death or recovery, as a means of leaving the reservoir of disease. For diseases where the number of new cases in a period of time exceeds the combined number who die or recover, then the prevalence of a disease will increase, e.g. as in the case of diabetes today. Similarly, as death and recovery rates overtake the incidence rate, the pot of disease will start to run dry. It is just this process in the real world, with the ebb and flow of disease incidence, that leads to the epidemic curves we see, particularly for infectious disease but also for diseases such as ischaemic heart disease.

We can take this analogy still further to understand how these terms may be used to describe certain diseases. Take, for example, Figures 4.5A, B and C, for a disease such as cancer of the lung, which despite modern advances in medicine, in the majority of cases, is rapidly fatal. Figure 4.5A depicts this by showing that few people recover from the disease, comparatively few live with the disease and the majority die. If we therefore wish to study changes in the incidence of this disease we could use deaths registered from cancer of the lung as a proxy measure. In the case of seasonal influenza (Figure 4.5B), deaths from this disease are extremely rare so the use of death registration would not be a good measure to use to plot the

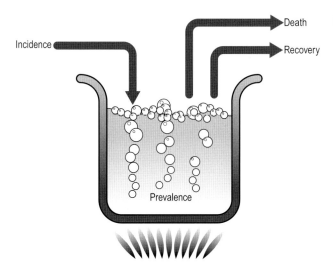

Figure 4.4 • Measures of morbidity.

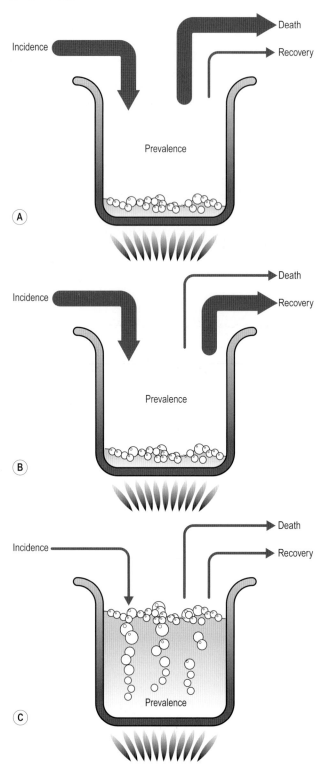

Figure 4.5 • Measures of morbidity for specific disease conditions. (A) A disease with a short life expectancy and high case fatality, e.g. cancer of the lung. (B) A disease of short duration, with high attack rates, low mortality and short recovery times. (C) A disease with low mortality and little or no remission that runs through the life course.

course of this disease. Influenza activity is monitored using sentinel practices that count the number of new cases of the disease they see in their populations, i.e. incidence; since this disease is self-limiting, in the majority of cases, and most people recover and do not die, the pot of disease in the population is quite small at any one time, but increases as the incidence rate rises and then diminishes as described above. For a chronic disease such as rheumatoid arthritis (Figure 4.5C), there are few new cases per year of the disease, few die and not many recover, with the result that there is almost a constant pot full of the disease over time. Since healthcare services need, in the case of rheumatoid arthritis, to be geared up to help those afflicted, prevalence data would be the correct measure used to specify population need.

Causation, treatment and effectiveness

Historically, the medical literature consisted, to a large extent, of case reports and careful observations made by health professionals of individuals afflicted by one disease or another. Looking back from these days of 'evidence-based practice' these case reports may look quaint and outdated at one level, yet at another they provide vital insights into the presentation, symptomatology and outcome, which can be vital for rare diseases. Were it not for such detailed case reports, in publications such as the *New England Journal of Medicine* in the early 1980s (Reinherz et al 1981) highlighting the range of symptoms seen at the outset of the epidemic in patients infected with HIV, AIDS as a disease entity would not have been recognized so quickly. The similarity of published cases of the disease afflicting young, male homosexuals, living in New York City and those thousands of miles away in San Francisco, led investigators to conclude that this syndrome must be related to an infectious agent. Epidemiological detective work based on this hypothesis predicted that it should be possible to link two unrelated cases of AIDS to a common infectious source. This finding led to the conclusion that AIDS and the immunodeficiency manifesting itself in cases was of infectious viral origin, which we now see in global proportions and not just as a niche disease.

Observational studies, and case reports, as described above, suffer with the difficulty of being able to contextualize one's findings. This is especially true for novel and/or rare diseases because one can never be sure how commonly such cases occur in the general population and that the symptoms, time course and outcomes observed would apply to all those with a particular disease. Even associations between cases and circumstance may be spurious; e.g. homosexual practices are not the cause of AIDS, as was first thought, but merely one mode of transmission, by sexual contact, in a group unfortunate enough to have one of its members contract the disease.

We saw from Box 4.2 that several conditions need to be satisfied before one can draw any conclusions about the strengths of association and possible causation between an agent and a disease condition. Box 4.5 now introduces the concept of a hierarchy of evidence in epidemiological study design. It will be noted, from Box 4.5 that observational studies, such as cross-sectional surveys, are the lowest level of evidence of association, while randomized controlled trials, RCTs, a true experimental design, are seen as the most powerful and are seen as the 'gold standard' for evaluating the effectiveness of interventional treatments.

In order to find the aetiology of a disease, or to define a causal relationship with a putative agent, we move up the hierarchy of evidence from observational studies, which can hint at potential relationships between risk factors and disease, through case-control studies, designed to explore this relationship in more detail, to cohort studies, where groups of individuals without disease are followed up until such time as they develop a disease of interest.

Cohort studies have the advantage, as set out in Table 4.1, that all the information needed to explore aetiology is collected, up front, before any disease develops. Cohort studies therefore allow causality to be explored, as well as allowing the incidence and prevalence of disease to be calculated. This causal relationship can be further evaluated using

> ### Box 4.5
>
> **Hierarchy of evidence**
> - Randomized controlled trials
> - Cohort studies
> - Case-control studies
> - Observational studies, e.g. case reports, ecological studies and cross-sectional surveys

Table 4.1 Epidemiological study – methodologies, uses, advantages and disadvantages

Study type	Design	Uses	Advantages	Disadvantages
Ecological studies	Group or population under consideration, not individual	Investigation of relationship between one population-based parameter and another	Uses available data Looks at effects on whole population, some of which may be difficult to measure at an individual level	Population-based data so factors of interest may not be related at an individual level Population unit selected can affect results of a study (Ecological Fallacy)
Cross-sectional surveys	Data collected across a population at one point in time	Prevalence studies of disease Look for associations in the population Collect information on populations relating to beliefs, behaviour, lifestyle or physiology at an individual level	Easy to do Useful for investigating common chronic conditions Allow methodology to be replicated easily and so comparisons in time and place can be made	Poor for acute conditions Uncommon conditions are not detected efficiently Association but not causality can be identified but the direction of this relationship cannot be investigated by this method Findings may be spurious
Case-control studies	Retrospective study where one starts with the effects of an entity of interest and looks back historically for a cause. Cases are selected that have a disease of interest and they are matched with similar individuals in whom the disease is absent to look for potential causal factors	Good to investigate the potential aetiology of a disease	Quick and easy to do Efficient method, especially for rare conditions Easy to replicate Relatively cheap to perform All the data of interest potentially already exist	Data often incomplete due to lapses in recall or loss of records Recollection may be biased by knowledge about the disease that cases have Interviewer bias due to knowledge about the presence or absence of disease. Controls do not represent the true disease-free population Can show association but not causality
Cohort studies	Longitudinal study, whereby a group selected from a population are followed over time with data collected at recruitment and then at predefined follow-up. Explicit outcome criteria often stated up front and designed into the study	Good to investigate disease aetiology and the strength of the association with causal factors Investigation of treatment outcomes such as hospital admissions and adverse health outcomes such as death Able to study the natural history of disease	Measures of risk and protection can be obtained Data recorded are unbiased by outcome Investigation of rare exposures	Expensive Often large and difficult to manage Not good for rare diseases due to infrequent occurrence and hence large cohort size required Follow-up of subjects can be difficult and costly and will lead to loss of participants Can investigate causality

Table 4.1 Epidemiological study – methodologies, uses, advantages and disadvantages—cont'd

Study type	Design	Uses	Advantages	Disadvantages
Randomized controlled trials	True experiments Participants are selected with strict inclusion criteria. Are randomized to either receive or otherwise the intervention of interest. Followed up periodically with explicit data being collected and outcomes defined	Investigate cause and effect Good to compare treatment options (pragmatic trial) Investigate dose response by comparing outcomes for different dosage regimes (explanatory trial)	Can be used to investigate the effects of changes in a single variable on outcomes The 'gold standard' for evidence of effectiveness	Not always feasible or ethical Difficult and costly to carry out Compliance can be difficult to measure or enforce Generalizability of results to the wider population can be difficult to interpret Study can be subject to bias

interventional study designs such as the randomized controlled trial (RCT), whereby individuals with explicit inclusion criteria for the study, e.g. males between the ages of 26 and 40 years who lead a sedentary life, are randomized to an exercise programme or no intervention to look at the effects of exercise on cardiovascular risk factors such as serum cholesterol, blood pressure and body mass index. In this example participants would be followed over time and the outcomes and measurements of interest recorded at predefined time intervals. At the end of the study period, the rate of occurrence of outcomes in the intervention group, or in this case the values of physiological parameters, are compared in the two groups. This type of study can experimentally explore questions about the effectiveness of interventions on risk factors, or disease occurrence, in this example exercise and cardiovascular risk factors, or drug therapy and the occurrence or progression of disease, e.g. triple drug therapy and the progression to AIDS of people infected with HIV. Table 4.1 takes each of the study designs of Box 4.5 and highlights the uses, advantages and disadvantages of each.

In order to further explain how one can use Box 4.5 and the hierarchy of evidence to take us closer to finding the cause of a particular disease, we will use the example of the relationship between cigarette smoking and lung cancer.

If we cast our minds back to the period soon after the end of the Second World War, doctors were starting to observe an increase in the number of cases of cancer of the lung that were occurring in middle-aged men presenting to them. On taking a careful history, it would seem that most, if not all, of the cancer sufferers were, or had been, moderate to heavy smokers of tobacco, this disease being rarely seen in non-smokers. The hypothesis is, therefore, that smoking causes lung cancer, based on case reports and anecdotal clinical experience.

It is therefore decided to carry out a large population survey, a cross-sectional study, of smoking behaviour and the occurrence of lung cancer. The problem with this type of approach, for this particular line of enquiry is that, since smoking has been and still remains a rapidly fatal disease, it is not very efficient in picking up a significant level of lung cancer sufferers in the population. Another way to tackle this problem might be to collect data, at a population level, relating to total consumption of tobacco per head of population and correlate this with standardized mortality rates for lung cancer. This approach is known as an ecological study and may be good for hypothesis forming, e.g. if we find that countries that have high population tobacco consumption rates, on average, also have high rates of lung cancer deaths, we might be encouraged in our thinking that there is, after all, an association between smoking and disease. However, this can also lead to what is known as an 'ecological fallacy', since we do not know, at an individual level, whether the deaths are occurring in those who have consumed the tobacco, or whether both tobacco use and death may be associated with some other factor which is the true aetiology of the disease.

Since we decide we are unable to depend on a cross-sectional study to pick up an adequate number of cases of lung cancer, we need, therefore, to adopt a different approach. It is at this point we turn to the case-control study design. In this type of investigation we start with our cases of disease, i.e. those with lung cancer, perhaps identified in an oncology clinic. We then match each case with one, or more, individuals, termed controls, who are cancer free but similar in most other ways to the cases in terms of age, sex, lifestyle, socio-economic grouping and possibly occupation. We would then take a detailed history from all cases and controls with regard to all those factors we feel important in the aetiology of the disease, in this case exposure to tobacco smoke and personal smoking history. Once we have collected all the data, we are able to calculate the proportion of smokers that are cases with lung cancer out of the total pool of smokers, which will be made up of both cases and controls. We are also able to calculate a similar proportion of non-smokers who have lung cancer, out of the total pool of non-smokers, drawn from cases and controls. The ratio of:

$$\frac{\text{Ratio of smokers in the study with lung cancer/smokers in the study without lung cancer}}{\text{Ratio of non-smokers with lung cancer/non-smokers without lung cancer}}$$

is termed the odds ratio of getting lung cancer if one is a smoker as compared to not smoking. If smoking offers no risk of developing disease, this ratio should be equal to one; if there is an increased risk of developing the disease there will be a greater proportion of cases of cancer in smokers than non-smokers and the odds ratio will be greater than unity; if it were protective, which it is not, then there would be a lower proportion among smokers and the odds ratio would be less than one. The greater the magnitude of the odds ratio, e.g. if it were 15, then the stronger the association between the risk factor and the disease. Since we are dealing with retrospective data, in which we start with cases of a disease, we are not able to prove causation in a case-control study. However, large odds ratios reassure us that we should progress to more expensive and elaborate studies to confirm our hypothesis. Table 4.1 tells us that case-control studies are good for investigating rare diseases, are relatively cheap to perform and can give results in a timely fashion, since all the data required for the study already exist. The disadvantages are that they can be prone to bias in a number of forms; for example, recollection bias is where individuals with a disease, suspect-

ing that it may be linked to the risk factor of interest, are more lightly to recall its use than those without the disease. Also the cases we choose to use in a case-control study may not represent the total spectrum of disease presentation; for example, a disease may be rapidly fatal and hence some individuals with the disease are not seen among the cases because they never make it to an oncology clinic.

The causal relationship between cigarette smoking and lung cancer was finally demonstrated in the 1950s by Sir Richard Doll using a cohort study design with British doctors as subjects. Doll used the register of the General Medical Council of the United Kingdom as a sampling frame to contact a cohort of doctors in medical practice who fulfilled his inclusion criteria for the study. Each doctor in the study cohort was contacted and asked to give consent to take part in the study; participation required them to consent to Sir Richard being contacted by the Registrar General if and when these doctors died, at which time cause of death would be recorded. The initial questionnaire survey included questions relating to lifestyle and smoking behaviour as well as other demographic data. The cohort was followed for a number of years and as deaths from both lung cancer and cardiovascular disease accumulated, it became clear that smoking was associated more frequently with these causes of death (Doll and Hill 1956, Doll et al 2004). The studies of Doll and others are now landmark success stories in the history of the development of epidemiology as a basic clinical science and demonstrated for the first time the causal link between smoking and several lethal diseases.

Cohort studies are able to answer questions about risk and disease incidence, demonstrate causality and plot the broad clinical course of a disease. However, they are expensive and time-consuming to conduct and require an onerous effort to ensure follow-up. Ensuring maximum follow-up rates is very important, since individuals lost from the study can bias the results. In the case of the cohort used by Sir Richard Doll, provided doctors remained on the medical register and resided in the UK until death, follow-up was relatively straightforward; deletions from the medical register, migration and death overseas were potential confounders to this study and could lead to bias in the results. In a cohort study one is able to quantify the relative risk associated with exposure to a noxious agent, by using the ratio:

$$\frac{\text{Proportion of the exposed}}{\text{population who develop disease}}$$
$$\frac{\text{Proportion of the population}}{\text{who are not exposed who develop disease}}$$

In a cohort study we know the true prevalence of disease in a defined population and we are able to ascertain exposure to an agent of interest, in this case tobacco smoke, so we are able to calculate the prevalence of disease in exposed and non-exposed individuals. This information allows us to calculate absolute risk with or without exposure and hence the relative contribution of a factor in increasing one's life chances of disease development. As with odds ratios, values greater than 1 represent harm, while those less than 1 represent benefit.

In order to understand the true impact of an agent on a population, i.e. the number of extra cases that occur in smokers as a result of their habit, it is necessary to take into account the absolute risk of developing disease, which, in this example, will be the number of cases of lung cancer occurring among non-smokers; only then can we understand the impact smoking has in terms of additional cases. This latter point is important since a relative risk of 2 would imply the doubling of the number of cases of a disease of interest on exposure to a noxious agent; this may, on occasions, have a less dramatic impact when one realizes this may only represent one extra case per 100 000 people exposed. Therefore caution is needed in interpreting relative risk when it appears in publications. Cohort studies also allow us to explore the dose–response relationship of cigarette intake and disease; it is possible in this type of study to stratify our cohort by exposure, i.e. heavy smoker, intermediate, light and non-smokers, and look at disease occurrence in each of these groups.

It is not ethically possible to design a randomized control study of smoking and its role in the development of lung cancer since we know already that smoking is harmful. However, for many disease/treatment interventions it is possible to construct such a study.

Any RCT has several steps that are crucial for its effective execution (Figure 4.6). Every RCT needs to make clear its explicit inclusion and exclusion criteria by which subjects for the study group are selected. Next there needs to be some effective mechanism that randomizes subjects to either the intervention or control arm, such that all individuals in the study group have an equal chance of being selected as a subject or control. Investigators need to identify before the start of the trial what outcome measures will be used, e.g. survival time if it is a new cancer therapy, treatment response such as lowering of blood pressure, etc. duration of the study follow-up period and type and duration of the review process along the way. Randomization, in this type of study, is introduced to eliminate selection bias, whereby individuals with differing disease risk are systematically selected for one or other arm of the trial. In order to minimize the results being biased by either the knowledge of the participants, or the investigators, that certain subjects are taking active therapy, a technique known as blinding is often introduced. This process of observer bias, as it is called, is often further eliminated by the introduction of a placebo. A placebo intervention, in a RCT, will be some modality not thought to influence the outcome of a study, e.g. in a drug trial, two identical looking tablets are often produced, one with active drug, and the other of inert base substance. With this methodology, study subjects will not know whether they are being treated with an active tablet. Inves-

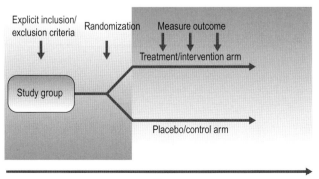

Figure 4.6 • Structure of a randomized controlled trial.

tigators can also be blinded by this methodology to having knowledge of which arm of the study group any individual has been allocated to until all the results have been collected and collated. RCTs can be costly and time-consuming. They do, however, allow one to quantify treatment effectiveness and absolute and relative risks of one intervention compared to another. Table 4.1 sets out some of the advantages and disadvantages in conducting an RCT. The same rigour applicable to cohort studies applies equally to RCTs, ensuring that 'drop-out' rates are minimized as these can severely bias a study's findings.

With the rise of the digital age, powerful desktop computing, complex software tools to manipulate and manage large databases, coupled with the Internet, affords international collaboration on a global scale and unprecedented access to the published literature and has led to the development of the techniques of systematic review of the literature and meta-analysis of clinical trials. Both techniques are beyond the scope of this chapter but interested readers will be able to find a wealth of material on both subjects elsewhere.

Conclusion

Epidemiology is a basic science for the clinical disciplines and the practice of evidence-based healthcare. The techniques and methodologies described in this chapter are essential for the understanding of disease causation and evaluating treatment effectiveness and today are used worldwide to elucidate disease aetiology and target therapy.

We have not covered the epidemiological principles that underpin the diagnostic process, nor have we addressed how these may be applied to screening, as this is beyond the scope of this chapter. The approach has been taken to concentrate on epidemiology and its application to practice and has deliberately sought to equip the reader with the necessary understanding, so that they may be able to read the published literature and interpret its findings, in order to provide effective evidence-based care. The material has been covered in a non-mathematical way. Knowledge acquired here can be built upon with reference to some of the more technical texts suggested below.

SUMMARY

- This chapter focuses on providing an understanding of the broad nature of epidemiological investigation.
- The section on quantifying health seeks to provide the reader with an understanding of the terms used in epidemiology and public health and how they may be used to compare and contrast the health status of a population over time and with others.
- Questions of causation, treatment and effectiveness are addressed, using the relationship between smoking and lung cancer to illustrate how the 'hierarchy of evidence' may be used. Strengths and weaknesses of various study designs are explored.

DISCUSSION POINTS

1. Discuss which measures of morbidity and mortality could be used to monitor the following diseases and conditions over time and what sources of data you would use:
   (a) asthma
   (b) cancer of the pancreas
   (c) hepatitis B
   (d) Crohn's disease
   (e) MRSA.
2. You are asked to examine the association/ causal relationship between the following pairs of risk factors. In each case discuss

which types of study design would be most appropriate, why you would use this methodology, the study population setting, and data sources that may be used:
   (a) brain tumours and mobile phones
   (b) bowel cancer and diet
   (c) accidental contamination of the water supply and memory impairment
   (d) Gulf War syndrome and congenital abnormality in offspring
   (e) alcohol consumption and liver cirrhosis.

References

Chadwick J, Mann WN 1950 The medical works of Hippocrates. Blackwell Scientific Publications, Oxford: 89

Doll R, Hill AB 1956 Lung cancer and other causes of death in relation to smoking. A second report on the mortality of British doctors. BMJ 233: 1071–1076

Doll R, Peto R, Boreham J, Sutherland I 2004 Mortality in relation to smoking: 50 years observations on male British doctors. BMJ 328: 1519–1533

Fone D, Jones A, Watkins J, et al 2002 Using local authority data for action on health inequalities: the Caerphilly Health and Social Needs Study. British Journal of General Practice 52: 799–804

Grimes DJ 2006 Koch's postulates then and now. Microbe 1: 223–228

Hill AB 1965 The environment and disease: association and causation. Proceedings of the Royal Society of Medicine 58: 295–300

Johnson S 2007 The ghost map: the story of London's most terrifying epidemic – and how it changed science, cities and the modern world. Penguin Group (USA)

Reinherz EL, Geha R, Wohl ME, et al 1981 Immunodeficiency associated with loss of T4+ inducer T-cell function. New England Journal of Medicine 304: 811–816

Vijayanand P, Wilkins E, Woodhead M 2004 Severe acute respiratory syndrome (SARS): a review. Clinical Medicine 4: 152–160

Webster's New World Medical Dictionary 2001 Foster City: IDG Books Worldwide

Recommended reading

Gillam S, Yates J, Badrinath P 2007 Essential public health: theory and practice. Cambridge University Press, Cambridge

Mayer D 2004 Essential evidence based medicine. Cambridge University Press, Cambridge

Sackett D, Haynes RB, Guyatt GH, Tugwell P 1991 Clinical epidemiology: a basic science for clinical medicine. Little Brown and Company, London

5

Social capital and health

Sarah Cowley

KEY ISSUES

- Social capital, health and health inequalities
- Criticisms of social capital theory
- Development of social capital as a concept
- Attributes of social capital
- A tripartite definition of social capital
- Examples from practice

Introduction

Social capital is of interest in a wide range of fields, including business, community relations, crime, economics, education, politics and health. It is a complex concept, which seemed to burst on to the scene in the 1990s, bringing enthusiasm and scepticism in almost equal measure. Although social capital is very important for health and health inequalities, it is also a highly contested concept within the field of social theory and its importance for public health is not well understood. The literature is voluminous and expanding exponentially, so selected examples are used in this chapter to provide an explanation of what it is and why it is considered so important to health. Then, the major criticisms will be outlined, before explaining the embedded meanings and confusions that have created controversy. Some of the responses that aim to unravel the tangle of critique will be offered, before concluding with some practical examples showing the value of social capital in practice.

Social capital: enthusiasm

The ownership of capital is considered an advantage, and social capital may be viewed as the advantage gained by an individual or a group of individuals (such as a community) as a result of being part of a social network (Hean et al 2003). At a common sense level, this straightforward definition seems logical and helpful; Cowley and Hean (2002) expand by offering examples from primary healthcare. An elderly patient being given a lift to a surgery by her daughter has received practical support by virtue of the fact that she is part of a family network, for example. Or an isolated parent, who has no friends to commiserate with the difficulties in coping with a young, crying baby, is at a disadvantage compared to the person who can tap into informational, emotional and social support; this is quite apart from (and in addition to) any practical help that may be available through a friendship network. At a more general level, there is an advantage for those living in communities where everyone knows and trusts their neighbours, extending a helping hand in times of need in the realistic expectation that, when the situation is reversed, the favour will be returned.

As well as networks, resources such as trust and support, norms of cooperation, reciprocity, participation and solidarity with community members are also considered central to the idea of social capital (Putnam 1993). In a qualitative analysis of two community projects, for example, Campbell et al (1999)

Box 5.1

Describing social capital

Characteristics of social capital in two communities (Campbell et al 1999)	Mechanisms: macro and micro (Putnam 2004)
Local identity: sense of 'belonging-ness'	Social support
Meeting life challenges	Communications patterns
Trust	Social identity and risk behaviour
Reciprocal help and support	Access to resources (medical and otherwise)
Attitudes to local government	Resolution of dilemmas of collective action
Formal and informal group memberships	Physiology (e.g. stress levels)
Subjective perceptions of 'community' including:	Disempowerment
Respect and tolerance	Isolation
Gossip	
Safety from crime	
Children's freedom of movement	
Neighbourliness	
Reciprocal help and support	
Local identity	
Living and working conditions	

---

identified certain key characteristics that marked the presence of social capital, while Putnam (2004) provides an updated list of mechanisms through which social capital may work (Box 5.1).

Similarly, Cowley and Billings (1999) recorded the 'resources for health' available to help promote positive health; these included being able to turn to family and friends for help and support, relying on neighbours and neighbourhood facilities like schools, nurseries and transport. Some of these resources are examples of what has been called the 'civic society'. This includes an expectation that there will be reliable services and facilities, although those in turn depend upon good government and the forms of participation (voting, political activity, democracy and so on) identified by Putnam (1993) in his seminal text about civic traditions in modern Italy.

Social capital and health

In this first text, Putnam (1993) suggested that health depended upon factors like diet and lifestyle, which are beyond the control of democratic government; he had reversed this opinion by the time his next book was published seven years later (Putnam 2000). There, he stated that, 'Of all the domains in which I have traced the consequences of social capital, in none is the importance of social connectedness so well established as in the case of health and well-being' (p. 326).

This enthusiasm is mirrored elsewhere. A discussion paper prepared for the British Cabinet Office (Performance and Innovation Unit (PIU) 2002) described the 'explosion of interest' and exponential growth in academic publications in social relationships, norms and networks since about 1995. In reviewing that massive literature, they concluded that 'overall, the evidence described in this paper from a range of sources using a variety of methods for the beneficial effects of social capital is impressive' (p. 5). In the fourth edition of *Health for All Children*, Hall and Elliman (2003) state that 'a growing body of evidence suggests that social capital is as important a predictor of health outcomes as absolute levels of wealth or poverty' (p. 32). The evidence continues to expand. Petrou and Kupeck (2008), for example, analysed data from a large, nationally representative sample (the 2003 Health Survey for England), and showed that poor measures of health status were significantly associated with low stocks of social capital across the domains of trust and reciprocity, perceived social support and civic participation. Comparing the 'social capital best case' with a notional worst-case scenario, they calculated that individuals from the 'worst-off' situations would be 79.5% less likely to report very good or good health status. This analysis draws attention to the significance of social capital for understanding health inequalities, which is one of the key areas of interest for this field.

Social capital and health inequalities

Health inequalities have become one of the major challenges to public health, as they are globally pervasive and the reasons underlying them are poorly understood. Much of the interest in the concept of social capital has come from researchers trying to explain why these arise, particularly within and between resource-rich countries.

It is clear that absolute poverty is a major cause of the different patterns of morbidity and life expectancy between the developed world and areas where inadequate food, poor or contaminated water supplies and lack of high-quality healthcare lead to disease and early death. However, once countries have passed beyond what Wilkinson (1996) terms the 'epidemiological transition', when they are sufficiently well developed to ensure basic physical requirements for health for their whole population, and starvation and death from major epidemics are no longer key concerns, a pattern of health inequalities remains. Even in the absence of absolute poverty, across the developed world, there is a social gradient in mortality from many illnesses, and in life

expectancy overall. The pattern of infant mortality, shown in Figure 5.1, illustrates this gradient; even though the absolute figures have improved overall, there is a persistent gap between babies born to managerial and professional groups (the best off) and those in families headed by a 'routine and manual' worker. The outlook for infants born to the poorest and most excluded groups, including students, unemployed people and those who have never worked (the worst off), is worse still. Similar patterns pertain for life expectancy.

In the USA, Kawachi et al (1997) analysed survey data from 39 states in terms, borrowed from Putnam, of social networks, trusting relationships and cultural norms that act as resources for individuals and facilitate collective action. Each of these elements of social capital showed a strong inverse correlation with all-cause mortality rates, after adjusting for age. Soon, a raft of studies emerged, each showing a similar pattern across the developed world, both within and between countries (Wilkinson and Pickett 2006). In each case, as well, mortality and morbidity follow a gradient, with people living longer, healthier lives at each step up in their status and wealth.

Poverty is a key mediator, and lack of sufficient money for good food, heat and housing matters immensely to people's health. However, to repeat the key point, inequalities are distributed across a gradient, with each step up showing an advance in health outcomes, right from the least to the most well off. This pattern cannot be explained by the

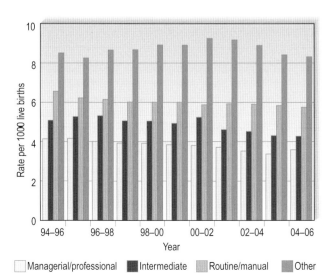

Figure 5.1 • England and Wales. Three-year average infant mortality rates by social economic group. Source: Office for National Statistics. NB; there was a change in the method for classifying social economic groups in 2001.

presence or absence of absolute poverty. Nor, Wilkinson (2006) argues, do the material privations of having a house with a smaller lawn to mow, or one less car, seem plausible explanations for these differences. Instead, there seems to be some way that health inequalities are related to psychosocial factors, affecting the whole population and not just those who are living in poverty. As Moore et al (2006) identified, a search for this explanation, encouraged by the ideas suggested by Wilkinson (1996) and Putnam (1993), led to public health interest in social capital. Studies using a variety of proxy measures, such as the extent of public participation or neighbourhood trust and relationships, began to emerge soon after.

Social capital: scepticism

Given the apparently immense benefits to be gained from social capital, it might seem churlish to raise any doubts or questions about it. However, there are a number of concerns, which have given rise to a rich and competitive literature, particularly in the economic and sociological journals, which can seem confusing to anyone outside those disciplines, or even within them. Some of the debates seem bitter and critical, while others build systematically and courteously upon what went before.

Lack of clarity

One of the main concerns is the lack of clarity and conceptual confusion that surrounds much of the work about social capital. Even the enthusiasm expressed by the Performance and Innovations Unit was tempered by the plethora of definitions encountered in their literature review, leading them to caution about the potential mis-specification or ambiguity in some of the models used in the empirical literature (PIU 2002). Opinions are divided about whether this is because social capital is a falsely inflated concept (Labonte 1999) or because of the lack of clear guiding principles underpinned by a sound theoretical base (Lomas 1998, Wall et al 1998). Whatever the reason, unclear concepts create problems for research.

Kawachi et al (2004), for example, identified 31 studies from across the world, which illustrate the wide variability of definitions and unclear concepts. The results showed that the presence of social

capital led to better health outcomes in the large majority of studies, but the indicators used varied widely (Box 5.2). The authors highlight a key difference: that some measures (mortality and crime rates, for example) relate to collectives or whole populations, while others relate to aggregated measures (such as self-rated health and self-esteem) drawn from individual respondents. This raises the question about who 'owns' social capital, and whether it is legitimate to measure it in a community, but apply it to individuals, or vice versa. Without theoretical and conceptual clarity about exactly what is being measured or why, it is hard to have faith in the results, and Hean et al (2003), among others, have called upon researchers to explain the mechanisms being measured in theoretical terms.

Lack of theoretical awareness

Concerns about a lack of clarity are linked with the second major area of criticism, which can be summarized as a lack of theoretical awareness. Critics suggest that much of the social capital literature is merely rewriting well-established theories; social capital is described as 'old wine in new bottles' or as a 'catch-all phrase' for social support and democratic theory (Berkman et al 2000, Edwards and Foley 1998, Labonte 1999, Muntaner 2004, Portes 1998). Such writers point out that we have known the importance of social circumstances on the quality of life and health since the work of 19th-century sociologist, Emile Durkheim. The collective impacts of social relationships and social trust on health have been very well documented, and there is an expansive empirical literature about both social networks and the different forms of community, including its cohesion. Social capital literature is viewed as naive and uninformed by these critics, who suggest it fails to take sufficient account of existing social theories. Szreter and Woolcock (2004) suggest that the majority of the literature about social capital and health can be divided under two headings: that which is concerned with how psychosocial mechanisms, such as social support, affect health and that which purports to explain health inequalities (as outlined above). These two large fields of interest were well represented in psychological and sociological literature long before social capital emerged as a concept of interest.

Box 5.2

Indicators and health outcomes: measures used across 31 studies of social capital, 1997–2004 (derived from Kawachi et al 2004)

Indicators of social capital (or lack)	Health outcomes: measures used
Social trust, social cohesion	Mortality rates and life expectancy
Social mistrust/distrust	Firearm violent crime; homicide rates
Civic engagement and/or participation	Self-reported sense of insecurity
Electoral/voting participation	Low birthweight
Community organizations	Self-rated health/poor health/physical health
Workplace cohesion	Teen birth rates
Crime rates	Adolescent sexual risk/protective behaviours
Membership of organizations or associations	Rates of sexually transmitted diseases
Density of association/local networking	Binge drinking
Volunteering	Food security
Social involvement	General health
Informal sociability	Mental health
Informal social control	Self-esteem, satisfaction and behaviour
Reciprocity	Proportion of residents/children receiving mental health services
Help from organizations	Psychiatric hospitalization
Lack of helpfulness	Alcohol and drug service use
Collective efficacy	Tuberculosis rates
Close-knit; shared values, get along with each other	Leisure time physical inactivity/walking activity
Parental attachment to community	Child behaviour problems
Parental sense of community	Medication: hormone replacement therapy; antihypertensive medication

In exploring psychosocial mechanisms, Stewart-Brown and Shaw (2004) carried out a study that differed from those taking the community as a starting point, instead bringing the family into sharper focus. They hypothesized that the roots of social capital were embedded in relationships in the home during childhood, which would influence health in later life. By comparing the results of two systematic reviews with published birth cohort data across three cohorts (born in 1946, 1958 and 1970), they were able to provide strong evidence that the quality of relationships in the home in childhood has an impact on both physical and (particularly) mental health in adulthood, regardless of socio-economic circumstances. This important analysis identifies issues such as warmth, relationships, social support and the developmental importance of children growing up in circumstances that are conducive to trust and networking, so that as adults they might both accept trust and be the kind of person, or neighbour, who is trusted by others.

Despite the value of the work, reflecting the criticisms outlined above, Stewart-Brown and Shaw's (2004) study of social trust and relationships would have been equally useful if the term 'social capital' had not been used. However, the study does underscore the potential for social capital to be both generated and used within relationships, which is the basis for the norms of reciprocity and obligation that arise in much of the social capital literature. In terms of measurement, it is important to know whether data are being drawn from a social capital user or generator, or from both (Hean et al 2003). This distinction is similar to one suggested by Snijders (1999) to distinguish between different social capital pathways. He suggested using the term 'complementary' to describe when one person has the social capacity to offer some element, such as support or information, from which another can benefit; and 'symmetrical' for when there is a collaborative or cooperative effort from which all parties can benefit equally. The distinction is important for researchers, so they know what to measure. In addition, it becomes important for practitioners and those interested in improving social capital in an area. Is it possible for an outside person, such as a health professional, to enable the generation of social capital through networks and groups, for example? Community development literature is divided on whether the activities of an insider or outsider, or lay or professional worker, are most effective; the social capital literature has not really engaged with these issues.

Negating power and poverty

Both a lack of conceptual clarity and the failure to specify the theoretical basis for social capital may be regarded as acts of omission. They are criticisms that have largely been taken on board by researchers in the field of social capital, with varying degrees of success. The third group of complaints represents more fundamental differences of opinion. Kanazawa (2006) is something of an outlier in the debates. He draws on evolutionary genetics to suggest that average intelligence quotient (IQ) as measured across countries provides a better explanation than social capital for international health inequalities, an idea that is given short shrift by Wilkinson and Pickett (2007), who reject the way he conceptualizes IQ.

A larger group of papers question the lack of attention in the social capital literature to social structure, particularly poverty, social class and power relations within society, at times portraying it as an almost wilful act of commission. Navarro (2004), for example, accuses Szreter and Woolcock (2004) of ignoring 'authors such as myself who have shown the uselessness (and even harm) of such a concept as defined by Putnam ... the authors seem unaware of the enormous importance of *politics and power relations* in explaining why the concept of social capital first appeared in the US in the 1980s' (p. 672, original emphasis). Navarro contends that social capital has been popularized so that politicians can avoid engaging with the more damaging aspects of capitalism. The failure to engage with inequities in the power base, as represented by social class (including race and gender), and a focus on analysing society through individuals rather than through the collective social structure, together mean that social capital literature cannot provide a meaningful explanation or understanding of our political realities, in

Navarro's view. While other writers use more temperate language, the idea that the psychosocial environment can explain health inequalities is widely disputed by those who argue that income inequality influences access to other resources (Lynch et al 2001). Historically, it is claimed, the availability of material resources and its impact on health can be measured through cohort effects over time (Davey Smith and Lynch 2004, Muntaner 2004), a point that will be missed by the form of data collected through cross-sectional, one-off surveys.

Further, the idea that social capital can be generated formally has been criticized as reflecting the perspective of the dominant cultural authority, with little consideration being given to either the norms or rules that govern such behaviours in a given context or the conflictual and dialectical facets of the concept (Forbes and Wainwright 2001).

Overall, the concerns of this critical group of writers are twofold. First, there are a range of explanations and theories about social class, poverty and power, which they fear are being neglected in favour of the friendlier and less challenging ideas promoted by social capital. Second, in practical terms, this can be used by politicians to avoid redistributive policies, or actions to ameliorate the effects of poverty. Instead of redressing the lack of money and power that is the heart of disadvantage, policies may concentrate on the cheaper alternative of community development projects or, worse, blame the poor health of individuals in deprived areas on their supposed lack of neighbourliness or failure to take part in group activities.

Social capital: theory and concept

To understand the basis of some of the criticisms of social capital writers and research, it is necessary to understand the development of the concept and how the work has progressed over the last two decades. Social capital is usually traced back to three main theorists, who each have different interests and ways of explaining the term.

The French sociologist Pierre Bourdieu (1997) described social capital within his wider theory about how society works. He was interested in a range of different forms of capital, including economic, symbolic, social and cultural capital. Social capital encompasses the range of resources that a person might accumulate and use in social relations, and it is described as 'fungible' in that it is inter-linked with the other forms and cannot always be entirely separated from them. He distinguished social capital by describing it as the aggregate of the actual and potential resources derived from being the member of a group or network. Bourdieu used social capital to explain the way that relationships within and between those groups both maintain status and set the terms for negotiation and compe-tition for resources, defining their value across dif-ferent fields of activity. His theory takes into account power relations, social structure and social values, as well as the collective actions through which they are developed and disseminated.

As part of a wider enterprise, Coleman (1988) aimed to draw together both sociological and eco-nomic perspectives in explaining social actions, and he saw social capital as a useful example in this endeavour. He described social capital, not as a single entity, but as a variety of different entities with two elements in common: they all consist of some aspect of social structures, and they all facili-tate certain actions of individuals who are within the structure. While networks feature in his theorizing, as well, productivity is more prominent than in Bourdieu's writing. Indeed, for Coleman, social capital is defined by its productive function, which helps make possible certain ends that would not be possible in its absence, and which generates some resources through relationships.

The political scientist Robert Putnam is, perhaps, the most prolific writer in the field, as well as being a highly charismatic speaker. He was credited with sparking a massive increase in interest and academic writing about the concept (Performance and Innova-tions Unit 2002) through his book about democracy and civic traditions in modern Italy (Putnam 1993). Here, he described the norms of reciprocity and networks of civic engagement that become embed-ded and enacted through moral resources, such as trust and cooperation across the whole social system and not only by individuals. Locality, neighbourhood and community all feature highly in Putnam's writ-ings, but relationships and networks less so. In later publications, Putnam (2000) identified the func-tions of *bonding* social capital, the so-called 'social glue' creating the strong bonds that form between family members or those belonging to a particular club, close friendship group or support network and of *bridging* social capital. The latter is characterized

as the 'social oil' that lubricates the less dense but more cross-cutting ties, perhaps with work col-leagues or acquaintances in a local community. The importance of ensuring the presence of both forms, along with a proposed third form of *linking* social capital (Szreter and Woolcock 2004) will be consid-ered further below.

These different theoretical emphases have had an impact on the way social capital is used in research and in practice. Much of the interest in social capital for health has derived from variations of Putnam's work. Moore et al (2006) traced the epidemiological and public health interest in the concept back to 1996, when two key publications appeared: Wilkinson's (1996) book about *Unhealthy Societies*, which devoted a whole chapter to the potential impact of social capital on health, and a *BMJ* paper which concluded that 'investments in human and social capital' parallel state level variations in income inequality (Kaplan 1996). A year later, Kawachi et al (1997) published the first empirical study to demonstrate the links between social capital, income inequality and health. All three of these publications cited Putnam; Moore et al suggested that they focused too heavily on generalized measures of trust and civic engagement, such as voting behaviour, or membership of clubs, instead of including the more relational aspects (like social support and having someone to turn to) emphasized by Bourdieu and Coleman. Stephens (2008), on the other hand, detects a recent swing towards Bourdieu's theories to underpin social capital research, beyond her own study, along with an awareness of the need to answer the many criticisms.

Social capital: progress

The need to clarify terms and definitions requires a focus on the underlying theory. Hean et al (2003, 2004), for example, concentrated on concept clari-fication and explaining which elements of social capital it would be appropriate to measure before developing an instrument to measure the generation of social capital within formal groups or networks. Szreter and Woolcock (2004), on the other hand, unravelled the general trends of thought across the literature to identify common ground and the basis for a tripartite definition which, they hoped, would be widely accepted and lead to a consensus about the nature of the social capital.

Attributes of social capital

Before developing an instrument to measure social capital, Hean and colleagues felt it was necessary, at the start, to try and understand what kind of concept it is overall, and how the different attributes fit together. First, they carried out an expansive review of the literature and concept analysis, to identify the various attributes and components embedded within the social construct (Hean et al 2004), described below. Then, these attributes were used to elaborate a model and description of the cycle for generating social capital within formal groups or networks (Hean et al 2003). This model informed the development, piloting and validation of their instrument, which is specific to those situations. They rejected the idea that it would be possible to produce a general instrument that could measure all aspects of social capital in any circumstances, because the concept is far too complex.

Box 5.3 lists the global and component attributes of social capital identified by these authors. Global attributes are properties that provide a generic description of the concept, while component attributes describe single and specific dimensions of social capital. A key issue revealed by this analysis is that some of the component attributes may generate an overall impression of the social capital available. While the individual components of social capital may be discussed, no single component can describe in full the advantage of having access to social capital. In line with critics of the loose definitions used in some research, Hean et al (2004) propose that a study that measures only social support and trust, for example, should not be regarded as a study of social capital. It is only when all the global attributes are measured with at least some of the component attributes that social capital can be said to be present. Further, they suggest that when measures of social capital are used, there is an onus upon the authors to spell out how those measures fit within the theory they are using.

The global attributes are well described across the social capital literature. As explained above, the idea that social capital exists in or through relationships is central to the way both Coleman (1988) and Bourdieu (1997) describe the concept. Those who are particularly interested in the psychosocial elements of social capital have taken up this idea. The quality, quantity, context and dimension of relationships are all considered important, as well as whether they occur between individuals, groups and social agencies (Gillies 1998). While relationships are largely associated with the social side of social capital, the dynamic and durable elements of the phenomenon are part of its 'capital' nature. Social capital, seen as a whole, has a tendency to increase with use and depreciate when neglected (Bourdieu 1997, Putnam 1993).

Social capital is also defined by its productive function (Coleman 1988); in short, what social capital generates is also what a person 'can get from it'. The functions of a network may be expressed in generalized terms such as facilitation, cooperation, learning from each other and generation of trust, gossip, reputation or regulation. A distinction should be drawn, however, between the function of social capital and its consequences. Being part of a student study group, for example, may allow a student to learn with and from her peers (the function), with improved grades being the consequence.

The final global attribute refers to the multidimensional nature of social capital, since it may serve several purposes simultaneously (Coleman 1988, Putnam 1993). Social capital generated in the same study group, for example, may provide members with the benefits of learning while also providing information and support (such as friendship) in relation to other needs.

The first of four component attributes is the network through which social capital is generated, which is particularly popular with those who take a communitarian view of social capital (Putnam 1993, 2000). However, the literature recognizes networks other than those based in communities, describing

---

Box 5.3

Attributes of social capital (derived from Hean et al 2004)

Global attributes	Component attributes
Within/through relationships Dynamic Durable Defined by its productive function Multidimensional	Network characteristics Resources Norms and rules Trust

social capital as occurring across a wide range of networks, from the informal (e.g. family, friend, work and neighbour networks) to the formal (e.g. health clubs, patient associations and support groups). They may be described in physical terms, such as network size and type, by affective characteristics, such as social cohesion and feelings of solidarity, or by behavioural measures like frequency of participation and level of involvement (e.g. as a group leader as opposed to a passive subscription payer).

Trust is another commonly quoted component attribute of social capital. It is defined as the belief in the goodwill and benign intent of others (Kawachi et al 1997). However, trust differs from one context to another, and varies according to whether or not the person concerned is known personally or not. Feelings about whether to trust friends, neighbours and colleagues from the same club or network differ in quality from those held about folk of whom individuals have no first hand knowledge; just 'people around here' or 'in my neighbourhood'. It can be very hard to envisage whether or not an individual can be trusted if they are not known personally. Levels of intimacy also influence the nature and extent of issues around which trusting behaviour is sought, prompting the question of 'trusted with what?'

The resources of the relevant network are also key component attributes in the social capital literature. Two forms of resources are relevant: those external or internal to the individual (Cowley and Billings 1999). External resources that exist outside of the individual are accessible only through interaction with others within that same network. They may take both physical (e.g. financial and other material resources) and abstract forms (e.g. a collective skill base of people in the network, informational support, willingness of members to offer assistance).

Norms and rules make up the fourth component attribute that creates the overall picture of social capital. Norms are the unstated rules or standards that govern actions during informal or spontaneous social relations. While deviation may be punished by socially imposed sanctions enforced by other group members, compliance with these norms may promote spontaneous cooperation between individuals. Also, while such cooperation may restrict or facilitate individual and group action for the benefit of the whole network (Coleman 1988), that does not necessarily mean that it benefits the whole of society. Terrorist networks and criminal gangs, whose solidarity and clear norms help them to maintain their membership, beliefs and behaviours, are examples that are often given to show the negative side of social capital (PIU 2002, Putnam 2000).

A tripartite definition of social capital

Szreter and Woolcock (2004) set out to address the analytical and political controversies around social capital, and to reduce the emerging divide that they detected between three different groups who:

- focus on the primacy of support networks
- emphasize economic and social inequality and
- argue that access to resources explains health outcomes.

Their article was published in the influential *International Journal of Epidemiology*, along with a series of responses and commentaries from leading authors across the spectrum of views about social capital and public health. While this was an attempt to move the debate on in a positive way, the authors maintained that social capital is and will remain (like class, gender and race) an 'essentially contested concept'. Such concepts reflect 'a consensus on the broad nature of the phenomenon they refer to and its great importance, without any agreed-upon closure on the terms of its definition' (Szreter and Woolcock 2004: 654). Instead of a single definition, therefore, they enlarged upon three equally important, but conceptually different, aspects of social capital: bonding, bridging and linking.

The bonding and bridging forms of social capital have been distinguished in the literature since the late 1990s. Bonding social capital is said to come from networks that generate trusting and cooperative relations between members who see themselves as fairly similar, perhaps because they live in the same area or work in the same team or a similar job. The sense of identity and solidarity that comes from community or neighbourhood networks, or through work associations or trade unions, may create very positive social capital. However, having a group, network or neighbourhood that is too closed and inward looking may follow exactly the same mechanisms, but create problems for society. This is not to detract from the importance of bonding social capital; it is only to suggest that it would not be helpful alone. Bridging social capital is equally

Case example 5.1 Bonding and bridging capital

Hendon is an area where many new mothers are professional women, who are both competent and capable, and demographically middle class. Even so, the birth of a new baby can be a stressful and isolating time, as the women are separated from their usual friendship networks gained through work; many are distant from immediate family and unfamiliar with the needs and demands of a new baby until the birth of their own infant. Recognizing their need for peer support, health visitor Mary Daly developed the Hendon Parents Support Group, which ran weekly in a room made available at the local clinic. The parents facilitated the group themselves, electing a Chairperson to welcome new members, identify discussion topics and specific areas of support and generally coordinate the group meetings. Each week, the health visitor was available in the clinic building at the start and end of the meeting; she would help them to identify suitable speakers, point them to information or serve as a resource herself.

At one point, a group of Kosovan refugees was housed in the area; initially they spoke little English and had specific health needs related to their own traumatic histories. The health visitor helped this group, too, to set up a peer support group for new mothers, introducing them to key members of the established parents support group. The existing group took the newcomers under their wing, helping them with invitations and administrative elements of the group, and advising them about health and obstetric services in this country. Both groups found they had a common grievance about the local maternity hospital, and worked together to lodge formal complaints that were eventually resolved. But for the parent support initiative, the recent arrivals might have felt discriminated against by their adverse treatment; and joining forces to sort out a shared problem helped to create solidarity between the groups in the local area.

Contact: Mary Daly, health visitor, Barnet Primary Care Trust, now at Mary.daly@haringeypct.nhs.uk.

important, in developing relationships of respect and mutuality between people who do not share obvious points of similarity, including age, ethnicity, social class and so on.

Putnam (2000) suggests there is a real decline in these forms of social capital. His biggest concern is the potential reduction in bridging social capital, with increasingly closed and segregated communities, along with an alleged loss of society's ability to reach out and support its members when they most need it. The existence of local neighbourhood networks, once common across both Britain and America, are reducing in type and number, perhaps because of increasing travel-to-work times, mothers returning to work soon after the birth of their babies and increasing household mobility, within and between countries. On the other hand, new forms of community groups are developing, through work associations, or developing mobile technologies (Internet, telephones) and social networking sites that create the ability to continue long-distance relationships that would have been impossible in years past. As shown in Case example 5.1, the kinds of group and networking activities encouraged by health visitors can help to improve both bonding and bridging social capital.

Szreter and Woolcock (2004) hoped that defining the different but complementary aspects of bonding and bridging would encompass the main interests of writers concerned with both the net-

working and the relational side of social capital. They were also very conscious of the criticisms that the social capital literature took too little account of social structure and power relationships. The third element of their tripartite definition, therefore, sets out the nature of linking social capital, which is defined as 'norms of respect and networks of trusting relationships between people who are interacting across explicit, formal or institutionalized power or authority gradients in society' (p. 655). There is a particular role here for professionals, who can serve as the link between individuals and public services, either by intervening to enable someone to access the official help they need, or by advocating for a particular form of provision to be made available for a group or area. Case example 5.2 sets out how this worked in one children's centre.

In both of the examples, it is easy to see that there is some overlap between the three forms of social capital identified within Szreter and Woolcock's tripartite definition, illustrating that at any one time bonding, bridging or linking may predominate. Following Hean et al's (2004) concept analysis, too, both examples describe the dynamic, durable and multi-dimensional nature of social capital, showing how it operates through relationships to produce the resources and trust by which it is defined. It is also clear that certain rules and norms (such as being client-led in Case example 5.1, and emphasizing consent, confidentiality and

Case example 5.2 Linking and bonding capital

Woodhouse Sure Start Children's Centre, in Kirklees, developed from a 5th Wave Sure Start Local Programme (SSLP). Aiming to establish integrated working with the SSLP, the health visitor team worked with a policy consultant and an information technology company that specialized in data integration to develop a meaningful Universal Needs Assessment (UNA). This evolved as the SSLP developed into a children's centre in 2002. The aims underpinning the UNA were twofold; first every family would be offered a service tailored to their own specific needs and aspirations, in which the practitioner could fully account for how subsequent resources were utilized. The second aim was to be able to assemble information about needs and services in a way that would enable extraction of anonymous, meaningful and live information to plan for and develop services in a defined area or for cohorts/groups of families with similar characteristics.

The UNA would, therefore, provide a baseline for local target setting and performance monitoring. Information from the assessment and subsequent use of services and activities has been integrated into a single database and management system, which has been expanded using a 'whole systems' approach to include all the families, staff and services encompassed in the children's centre. As part of the health visiting service at the first contact, families are offered the opportunity to register with the children's centre, and receive an explanation and a leaflet, which provides information required to be compliant with the Data Protection Act. This covers a basic data set of personal information as applicable, such as details regarding ethnicity, current pregnancy, asylum/refugee or single parent status. Agreement is sought to their information being shared for the purposes of monitoring and developing services.

The UNA takes place after the families have had time to build a relationship with their health visitor, and to feel comfortable with the assessment, which is carried out though a personal interview. The UNA was developed by drawing together information from three main sources: the expertise of health visitors used to carrying out family health needs assessments, published research about risk and resilience factors affecting families, and policy documents setting out requirements for assessments. The process has been continually refined and developed as a result of feedback from those using the system (families, professionals and service managers).

The 'whole systems' element enables full accountability. It is possible to monitor whether individuals take up the services or packages of care offered by the lead professional, both to reassess their progress and continued needs, or to find out why if this has not happened for any reason (perhaps a change in circumstance, for example). It is also possible to request a wealth of anonymized information including evidence of performance against national and local targets and outcomes. The system is also designed to enable full costings to be determined for each individual package of care. The system allows a community view of what is happening across the area, by aggregating anonymized details from all families registered at the children's centre, enabling services to develop flexibly according to changing needs across the area. These sources of information proved invaluable, and ensured that service planners and commissioners could have meaningful information about needs and provision to meet them.

However, there remained a stubborn gap between the recorded need and level of vulnerability, and that perceived by both experienced health visitors and the families they were assessing. Some families appeared somewhat more vulnerable than the formal assessment suggested, while others seemed less so. The introduction of a small module of questions relevant to social capital solved this problem. Seven questions were developed by consulting the Social Capital Question Bank (Ruston and Akinrodove 2002); one question was selected from each of the five aspects of Blaxter et al's (2001) typology (social participation; civic participation; social networks and social support; reciprocity and trust; views of the local area and physical environment) with two more specifically included at the request of health visitors. The questions were printed onto laminated cards for ease of use, and were piloted with 204 families. Before asking these questions, the health visitor recorded her professional judgement about the family's level of vulnerability, to assess against the level of individual social capital revealed. In all but five cases, the two assessments matched, so this module was incorporated into the overall UNA from then on. Social capital appeared to be the missing link, showing resilience as well as vulnerability, and allowing a more accurate assessment of need to be made. The answers to questions also gave invaluable information about where the efforts of the service needed to be directed, to enhance the overall experience of living in the area and recorded social capital for all.

Contact: Margaret Hornsby (who developed the social capital module for the UNA), Margaret.hornsby@ntlworld.com, or Kirklees Council Early Years Services, www.Kirklees.gov.uk.

accountability in Case example 5.2) have been established, along with specific network characteristics in each case.

Conclusion

Social capital is a complex and contested concept but, as this chapter has shown, there is emerging agreement about its major attributes and function, and about its importance to health and health inequalities. It is not only found in local areas or generated through geographical communities, but these are a major focus. Support groups and associations, along with trust relationships and networks of any kind, can help to contribute to the development of social capital and thence to health improvement. Social capital, therefore, offers an important framework for everyday community practice.

SUMMARY

- Social capital is a complex concept, of interest across a wide range of fields.
- Social capital is of interest to health practitioners, because of its potential to ameliorate health inequalities and support positive health.

- There are various theoretical roots, which each emphasize different aspects, such as relationships, trust, social networks and community participation.
- Social capital is a concept that excites both enthusiasm and scepticism. Both viewpoints are explored and explained.

DISCUSSION POINTS

1. Think about your own social capital: which networks are most important to you? How do you support them? Have they changed with life transitions, like moving house, getting married, having children, changing jobs, growing older?

2. Which clients on your caseload are least likely to have access to social capital? How could you help change this?

3. What are the main difficulties with trying to measure social capital? Do these problems mean the concept is too flawed to be useful, or is it a valuable way of thinking about how some people get more benefits from social contacts than others?

References

Berkman L, Thomas G, Brissette I, Seeman TE 2000 From social integration to health: Durkheim in the new millennium. Social Science and Medicine 51: 843–857

Blaxter M, Poland F, Curran M 2001 Measuring social capital: qualitative study of how older people relate social capital to health. Final Report to the Health Development Agency. London

Bourdieu P 1997 The forms of capital. In: Halsey AH, Lauder H, Brown P, Stuart Wells A (eds) Education: culture, economy, and society. Oxford University Press, Oxford

Campbell C, Wood R, Kelly M 1999 Social capital and health. Health Education Authority, London

Coleman JS 1988 Social capital in the creation of human capital. American Journal of Sociology 94: S95–S120

Cowley S, Billings J 1999 Resources revisited: salutogenesis from a lay perspective. Journal of Advanced Nursing 29(4): 994–1005

Cowley S, Hean S 2002 Social capital in primary health care (editorial). Primary Health Care Research and Development 3: 207–209

Davey Smith G, Lynch J 2004 Commentary: Social capital, social epidemiology and disease aetiology. International Journal of Epidemiology 33: 691–700

Edwards B, Foley M 1998 Civil society and social capital: beyond Putnam. American Behavioral Scientist 42: 124–139

Forbes A, Wainwright S P 2001 On the methodological, theoretical, philosophical and political context of health inequalities research: a critique. Social Science and Medicine 53: 801–816

Gillies P 1998 Effectiveness of alliances and partnerships for health promotion. Health Promotion International 13(2): 99–120

Hall D, Elliman D 2003 Health for all children, 4th edn. Oxford University Press, Oxford

Hean S, Cowley S, Forbes A, Griffiths P, Maben J 2003 The M-C-M' cycle and social capital. Social Science and Medicine 56: 1061–1072

Hean S, Cowley S, Forbes A, Griffiths P 2004 Theoretical development and social capital measurement. In: Morgan A, Swann C (eds) Social capital for health: issues of definition, measurement and links to health. Health Development Agency, London: 41–68

Kanazawa S 2006 Mind the gap … in intelligence: re-examining the relationship between inequality and health. British Journal of Health Psychology 11: 623–642

Kaplan GA 1996 Inequality in income and mortality in the United States: analysis of mortality and potential pathways. BMJ 312: 999–1003

Kawachi I, Kennedy B, Lochner K 1997 Social capital, income inequality and mortality. American Journal of Public Health 87: 1491–1498

Kawachi I, Kim D, Coutts A, Subramanian SV 2004 Commentary: reconciling the three accounts of social capital. International Journal of Epidemiology 33: 682–690

Labonte R 1999 Social capital and community development: practitioner emptor. Australian Journal of Public Health 23: 430–433

Lomas J 1998 Social capital and health: implications for public health and epidemiology. Social Science and Medicine 47: 1181–1188

Lynch J, Davey Smith G, Hillemeier M, et al 2001 Income inequality, the psychosocial environment, and health: a comparison of wealthy nations. Lancet 358: 194–200

Moore S, Haines V, Hawe P, Shiell A 2006 Lost in translation: a genealogy of the 'social capital' concept in public health. Journal of Epidemiology and Community Health 60(8): 729–734

Muntaner C 2004 Commentary: social capital, social class, and the slow progress of psychosocial epidemiology. International Journal of Epidemiology 33: 674–680

Navarro V 2004 Commentary: Is *capital* the solution or the problem? International Journal of Epidemiology 33: 672–674

Performance and Innovation Unit (PIU) 2002 Social capital: a discussion paper. Cabinet Office, London

Petrou S, Kupeck E 2008 Social capital and its relationship with measures of health status: evidence from the health survey for England 2003. Health Economics 17: 127–143

Portes A 1998 Social capital: its origins and applications in modern sociology. Annual Review of Sociology 24: 1–24

Putnam RD 1993 Making democracy work: civic traditions in modern Italy. Princeton University Press, Princeton, NJ

Putnam RD 2000 Bowling alone. The collapse and revival of American community. Simon and Schuster, New York

Putnam RD 2004 Commentary: 'Health by association': some comments. International Journal of Epidemiology 33: 667–671

Ruston D, Akinrodove L 2002 Social capital question bank. Office for National Statistics, London

Snijders TAB 1999 Prologue to the measurement of social capital. The Tocqueville Review 20: 27–44

Stephens C 2008 Social capital in its place: using social theory to understand social capital and inequalities in health. Social Science and Medicine 66: 1174–1184

Stewart-Brown S, Shaw R 2004 The roots of social capital: relationships in the home during childhood and health in later life. In: Morgan A, Swann C (eds) Social capital for health: issues of definition, measurement and links to health. Health Development Agency, London: 157–186

Szreter S, Woolcock M 2004 Health by association? Social capital, social theory and the political economy of public health. International Journal of Epidemiology 33: 650–667

Wall E, Farrazzi G, Schryer F 1998 Getting the goods on social capital. Rural Sociology 63: 300–322

Wilkinson R 1996 Unhealthy societies. Routledge Press, London

Wilkinson R 2006 The impact of inequality: the empirical evidence. Renewal 14: 20–26

Wilkinson R, Pickett K 2006 Income inequality and population health: a review and explanation of the evidence. Social Science and Medicine 62: 1768–1784

Wilkinson R, Pickett K 2007 Economic development and inequality affect IQ: a response to Kanazawa. British Journal of Health Psychology 12: 161–166

Recommended reading

Castiglione D, Van Deth J, Wolleb G (eds) 2008 The handbook of social capital. Open University Press, Oxford
This text offers discussions about the concept of social capital and the way in which it has been applied in *empirical research. This will be a useful resource for students wishing to learn more on this topic.*

Field J 2008 Social capital: key ideas, 2nd edn. Routledge, London
This second edition provides a current overview of the continuing *debate surrounding this subject. This clear and comprehensive text helps the reader understand the theoretical underpinning of the subject, and the influence that it has on public policy and practice.*

6

Needs assessment, public health and commissioning of services

Nigel Monaghan

KEY ISSUES

- Identification of need
- Strengths and weakness of evidence
- Integration of diverse evidence
- Prioritization
- Implementing change

Introduction

This chapter explains a major public health contribution to commissioning and the identification and analysis of needs. It includes an explanation of how the process of needs assessment has evolved. A range of approaches to assessing need are described with an explanation of their advantages and disadvantages and how to choose the most appropriate approaches.

Need, demand and capacity

What people desire or request from a healthcare system may not be what they actually require. Although there is a need for treatments to be developed for incurable diseases, in the absence of a cure it cannot be argued that there is a current need for a particular treatment to be provided. This is captured in the definition of need for healthcare used by Stevens et al who define needs assessment as 'the population's ability to benefit from healthcare' (Stevens et al 2004).

The fact that healthcare resources, whether hospital beds, appointments, healthcare professionals'

time or money, are finite means that it is possible for capacity to be inadequate to meet the need in the population. In addition, there is scope for demand to outstrip the capacity of the system. Healthcare needs assessment is a key element in ensuring that there is sufficient and appropriate capacity to address need. However, once needs are defined, demand management measures will also be needed to ensure capacity is used appropriately.

Need that is being addressed by services is met need. Need that is not being addressed by services is unmet need. Similarly demand associated with need is appropriate demand whereas demand that is not associated with need is inappropriate. Managing inappropriate demand will help to protect resources that are required for others with real needs. However, converting unmet need into met need requires further action. Many people in need are not aware that they are in need, and often many of their carers, paid and unpaid, are not either. Describing the full extent of need and potential responses to it is an early step to converting unmet need into met need.

Further definitions of need which are widely used were proposed by Bradshaw. He suggested four different types of need: normative need, expressed need, comparative need and felt need (Bradshaw 1972). In Bradshaw's view, normative need is what expert opinion based on research defines as need. This roughly equates to a professional expert opinion on the ability to benefit from healthcare.

Comparative need is an extrapolation of the principle of distributive justice: those in equal need get equal response, those with greater need get greater response. Comparative need seeks validity not from expert opinion based on research but from extrapolation from one community to determine the services required in another area with a similar population. This assumes that the service provision in the first area is appropriate. Comparative needs assessment is sometimes undertaken by professionals, and also by communities or individuals, who compare the service they receive with that of another community or individual. Examples of this include people comparing differences in treatment for cancer across geographical areas.

Expressed need is estimated by observation of the community's use of services. The interplay of capacity and demand can confuse this. There may be no evidence of demand for a treatment which is not provided, for example. Again therefore this assumes a comprehensive range of appropriate services in the first place. Naidoo and Wills (2000) indicate that expressed needs are those that are articulated by service users and public health workers may empower people to turn felt needs into expressed needs in an effort to promote action to enhance health.

Felt need refers to what communities and individuals may feel they need in order to improve their health. Sometimes this is articulated; however, at other times felt needs may remain suppressed. Views from those in the community may be solicited in a comprehensive formal manner such as from a survey, or may be offered spontaneously. Felt needs may be constrained by beliefs, or by a lack of knowledge, assertiveness or confidence. For example, communities may think that an increase in hospital beds offers a solution to addressing a health need better than community-based services or preventive public health activity. People are more likely to express strong feelings about services they believe they will use in future. Public health workers may work with communities using community development approaches to try to identify felt needs.

While great weight will inevitably be given to normative needs, these other dimensions of equity and of service users' experiences are important aspects of need and service responses. Communities are more likely to accept findings of needs assessment which capture these wider dimensions of need as part of a holistic picture of community problems and appropriate responses.

Defining needs assessment

A definition can describe the nature or purpose of something. Those grappling with the concept of needs assessment for the first time require an understanding of both the reasons why needs assessments are undertaken and what is done during a needs assessment. Given the definition of need used by Stevens et al (2004) it would seem reasonable to suggest that they might define needs assessment as 'assessment of the population's ability to benefit from healthcare'. Two definitions of needs assessment are shown in Table 6.1.

For educational purposes, Montana North Central Education Service Region describes needs assessment as 'a systematic exploration of the current situation of how things are and the way they should be' (Montana North Central Education Service Region 2006). Within this definition is the concept of a systematic exploration which implies a holistic and thorough analysis within defined limits. It also explores a potential direction for change.

Hooper (1999) described needs assessment as the process of measuring the extent and nature of the needs of a particular target population so that services can respond to them. The definition of needs assessment which follows draws on both of these. Needs assessment is a systematic exploration of the extent and nature of the needs of a particular target population which seeks to effect change in services to maximize benefit from healthcare. Needs assess-

Table 6.1 Definitions of needs assessment

Definition	Source
Systematic exploration of current situation of how things are and the way they should be	Montana North Central Education Service Region (2006)
Process to measure extent and nature of needs of target population so that services can respond	Hooper (1999)

ment involves collection of information on the needs of a defined population or group who could benefit in some way. The process should identify current resources available to meet those needs and determine what gaps in care provision or in services exist.

This requires obtaining information from a variety of sources about current conditions, problems and circumstances and the resources and approaches being used to address these needs. The findings should support prioritization, development of strategies to address these needs and development of plans for the general population and for groups within the population.

A brief history of healthcare prioritization in the UK

In the UK the National Health Service (NHS) was founded on the principle of care being made available to all, free at point of delivery, on the basis of need. The approaches to assessing and responding to need have evolved over time and are worthy of consideration. There are differences across the countries of the UK which reflect the different legal system in Scotland, and a process of devolution which effectively commenced in the late 1970s, taking 20 years to be achieved. The content of this chapter is focused mainly on the approaches used in England and Wales, summarized in Table 6.2.

Needs assessment is a process intended to bring reason to decisions about which elements of care are and are not provided. If resources were unlimited then all needs and desires could be addressed and no decisions would be required. Thus needs assessment is used in many publicly funded healthcare systems to balance benefits against costs. High-cost and low-benefit elements of care are unlikely to be funded.

When the NHS was established in 1948 the provision of hospital care came from the hospitals which chose to join the new NHS. Most of these had previously relied on private care and charitable donations and were located in large urban areas. Attempts to address healthcare need on a more equitable basis commenced in the 1960s with efforts to improve access to hospital care outside large metropolitan areas through the Hospital Plans (Department of Health for Scotland 1962, Ministry of Health 1962). The Hospital Plans recognized the need to improve access outside large metropolitan areas and this was delivered through building district general hospitals typically to serve 125 000 to 250 000 population. In the late 1970s the emphasis moved from building of hospitals to moving of financial resources, although the building of new hospitals continued. In fact the building of the new hospitals had been slower than planned because of underestimates of costs that continued into the 1980s and 1990s. Within England the Resource Allocation Working Party examined NHS spend per head of population and sought over a period of years to allocate funding to regions on the basis of need (Department of Health and Social Security 1976). Within this formula need was assessed on the basis of mortality.

This process was not applied across the UK. However, in 1978 the Barnett Formula was introduced as a short-term measure to create a steady process of change to equalize public spending (including health spending) across the UK (Twigger 1998). The process was designed to produce a slow change. In recent years the higher levels of public spending in Scotland, Northern Ireland and Wales resulting from this formula have been defended on the basis of greater deprivation and need in those countries.

Table 6.2 Healthcare prioritization initiatives in England 1948 to 2003

Year	Initiative	Intent
1948	NHS established	Match previous private and voluntary facilities
1962	Hospital Plan	Build new hospitals in areas of lower provision
1976	Resource Allocation Working Party	Provide more resources to areas of high mortality
1991	Resource Allocation Formula Updated	Provide more resources based on broader range of indicators
1991	NHS & Community Care Act	Promote needs assessment as the basis for local decisions on care provision

The Resource Allocation method used in England was updated in the period from 1991 to 1995 incorporating a broader weighted capitation formula (NHS Management Board 1988), to recognize need broader than mortality; however, this model was criticized (Judge and Mays 1994, Raftery 1993, Sheldon et al 1993). It was not until 1991 that a more detailed local assessment of need was formally put at the heart of NHS planning and decision-making in England and Wales as a result of the NHS and Community Care Act 1991.

The evolution of needs assessment

Detailed needs analysis as conducted currently would not have been possible in the early 1960s or in the mid 1970s as techniques were less developed than they are now. However, by the early 1990s a range of indicators to measure disease, health status and social impact had been developed which were not available a quarter of a century earlier. There were also developments in critical appraisal and in accessing the scientific literature that facilitated needs assessment. Table 6.3 summarizes these changes.

The separation of contracting services from provision of care was intended to help contain costs. Partly this was intended to be through the use of market forces to create downward pressure on costs and partly through more critical decision-making about what would and would not need to be provided. The separation of contracting from provision of care was seen as advantageous because in the

preceding years many decisions had been made in response to shroud waving and lobbying. The problem with shroud waving and lobbying are that the voices of the most vocal and politically adept are more likely to be heard and hence their demands addressed. This was one of the contributing factors to the 'inverse care law'. Julian Tudor Hart used this phrase to describe the perverse outcome where more deprived populations in greater need of care generally have poorer access to care and poorer quality services (Hart 1971).

Thus one of the principles upon which needs assessment was established by the 1990s was that the assessment of need should be undertaken by a third party and not by a provider or beneficiary of care (Liss 1990). General medical practitioners had often been described as gatekeepers to hospital care for individual patients and to some degree were a third party although not a completely disinterested one. For decisions on the commissioning of services in the 1990s the third party was typically a public health trained individual, expected to review and appraise a range of information on need and the evidence base for responses to that need and to provide advice based on analysis.

Epidemiological tools to measure health have developed since the 1960s and made it easier to describe need in a range of ways, not just through mortality figures. During the 1990s critical appraisal also evolved. Initially an art practised by a few it became more of a scientific approach practised by many. As computers became commonplace, the indexing of evidence moved from books to electronic databases which could be searched rapidly. Once access to the evidence was easier there was a need to improve skills in appraising the evidence. Evidence-based practice was rolled out from academic centres to the heart of public health working and it has made a contribution to NHS decision-making. It combined a description of need and a critical appraisal of potential responses to that need.

These changes came quickly and needs assessment rapidly moved from being an art to being a science. The pace of change can be seen in the content of public health texts. The second edition of the *Oxford Textbook of Public Health* was published in 1991 and made no reference to need or needs assessment in its index. The third edition published in 1997 had indexed references and a chapter on measuring health need. During the intervening period, in 1994 Volume 1 of the first edition of *Health Care Needs Assessment* edited by Stevens

Table 6.3 Developments which have enabled needs assessment

Development	Impact
Information technology	Improved access to information
Better understanding of disease processes and causes	Better able to focus on key points in disease process
Evidence-based practice	Better able to quantify effectiveness of interventions
Separating commissioning from providing	Forced a more open decision process on interested parties

and Raftery was published. This comprehensive document described a standard approach to needs assessment for a series of common conditions. It was sponsored by the NHS Management Executive and circulated to health authority public health departments.

The NHS Management Executive sponsored the publication to support the development of the role of the health authorities in line with guidance they had published (National Health Service Management Executive 1989). This guidance highlighted the need to implement the following tasks in order:

- assessment of health needs
- appraisal of service options to meet those needs
- specifying services to be provided
- choosing between providers and placing contracts
- monitoring the contract
- controlling finances within cash limits.

The assumption was that a detailed needs assessment was the foundation upon which commissioning of services would be constructed.

In the 1990s public health professionals attached to purchasers of healthcare conducted needs assessments. They produced reports which either influenced the care process or gathered dust on shelves. To those not trained in public health the assessment of need often seemed to be something of a black art practised behind closed doors. Over time, needs assessment was demystified. Critical appraisal allowed more people to understand the strengths and weaknesses of evidence. As the process of needs assessment uses standardized approaches, models or techniques, the process became more transparent.

Now needs assessment is less likely to be conducted by a third party in isolation; it is becoming common for needs assessment to be conducted in partnership, engaging commissioners, providers and users of care. An open process using standardized approaches, quality assured with public health support and with a partnership or community contributing or leading the work, combines objectivity and inclusion, meaning findings are more likely to be implemented by all parties.

Types of needs assessment

Stevens et al (2004) describe three types of needs assessment: comparative, corporate and epidemiological. The former two are less labour intensive.

Comparative needs assessment compares services in one area with those elsewhere. This relates closely to the comparative need described by Bradshaw (1972). The underpinning assumptions are that difference justifies investigation and, if the differences are to continue, justification. The comparisons which can be made are limited by the availability of relevant data.

The corporate approach to needs assessment is a process of engagement of relevant stakeholders. Inevitably demand is blended with need and vested interest with science. This approach has the advantage that information from all parties and perspectives is engaged in the process to create a corporate view.

Epidemiological needs assessment, according to Stevens et al (2004), includes eight stages. The elements in summary form are:

- statement of the problem
- defining subcategories according to care requirements
- defining prevalence and incidence: who would benefit from treatment
- describing currently available services and costs
- applying the evidence base to describe effective and cost-effective services
- defining a future model of care based on the information collected to date
- defining outcome measures, audit methods and targets
- identification of information and research gaps identified by the needs assessment.

Much of the epidemiological approach is objective and factual. However, there are key judgements to be made. At the commencement, the statement of the problem will need to be carefully considered, and a corporate approach to defining the problem is commonly used by the author at the outset of needs assessment and other tasks. If the wrong problem is addressed or a key element of the problem is ignored, the outcome is unlikely to address the problem effectively. Models of care are another element where judgements have to be made. The evidence base in professional journals is weak in this area. Often the greatest potential gains in cost-effectiveness come from developing a skill mix, allowing staff to take on new roles. However, implementing these for the first time is something of a leap of faith and not all are willing to leap. Care pathways are one way to delegate but they are not commonly used in the UK.

To ensure that the epidemiological approach can take all stakeholders on the journey, it is common to combine the epidemiological approach with the corporate approach. Frequently the comparative approach is also used in the same needs assessment process to throw some challenge into the process, using as a comparator known examples of modern practice used elsewhere. For a major piece of needs assessment work the approaches recommended by Stevens et al (2004) are a useful framework. For the first timer working in, for example, a primary care setting, the approach may be too academic or comprehensive. For that setting there may be other more appropriate tools.

Needs assessment in primary care

The Scottish Needs Assessment Programme published a guide to needs assessment in primary care (Scottish Needs Assessment Programme 1998). This was drafted to support needs assessment conducted by teams working in practices or localities. Because it explains many of the principles underpinning needs assessment combined with advice on how to focus and conduct simple needs assessments, it is considered in some detail here. It proposes that there are at least seven potential aims and therefore types of needs assessments. A summary of these is shown in Table 6.4.

The rough guide document is a helpful step-by-step guide. It proposes a number of principles which shape the approach used:

- clarity on the aims of a needs assessment
- clarity on the definition of need being used
- the compilation of information to build up a picture of need
- understanding advantages and disadvantages of different methods of needs assessment
- the importance of ownership of needs assessment findings among those who need to implement the findings.

In addition, the document includes principles which should increase the likelihood that the effort put into a needs assessment has the intended impact:

- the placement of needs assessment within a planning framework
- preparation for before and follow through after a needs assessment
- following through the findings with an action plan
- repeating the needs assessment within the planning cycle to examine whether the actions have addressed the needs and assessing needs not met by these actions.

This guide proposes a three-stage approach. In stage 1, decisions need to be thought through and taken on:

- who will conduct a needs assessment
- the population, health issue and services to be examined; resources required to conduct the needs assessment
- the period over which the needs assessment should be conducted to influence the decisions it needs to.

Table 6.4 Seven aims and types of needs assessment

Type of needs assessment	Aim
Global priority	Identify high-level priorities for further work
Focused	Exploration in depth of a problem
Guideline based	Applying evidence base to local services
Community development	Engaging communities in service planning
Health alliances	Partnership exploration of and action to address determinants of health
Advocacy	Identifying and assessing particular needs of vulnerable groups
Economic	Ensuring best use of resources

Adapted from Scottish Needs Assessment Programme (1998).

Stage 2 consists of a decision on the aims of the needs assessment. This will shape the method used. There is a range of options and these options can be combined.

Global information-based needs assessment consists of using readily available information to describe the population, morbidity, mortality and use of services. Focused needs assessment looks in more detail at a problem, examining data on the local population and general information which can be applied to that population and information on effective interventions to respond to the problems identified. Guideline-based needs assessment seeks to improve the effectiveness of care by application of a guideline. When applied to local practice and population it can highlight the number of individuals whose care may change, resulting in an increase in the resources required.

The community development approach can either get people to describe their own problems and solutions, or share with them the findings of a global or focused needs assessment, and engage them in developing and prioritizing responses. The healthy alliances approach such as that proposed by Dahlgren and Whitehead (1991) uses a broad model of health that identifies determinants. Typically this examines a range of social and economic determinants, environmental and lifestyle factors by partners working together to ensure that the positive health impact of actions of the various agencies is maximized. The economic approach examines a range of approaches to address a need and to identify how the benefit is maximized from the resources available. The resources are limited, therefore maximum benefit comes from the choices that deliver most health gain for the resources used. Cost–benefit analysis helps to make these decisions.

Having made decisions on the approach or approaches to be used, the third stage consists of following one or more of the step-by-step guides. The strength of this Scottish Needs Assessment Programme approach to needs assessment partly lies in its focus and resulting simplicity, and partly in the potential to combine elements depending upon what is required at the time. If global information-based needs assessment has already established global priorities it is possible to:

- conduct a more detailed needs assessment
- look to address the need based on findings from the evidence base
- combine this with communities' views on existing and proposed evidence-based services

- work with partner organizations to address health determinants and service integration
- consider issues associated with inequalities and vulnerable groups
- define the necessary costs for the resulting service.

This journey from needs assessment to business case uses information from a variety of different types of needs assessment in a structured and easily explained approach.

Types of evidence and choosing appropriate evidence

Data and information which can be used in a needs assessment may come from routine data sources as a by-product of service management or from specially commissioned studies. In addition to locally collected routine data, there is information such as cancer incidence and census data which is collected and reported on nationally and reported on for smaller geographical units.

Routine data include census data, data on deaths and births (mortality and fertility), hospital activity and cost data, data from primary care practice management systems and equivalent data from a range of other provided services which may be either reported on already or may be made available for analysis. Making sense of the data and information and deciding what is appropriate to utilize commences with an understanding of how the evidence relates to the problem. An underpinning theoretical model or framework will assist in this. Often there will be a problem of absence of local evidence. Evidence from elsewhere may help give a feel for the position locally.

When conducting a needs assessment it is not unusual to start by indicating the sort of local information which you would like to have. You may find this is unavailable or may not be in the format you would desire and you may need to 'make do' with the available evidence and add value to that information, by linking it to other relevant data. Published surveys are a common example where findings from elsewhere may be extrapolated to the local situation.

Published surveys may give an indication of the prevalence or incidence of a disease or of risk factors for diseases. Applying these to a practice or locality population allows an estimate of the number of people in that population in need where that information is not collected. Similar populations can be expected to have similar findings, but findings from dissimilar populations may not be transferable and should be applied with caution. The range of published surveys is large. Some are routine data collection on a sample of service providers. An NHS example is general practice morbidity data. Many surveys are reported in peer-reviewed scientific journals and may be identified by searches of appropriate databases (see Chapter 4 for further information on measuring health).

Strengths and weaknesses of evidence

Whatever the evidence, it will have strengths or weaknesses. Quantitative evidence is evidence which attempts to measure the size of something. This can be useful to measure the scale of a problem. This type of evidence is easily subjected to tests of statistical significance which assist in accepting or rejecting it. It can be useful to prove differences. Qualitative evidence does not attempt to measure the scale of something or to prove something. Rather it explores the dimensions which are associated with something and has the potential to highlight relationships or dimensions which may be of importance. It may suggest possible explanations of why things are the way they are. It may suggest an explanation of how people are affected by a problem or services provided. Both of these types of evidence are important; separately they have limits, used together each can compensate for the other. Quantitative evidence may explain how common something is. Qualitative evidence may explain why what is measured in a quantitative study is important for those living in those circumstances.

Socio-medical indicators have been developed in an attempt to measure the impact on quality of life of various medical conditions. Often they assess ability to perform everyday tasks. They are sometimes used to assess the impact of interventions on improving quality of life. While these have value, for example in comparing outcomes for two different treatments for the same condition and in highlighting the important roles of social and nursing care support, they do not facilitate easy comparison of treatments for different conditions.

The peer review process is one mechanism which is intended to ensure that evidence is of good quality. Evidence from sources such as the Office for National Statistics is not subject to peer review. However, the processes used to sample the population, gather the data and correct the findings for non-participating subjects are made openly available in reports and thus subject to scrutiny. These sources of data tend to be expensive to collect, so although they are reliable, they are limited in scope.

Routinely collected data potentially allows for trends to be measured over time and for one area to be compared with another. In a few key areas such as cancer registry data collection, there may be quality assurance processes to standardize and clean data so that such comparisons can be made with some confidence. However, for most routinely collected data there are no such mechanisms. Differences that analysis suggests may in fact be real, but they may be the result of differences in the way data are coded or the completeness of data captured. This does not mean these data cannot be used to support needs assessment, rather it means that the data should be treated with some caution. Other independent data can be sought to confirm or refute such evidence.

The data and information which are sometimes necessary to consider but whose quality is likely to be lowest include both the informal survey and the anecdotal report. An informal survey has the potential to lack quality assurance which other sources include. It may ask questions about only part of the issue, that of interest to the person who designed the survey with their own agenda in mind. It may lack a sampling frame so that there is no indication of non-response bias. If the subjects are enticed into responding on the basis of their existing interest in the subject of the survey then there is a very good chance that those responding will be more interested in the topic than the wider population.

Complaints mechanisms fall between routinely collected data and anecdotal reports. Where complaints (and compliments) are encouraged and regularly used by an organization, they may be a form of routinely collected data. Where arrangements are less encouraging of complaints, those which emerge may or may not be representative of the bigger picture. This illustrates the need to understand the way data are collected and processed before using them.

Anecdotal reports may include a single opinion or the collection of views of a few. When a few rare events (e.g. cases of childhood leukaemia) happen within a small locality, concerns may be raised. This evidence does not mean that there is a local problem, but it may result in statistical analysis to clarify whether there may be problem and if so further analysis of what might be the cause.

To summarize, more weight should be given to information from more reliable sources. When information comes from less reliable sources, additional data or information should be sought if possible. If different data suggest the same conclusions then more confidence is associated with these conclusions.

Participative or third party approaches

In the past a 'third party' approach, where a third party conducts the needs assessment as neither a provider or recipient of care, has been promoted as objective. However, as many of these third parties are attached to funders of care they are not a true third party. Poor engagement of providers of care by the process may lead to recommendations not being implemented. As a result, partnership approaches to these tasks are now commoner.

Partnership approaches can be conducted using the scientific approaches to evaluation of evidence which have emerged over the last 20 years. Thus the quality assurance comes from the scientific approaches used. A further option is to ask a third party to quality assure (rather than conduct) the needs assessment process. Similarly third parties can be asked to lead, advise or provide technical support such as cleaning and analysing data.

The advantages and disadvantages of partnership approaches compared with third party approaches are:

advantages:
- local knowledge of problems and their context,
- buy-in of parties in a position to address the problem

disadvantages:
- there can be potential for vocal minorities to distort the process to suit their own agenda.

Conducting a needs assessment

Irrespective of the type of needs assessment conducted there are common themes and principles among the various approaches.

The first step is the most important because this sets the direction of all that follows. It is to understand and define the problem or problems which the needs assessment is intended to address. This is usually done in the form of a series of questions which the needs assessment is seeking to answer. This immediately raises the question of who is engaged in understanding and defining the problem. Somehow the views of a range of parties (commissioners, care providers, service users, providers of supporting and complementary services) need to be captured so that the needs assessment addresses the problem or problems identified by all parties. Approaches to assist in this include establishing a steering group to oversee the work or using a participative approach.

The second step is to define limits for the needs assessment. A needs assessment requires a defined population, and definitions of what it does and does not cover. These will vary according to the problem under study. Narrower needs assessments are easier to conduct and likely to give results sooner. Other needs assessments may have covered some of the territory of interest. An underpinning theoretical framework is helpful in defining limits and justifying them.

The third step is identifying readily available data and information to be used. The theoretical framework and limits of the needs assessment may help with this. Health librarians and other health knowledge management staff are useful people to engage to identify data and information sources.

The fourth step is collecting readily available data. Some data may only be releasable for the needs assessment if supplied in a particular way, for example anonymized. Data specially collected to inform the needs assessment may take time to collect. Assessing the quality of the data and information as they are collected is important in helping identify further supporting information and data where evidence available is not as strong as desired.

The fifth step is to examine the data and information and to interpret them against the questions which your needs assessment is seeking to answer.

The sixth step is to draw some conclusions from this interpretation. These will include actions to be taken if the needs assessment is more than a descriptive task.

The seventh step is to draft a report based on the interpretation setting out the approach used, limitations on the task, any theoretical framework used, the questions to be answered, the data used and sources, the interpretation of the data and the conclusions drawn.

The final steps will depend on the local circumstances. Their objective is getting the message across to those who can make the decisions which the report is recommending. Sign-up from a range of partners may assist. To facilitate this, the report may be circulated in draft form for comments before being finalized. The phrase to bear in mind here is 'How do I land the message?' The latter stages need to keep all parties on board in a manner that ensures actions will be implemented rather than ignored.

The commissioning cycle

The NHS is still struggling with commissioning of services. More frequently services are contracted for on the basis of what has previously been provided, often with little consideration of whether what is traditionally provided is what is needed. The Department of Health has a large area of its website devoted to commissioning (Department of Health 2007). The commissioning cycle is based on the four-stage planning cycle: analysing, planning, doing and reviewing (Richardson 2006).

It is common to describe the commissioning cycle as starting with needs assessment. If you were starting to provide care from scratch then this would be entirely logical. However, in most countries most healthcare resources are already committed. Thus it is equally rational to start by asking whether existing services are as well designed and efficient as they can be and whether they are addressing prioritized need. Then when efficiencies have been found, an analysis attempting to highlight unmet need can be conducted and the freed resources can help to address these needs. Thus needs assessment within the commissioning cycle can include elements of asking whether existing services are effective, efficient and targeted appropriately in addition to highlighting unmet need and possible responses to unmet need.

The public health role in commissioning

Needs assessment is a key part of the commissioning process and is therefore a key contribution made by those engaged in it. If considering information on need leads to the need being better targeted and if reviewing the evidence and consideration of cost-effectiveness ensures that the most effective and cost-effective solutions are commissioned, then the resulting improvement in health should be maximized. In addition, consideration of what can be done to prevent health problems through the work of the various agencies can be included in a focused needs assessment.

There are other public health contributions to commissioning. Provision of advice on performance indicators and contributing to reviews of service performance are other technical contributions. These draw on a combination of information processing skills, understanding of the distribution of disease and well-being in the population, and preventive and curative responses.

Public health is defined as improving the health of the population through the organized efforts of society (Acheson 1998). To effect change means taking the hearts and minds of others with you when considering need. Individuals are more likely to be convinced by conclusions of a needs assessment if they have been part of the process developing those conclusions.

In the early 1980s health needs assessment was a science practised by a few public health professionals. Often they would process information and draw conclusions, circulating their findings to those responsible for implementing them. A quarter of a century later it is becoming common for needs assessment to be conducted by a community or partnership. These needs assessments use underpinning theoretical frameworks, comprehensive searching strategies and scientific methods of appraising the evidence supported by advice from public health staff with expertise in needs assessment. This type of open, inclusive scientific approach has the advantages of both epidemiological and corporate methods of needs assessment.

This type of approach is consistent with one of the principles of the Ottawa Charter for Health Promotion, empowering community action (World Health Organization 1986). Putting information and decision-making into the hands of people in this way can build the confidence of the statutory bodies charged with commissioning services, their partners and the public.

Values in decision-making

Most of this chapter has covered the scientific approach to needs assessment. However, all decisions are made on values as much as they are on evidence. The reasons why low-cost and high-effectiveness treatments are sought is that these match values of providing care for all (from limited resources) and providing effective care. The scientific approaches proposed in this chapter make it easier to highlight key information against shared values.

Different values can result in different decisions being made on the same evidence. Where partners come together to conduct a needs assessment and have little experience of working together, a little time spent expressing the values which each party treasures can go a long way to developing a shared value base and later consensus on what the need is and how to respond to it. For example, for needs assessment in relation to substance misusers there may be different values underpinning the work of the police, voluntary and health services. A major advantage of partnership approaches to needs assessment is the potential to ensure that the values of the various stakeholders have been engaged during the process.

The assessment of the nature of any need may be a little easier than deciding how to respond to that need from the resources available. When resources are spent on one area they are not available for another. Deciding what not to do is as important as deciding what to do. Just because there is some potential to benefit from spending on an intervention does not mean that intervention has to be funded without regard to wider implications. An understanding of stated values and how the proposed action should deliver against them can assist in making a case for change.

Conclusion

Once a nation has put in place clean water supplies and sewerage systems to manage common infectious diseases, a myriad of health challenges are compet-

ing for the remaining resources. Needs assessment is an approach intended to ensure that limited resources are targeted to need. Needs assessment has developed alongside evidence-based practice and epidemiological tools to measure social impact of medical conditions. These approaches help to target the key issues and highlight key information. Ultimately needs assessment supports decisions about what will and will not be done and values are important in this process.

SUMMARY

- When issues such as clean water supplies for the population have been addressed there are many challenges to health yet only limited resources to respond.
- Needs assessment builds on the evidence base and understanding of relationships between determinants of health, disease and social impact of disease to highlight key information upon which decisions can be made.
- Using recognized approaches in partnership appears to offer the best blend of engagement and scientific approach.

DISCUSSION POINTS

1. What sort of problems would and would not be suitable for a needs assessment approach?
2. You are planning a local needs assessment in partnership. What issues need to be on the agenda of a first meeting?
3. When a needs assessment is completed how do you ensure changes it proposes will be implemented locally?

References

Acheson D 1998 Report on the Committee of Inquiry into the Future Development of the Public Health Function. Public health in England. HMSO, London

Bradshaw JR 1972 The concept of social need. New Society 496: 640–643

Dahlgren G, Whitehead M 1991 Policies and strategies to promote

social equity in health. Institute of Future Studies, Stockholm

Department of Health 2007 Commissioning. Online: http://www.dh.gov.uk/en/

Managingyourorganisation/
Commissioning/index.htm

Department of Health for Scotland
1962 A hospital plan for Scotland.
Cmnd 1602. HMSO, London

Department of Health and Social
Security 1976 Sharing resources
for health in England (Report
of the Resource Allocation
Working Party). HMSO, London.
Online: http://www.dh.gov.uk/
en/Publicationsandstatistics/
Publications/
PublicationsPolicyAndGuidance/
DH_4121873

Hart JT 1971 The inverse care law.
Lancet 1: 405–412

Hooper J 1999 Health needs
assessment: helping change happen.
Community Practitioner 72(9):
268–288

Judge K, Mays N 1994 Allocating
resources for health and social care
in England. British Medical Journal
308: 1363–1366

Liss PE 1990 Healthcare need: meaning
and measurement. Linkoping
University, Linkoping

Ministry of Health 1962 A hospital plan
for England and Wales. Cmnd 1604.
HMSO, London

Montana North Central Education
Service Region 2006 Needs
assessments. Online: http://mncesr.
org/nsdc.htm (accessed 27 June
2007)

Naidoo J, Wills J 2000 Heath
promotion: foundations for
practice, 2nd edn. Baillière Tindall,
Edinburgh

NHS Management Board 1988 Review
of the resource allocation working
party formula. Department of
Health and Social Security, London

National Health Service Management
Executive 1989 Role of District
Health Authorities: analysis of issues.
Department of Health, London

Raftery J 1993 Capitation funding:
population, age, and mortality
adjustments for regional and district
health authorities in England. British
Medical Journal 307: 1121–1124

Richardson F 2006 The commissioning
context: introduction. Online:

http://www.cat.csip.org.uk/_library/
eBook/Chap1FRichardson.pdf

Scottish Needs Assessment Programme
1998 Needs assessment in primary
care: a rough guide. Online:
http://www.phis.org.uk/PDF.
pl?file=publications/roughguide.PDF

Sheldon T, Davey Smith G, Bevan G
1993 Weighting in the dark: resource
allocation in the new NHS. British
Medical Journal 306: 835–839

Stevens A, Raftery J, Mant J 2004
An introduction to health needs
assessment. In: Stevens A, Raftery J,
Mant J, et al (eds) Health care needs
assessment: the epidemiologically
based needs assessment reviews.
Radcliffe, Oxford: 1–16

Twigger R 1998 The Barnett Formula.
House of Commons Research
Paper 98/8. Online: http://www.
parliament.uk/commons/lib/
research/rp98/rp98-008.pdf

World Health Organization 1986
Ottawa Charter for Health
Promotion. WHO, Geneva

Recommended reading

Diderichsen F, Varde E, Whitehead
M 1997 Resource allocation to
health authorities: the quest for an
equitable formula in Britain and
Sweden. British Medical Journal
315: 875–878
*This paper describes the background
to approaches in the UK and Sweden
to funding of healthcare on a fair
basis.*

Stevens A, Raftery J, Mant J, et al (eds)
2004 Health care needs assessment:
the epidemiologically based needs
assessment reviews, 1st series, 2nd
edn. Radcliffe, Oxford
Stevens A, Raftery J, Mant J, et al
2007 Health care needs assessment:
the epidemiologically based needs
assessment reviews, 3rd series.
Radcliffe, Oxford

*These two books were funded by the
Department of Health to assist those
involved in the commissioning and
strategic planning of health services.
They detail approaches to needs
assessments for a series of topics and
contain information which could be
helpful when scoping a needs
assessment project.*

Website addresses

Department of Health 2007
Commissioning: http://www.
dh.gov.uk/en/Policyandguidance/
Organisationpolicy/Commissioning/
index.htm

Institute of Public Care 2006 The
Commissioning eBook: http://
ipc.brookes.ac.uk/publications/
commissioning_ebook.htm

Chapter Seven

7

Public health and health promotion – frameworks for practice

Dianne Watkins

KEY ISSUES

- The emergence of health promotion and the new public health movement
- Defining health promotion
- Health promotion approaches and models and their application to public health in nursing practice
- Psychological theory and its application to behaviour change

The emergence of health promotion and the new public health movement

The term health promotion and its underlying theory have received much interest from 1978 up until the present time. Much of this has been fuelled by global policy, in particular the Alma Ata Declaration (World Health Organization (WHO) 1978), the Ottawa Charter for Health Promotion (WHO 1986) and the Health for All Policies which emerged from these documents. The move from cure to prevention gained momentum during the 1990s, with policy makers, governments and subsequently healthcare providers striving to take forward health-promoting initiatives in an attempt to reduce inequalities in health and reduce the burden of preventable diseases. Some activity was under the guise of public health medicine, while other work came under the remit of health promotion. Historically there has been confusion and overlap between health promotion and public health and the lack of distinction between these terms hindered collaborative working during the latter part of the 20th century. Fortunately a unity of health promotion and public health under the overall umbrella of what was called the 'new or modern public health movement' emerged in the 21st century with increased clarity over roles and responsibilities. The new public health is seen to comprise three overlapping spheres of activity: health improvement, health protection and health and social care quality (Gillam et al 2007). Health promotion now fits primarily under the remit of health improvement. However, for ease of reading and understanding, the term 'health promotion' will be used throughout this chapter recognizing its fit under the remit of health improvement, and public health. Figure 7.1 illustrates the new public health and its various dimensions.

The overlapping spheres of health improvement, health protection and health and social care quality allow for enhancement of the health of populations to be addressed through a number of different avenues. Health improvement is seen to encompass work to tackle inequalities and the socio-economic influences on health. Its emphasis is on health promotion, promoting individual, family and community health, lifestyle education and the psychosocial aspects of health (Gillam et al 2007, Griffiths et al 2005). Health protection is concerned with the control of communicable diseases, environmental issues such as clean air and water, any threats to health imposed by war, chemical or radiation, preparation to deal with disasters and occupational health. The domain of health and social care quality seeks to address issues associated with determining the quality and efficiency of health and social care

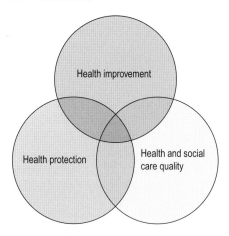

Figure 7.1 • The domains of public health (Griffiths et al 2005).

systems and organizations, the enhancement of quality standards in health and social care provision, the promotion of evidence-based practice, research, audit and evaluation, with an ultimate aim of promoting clinically effective practice (Gillam et al 2007, Griffiths et al 2005). The overlapping nature of the Venn diagram in Figure 7.1 illustrates that each dimension influences the others and there is a degree of common ground between each sphere.

This chapter will concentrate primarily on the sphere of health improvement, while recognizing the other dimensions and how they influence each other. The focus within health improvement is on 'health promotion', which incorporates education and the influence of socio-economic factors on health. Those working to improve health need to be aware of the effects of economic disadvantage, poverty, employment and unemployment, social class, education, housing and lifestyle on health achievement. Many of these elements are often beyond the control of the individual and will influence lifestyle choices and behaviours. The chapter now moves on to define the meaning and dimensions of health promotion.

Defining health promotion

It is acknowledged that health promotion does not sit alone as a concept, and is influenced by the disciplines of sociology, psychology, epidemiology, education, medicine and biological science, econom-

ics and statistics, to name but a few. This eclectic mixture of theories makes health promotion an interesting and challenging area, and means that those working to promote health should not do so without analysing and synthesizing how these theories fit together, how they influence practice and how they underpin the skills required to promote health effectively. Other chapters within this book make reference to some of these theories (e.g. Chapter 4). Health promotion theory is relatively new with a short history associated with its development, unlike theories associated with areas such as relativity or epidemiology. Much of the theory generation was initiated following developments in the 1970s, particularly Alma Ata (WHO 1978) and the Ottawa Charter for Health Promotion (WHO 1986), as previously mentioned. It is worth examining the latter as a starting point to discussions surrounding theoretical concepts and definitions. The WHO (1986) defines health promotion as:

> *the process of enabling people to increase control over, and to improve their health. To reach a state of complete physical, mental and social well-being, an individual or group must be able to identify and to realize aspirations, to satisfy needs, and to change or cope with the environment. Health is, therefore, seen as a resource for everyday life, not the objective of living. Health is a positive concept emphasizing social and personal resources, as well as physical capacities. Therefore, health promotion is not just the responsibility of the health sector, but goes beyond healthy life-styles to well-being. (WHO 1986: 1)*

The Ottawa Charter determines that this philosophy may be achieved through the areas of advocacy, enablement and mediation and is linked to specific areas associated with building healthy public policy, re-orientating health services, creating supportive environments, strengthening community action and helping people develop their personal skills. These broad areas illustrate the enormous task associated with health promotion and its emergence into a full public health framework (as previously outlined) allows for these issues to be addressed through maximum collaboration with multiple partners. For example, building public health policy and creating supportive environments may require working with governments, politicians and local councillors, environmental health departments and transport to develop local infrastructures and to address the social determinants of health. In the context of the wider public's health, nursing plays only a small part, and the profession cannot work in isolation when working to influence the overall health of individuals, communities and populations. Other chapters within the book expand on collaboration and partnership working for health in greater detail (see Chapter 21).

One of the early definitions of health promotion was offered by Catford and Nutbeam (1984). They characterized health promotion as incorporating any activity that set out to improve or protect health and this may be based on promoting behavioural, biological, socio-economic or environmental changes. This reasoning is based on the Lalonde Report (1974), which reported on the health of Canadians, and advocated that health promotion should be based around a health field concept that included four areas; human biology, environment, lifestyle and healthcare organization. The biological dimension includes aspects of physical and mental health inclusive of hereditary factors, diseases and disabilities which adversely affect health. Environment refers to those factors which individuals may have little personal control over and are outside the human body. Much of this is related to the area of health protection mentioned earlier in the chapter such as radiation, clean water, air pollution, war, socio-economic factors, etc. Lifestyle refers to individuals making choices which may adversely affect their health, such as smoking, drug/alcohol misuse, diet, exercise patterns, etc. These are primarily seen to be within the control of the individual; however, the other dimensions of a person's life may well influence lifestyle decisions. The fourth area of healthcare organization incorporates the quality aspects of healthcare delivery and organization and focuses on the delivery of cure and treatment. The health field concept has influenced much of the work around health promotion in the United Kingdom.

The meaning of health promotion has consistently been hampered by efforts to differentiate between health promotion and health education. One of the most recent conceptual analyses by Whitehead (2004) makes a clear distinction between these two terms. He states that health promotion is 'the process by which the ecologically-driven socio-political determinants of health are addressed as they impact on individuals and the communities within which they interact' (Whitehead 2004: 314).

The emphasis in this definition is on political endeavours and empowering communities to make a contribution to influencing the wider determinants and their detrimental effects on health. He describes health education as 'an activity that seeks to inform the individual on the nature and causes of health/illness and that individual's personal level of risk associated with their lifestyle behaviour. Health education seeks to motivate the individual to accept a process of behavioural change through directly influencing their value, belief and attitude systems, where it is deemed that the individual is particularly at risk or has already been affected by illness/disease or disability' (Whitehead 2004: 313). This interpretation suggests that health promotion involves working at a population or community level to influence health, while health education concentrates on working with individuals to try to improve personal health and well-being.

Other authors support the notion put forward by Whitehead. For example, Tones and Tilford (2001: xiii) state that health promotion = health education × healthy public policy. The personal opinion of the author of this chapter is that health promotion is an umbrella term that involves all activity that works to enhance health. This may involve working at a population or community level to improve social/environmental issues or develop healthy public policy, or working with individuals in one-to-one interactions to promote health-enhancing behaviour. Dividing these activities into the two separate areas of health promotion and health education may distract nurses from considering the broader issues that can influence health. Health education has a history of 'blaming the victim' and nurses are still criticized for not considering the influence of environmental and social factors on health achievement (Smith et al 1999, Whitehead 2003). Authors discuss the importance of ensuring that health promotion incorporates the socio-political dimensions, as well as behavioural aspects, thus ensuring that structuralist and individualistic aspects are considered (Tones and Tilford 2001, Naidoo and Wills 2000). The following section outlines briefly the impact of socio-economic and environmental factors on health to try to promote an awareness of why these are important to consider in health promoting practice.

The influence of environmental and social factors on health achievement

There is a wealth of evidence that documents the effects of environmental and social factors on health and people's decisions about their health and lifestyle (Acheson 1998). It is beyond the scope of this chapter to explore these determinants of health in great detail; however, an awareness of their impact is essential to be able to promote health effectively (Chapters 3 and 4 also make reference to these issues).

Environmental factors such as the geographical location of residence, natural disasters, war, famine, unsafe water, pollution, and working and living conditions can adversely affect people's health. These can be categorized into influences that occur at a macro, meso and micro level. Macro refers to the country or regional level. Examples of influences on health at a macro level include natural disasters such as the 'tsunami' (December 2004) or the tropical cyclone which hit Burma (May 2008); war and its effects such as the Somali civil war; political unrest, for example Robert Mugabe's campaign of terror against the people of Zimbabwe where people were brutally attacked and even murdered if they did not comply with his views and voted against him. The meso level refers to workplace, communities, schools, etc. which can influence health. Examples of adverse influences at a meso level include occupational hazards, for example excessive noise, operating complex machinery, labouring, shift patterns and their influence on health (Cooper and Starbuck 2005); the job one engages in makes a difference to health and is a known determinant that affects health achievement (Naidoo and Wills 2000) (for further information relating to the effects of work on health see Chapter 8). Geographical location of residence, the neighbourhood and community in which people live also influences health (Drever and Whitehead 1997, Wilkinson and Marmot 2003). It is well documented in the United Kingdom that there is a north–south divide in the country's health (Wilkinson and Marmot 2003) and examples of this have been demonstrated in Chapter 3. At a micro level environmental influences on health relate to peer group and family norms and values influencing health and health choices (Tones and Tilford 2001).

People's lifestyle choices may be dependent on environmental constraints and this should be considered when promoting health. Part of the role of the nurse working in a public health role should be to work to address environmental issues where possible, such as campaigning for safer roads and transport, community green areas and play facilities for children, better housing, workplace conditions or the school as a healthy environment for children.

Poverty and its influence on health and health choices have been repeatedly reported in numerous studies and there is a direct correlation between social class and health (Acheson 1998, Department of Health 2005). Before looking at the evidence base on the differences in health between social classes, it is worth identifying how social class is differentiated. The following outlines the National Statistics Socio-economic Classification (Office for National Statistics 2002). It supersedes the Registrar General's Social Class classification:

1. Higher managerial and professional occupations
   1.1. Large employers and higher managerial occupations
   1.2. Higher professional occupations
2. Lower managerial and professional occupations
3. Intermediate occupations
4. Small employers and own account workers
5. Lower supervisory and technical occupations
6. Semi-routine occupations
7. Routine occupations
8. Never worked and long-term unemployed.

It is important to note that many of the studies which provide the evidence base for the differences in health between social groups are based on the old Registrar General Classification of Social Classes I–V: Social Class I – professionals; Social Class II – managerial and technical; Social Class III – skilled manual and non-manual (white collar) workers; Social Class IV – semi-skilled workers; and Social Class V – the unskilled labourer. The social class of a family is based on the occupation of the head of the household and does not consider other workers within the family who may make a contribution to the household income. This is a limitation of taking only social class as an indicator of health. Wilkinson and Marmot (2003) have investigated other materialistic variables other than social class, such as possession of a car or being a house owner. In all circumstances it has been proven that more affluent people generally experience better health (Acheson

1998, Wilkinson and Marmot 2003). Material disadvantage makes a difference to health and social class provides some indication of ways of life and income experienced. The following outlines the original theories presented for the inequalities in health that exist between social groups.

Reasons for inequalities in health between social groups

(Adapted from Acheson 1998, Townsend and Davidson 1982.)

- Artefact.
- Natural and social selection.
- Cultural/behavioural.
- Materialist/structuralist.

Artefact and the natural and social selection explanation

This theory originally suggested that inequalities in health across the social strata were artificial and flawed and related to the way in which health was measured and defined. It argues that the data used to define differences in health between social groups present only 'ill health' and 'death' and do not present measures of health. The theory argues that while it is accepted that comparing the life chances of individuals in the highest and lowest strata of society leads to the finding that better health and longevity appear to be enjoyed by the wealthy, the comparison of life chances, between rich and poor, over time, is flawed. It is contended that this widening gap identified by 'The Black Report' and reinforced by others (Acheson 1998) is an artefact in that statistics have been collected over time and so do not reflect true difference. The artefact theory asserts that, in a society such as the UK, there has been great social upheaval over the past 100 years and that the social class structure itself is in a constant state of flux. It maintains that Social Class V in more recent times, for example, has little or no similarities to Social Class V, as defined, in bygone eras. The massive growth seen in the middle classes in post-war Britain and the rapid expansion in opportunities for higher education mean that this group has changed beyond recognition, making comparison over time impossible. The general trend in the gentrification of society means that the lower

social classes ultimately become a refuge for the old, weak and disabled living on the margins of society. Within these groups of people there will be a greater chance of death and ill health sooner or later and this explains the natural and social selection theory, inevitably leading to the poor health statistics found in the lowest social classes.

Cultural/behavioural explanations

This theory suggests that people in lower social classes engage in more adverse lifestyle behaviour, that their behaviour is irresponsible and their ill health is a product of this. In essence this theory blames people for their own ill health. It also suggests that there is a certain subculture present in different social groups which is either harmful or beneficial to health.

There are several theories which try to explain why people indulge in adverse lifestyles that affect their health and it is beyond the scope of this chapter to present the known evidence base on the links between smoking and health, drug misuse and health, poor dietary patterns and health, obesity and health, lack of exercise and health, stress and health, to name but a few. Tones and Tilford (2001: 27) suggest adverse lifestyles may be down to 'learned helplessness' resulting from chronic exposure to debilitating social conditions and lack of money. This suggests that people from lower social groups living in poverty may well search out lifestyle behaviours that help them to cope with the difficulties they continually encounter in their life. For example, there is evidence to suggest that women from lower social classes smoke to help them cope with their life in poverty (Graham 2000).

Other authors suggest there may be differences in the social norms, values and beliefs across the social class strata, with people from middle classes feeling they have more control over their health than those from lower social classes who do not believe they influence their own health. These beliefs are passed from generation to generation and hence the cycle of poverty and feeling helpless is perpetuated (Naidoo and Wills 2000).

There is a theory that postulates people influence and have control over their lifestyle, whoever they are. This 'victim blaming approach' blames people for their own ill health and proposes that people from all social classes are in control of their own lifestyle. There is contradictory evidence to dispute this theory based on the work of Acheson (1998).

Materialist/structuralist explanation

This theory suggests that ill health among the poorest is attributable to social and economic factors. For example, those with less money experience material disadvantage in relation to housing, diet, occupational hazards, transport, access to healthcare, etc. These factors adversely influence their health.

Some postulate that the unequal burden of illness and death experienced by the poorest in society is directly related to the distribution of wealth and resources. It is argued that due to poverty, people are forced to live in poor, cramped housing conditions. It is often those who live in poverty who are forced by their life circumstances to leave school early and consequently, due to a lack of education, are forced to take up low-paid, often hazardous employment. This lack of education and money can impact on lifestyle, life choices, material possessions such as adequate transport, house ownership and access to healthcare. In relation to health provision for the poor, the South Wales general practitioner Julian Tudor Hart made the observation that those with the greatest need often received the worst service, an observation that is now universally known as the inverse care law (Tudor Hart 1971).

This brief overview of inequalities in health is further expanded upon with examples from the Caerphilly Health and Social Needs Study in Chapter 3 and in Chapter 4 on epidemiology and its application to practice. It is suffice to conclude in this chapter that social class continues to be used as an indicator of health status and it is recognized that people from higher social classes experience better health compared to those from lower social classes (Acheson 1998, Department of Health 2005).

It is crucial for nurses to understand the impact of factors such as unemployment, social exclusion, poverty, gender, stress, violence, inadequate housing and workplace hazards on health and to consider how their roles can contribute to reducing inequalities in health. The Canadian Nurse Association (2005) states that nurses, through a re-orientation of their existing practice, can influence determinants that affect individual and population health through, for example:

- comprehending how determinants of health, for example age, gender, ethnicity, income, housing and social support, affect individual and population health and well-being
- incorporating questioning on the wider determinants that affect health when undertaking health assessments
- collaborating with partner health and social care agencies, e.g. citizens' advice bureaux, advocacy groups, housing departments, to raise awareness of need and mobilize resources
- working to inform and empower individuals, groups or communities to express felt needs
- being knowledgeable on the availability of local and national resources
- advocating for universal access to basic health programmes such as dental care
- campaigning for health improvement initiatives such as ending the physical punishment of children.

Assessing health needs using a social model of health recognizes the negative impact of deprivation and disadvantage on health. This can assist nurses in their public health role by alerting them to factors that could influence individual and family health (Watkins 2003).

To conclude this part of the chapter, it is important to recognize and understand the determinants of health and their influence on health and health choices and there is now uncontested evidence that there are gross inequalities in health between the rich and the poor, an issue now recognized by governments in the United Kingdom. The following health promotion approaches and models presented link back to the theory that has been covered in this section.

Approaches to promoting health

There are numerous approaches available to promote health. These have been defined as:

- medical/preventive
- behaviour change
- educational
- empowerment
- social change.

(Adapted from Ewles and Simnett 2003 and Naidoo and Wills 2000.)

The medical/preventive approach

The aim of the medical/preventive approach is to prevent disease (morbidity) and premature death (mortality) through the use of medical knowledge and persuasion. Work to promote health using a medical/preventive approach can be divided into three elements: primary prevention, secondary prevention and tertiary prevention. Primary prevention aims to prevent the very onset of disease. Examples of primary preventive measures include immunization and vaccination programmes, some screening programmes which aim to prevent the onset of disease, rather than detect disease, antenatal classes, new patient screening by practice nurses, parenting programmes and health education in schools that aim to promote well-being and healthy lifestyles, building self-esteem and teaching children to cope with and resist peer pressure, etc. Secondary prevention aims to prevent or halt the progression of disease, for example hypertension treatment, cholesterol-lowering agents, diabetes management, cervical cytology screening. Tertiary prevention aims to reduce further disability or reoccurrence of disease. Examples of this include cardiac rehabilitation programmes or palliative care. The medical/preventive approach and the behavioural approach are often used in combination and are based on a biomedical model of health.

The behavioural approach

The behavioural approach is based on persuading people to change their behaviour and adopt healthy lifestyles. There is some overlap between the medical approach and the behavioural approach in that it uses persuasion as its method and assumes that people are in a position to be able to change their behaviour, that they have the right skills and knowledge and that their social circumstances do not impact upon decisions they make regarding their lifestyle. Naidoo and Wills (2000) comment that this approach ignores the complexity associated with behaviour changes. Examples where a behaviour change approach can be seen in action include interventions that aim to help people stop smoking, exercise and healthy eating promotion, and safe sex. It presumes that behaviour change is within personal control and is not influenced by external factors.

There are advantages and disadvantages of using the medical/preventive and the behaviour change approaches. These approaches are usually based on sound epidemiological studies and research that has proven cause and effect relationships. Professionals utilize this information and provide expert advice to clients/patients. The view is that providing this knowledge to others will result in people changing their behaviour. If the advice given is followed then it can result in savings to the National Health Service and there have been some excellent examples of reductions in morbidity and mortality from using these approaches. An example of this is immunization and vaccination programmes. The disadvantages of these approaches are that they usually take away client choice and remove responsibility for health decisions away from individuals to health experts. These approaches are not always successful and changes in behaviour may be only short term, as the client/patient may not have been truly involved in the decision-making process and taken ownership of lifestyle decisions made. These approaches take a 'top down' style that ignores the social and environmental influences on health and health decisions. Those who adopt these approaches in their practice are at risk of adopting a 'victim blaming approach' and health professionals are constantly accused of this. Experts believe that a change in behaviour or a medical intervention is in the best interests of the client/patient and so will persuade and cajole people to comply, even if it is against their personal wishes. One of the ethical difficulties facing health professionals is that medical evidence may identify particular risks to health which patients/clients choose to ignore. The professional may feel it is their role to advise the patient and that free choice will adversely affect their personal health and maybe that of others. Examples of this include the mother who continues to smoke in the same room as her asthmatic child, the parent who refuses to have their child immunized, and the diabetic patient who refuses to follow dietary advice. The medical/behavioural approach is commonly used by nurses who are ideally placed to provide advice and support to well and ill people. Nurses are, however, criticized for not understanding the other elements of a patient/client's life that will inevitably influence their health-related decisions.

Educational approach

The educational approach aims to provide people with information on how they could improve their health. The focus is on increasing knowledge levels and developing people's skills, so that they are able to make health-enhancing changes (Naidoo and Wills 2000). This approach does not set out to persuade or cajole people into making decisions and respects the fact that people have free choice. It is supposed to present information in an unbiased manner, although health professionals may have their own agenda. This approach is criticized on the grounds that it makes an assumption between the acquisition of knowledge and consequent behaviour change. Those who utilize this approach in practice may ignore social and psychological factors that can influence decision-making. There are many examples which inform us that an increase in knowledge may not necessarily result in behaviour change. For example, smokers are made aware of the effects of smoking on health from the information available on cigarette packets. This knowledge does not, however, always result in smokers changing their behaviour to that of non-smokers. It is important to note that the relationship between the provision of knowledge and behaviour change is not a linear process and that limited success will be achieved from using the educational approach alone (Bunton and MacDonald 2002).

When using the educational approach, attention should be given to the three aspects of learning: the cognitive dimension which is about increasing information and understanding, the affective domain which relates to attitudes and feelings, and the behavioural which is about learning the skills to be able to implement a behaviour change or a task. People often need to move through this continuum before they are able to make a change in behaviour. For example, an adolescent may possess knowledge regarding safe sex and the use of condoms; however, when faced with this situation in real life, they may not have explored what their own feelings and attitude would be during a sexual encounter. They may lack the skills of assertion to demand the use of a condom and the actual know-how of how to apply a condom to a penis, resulting in indulgence in unsafe sex. Sexual desire may also overpower using a condom when faced with a real life experience. This demonstrates how behaviour may not always be congruent with knowledge and information. It may be more beneficial to combine the educational and the empowerment approach when engaging in health promotion practice.

Empowerment approach

The aim of the empowerment approach is to help people identify their own concerns and work with them to help achieve positive health outcomes. As previously mentioned, 'enabling' people to increase control over their health, as advocated by the WHO (1986), is a central component of health promotion. Definitions of 'enable' overlap with those of 'empower'. Enable is defined as 'to provide somebody with resources, authority or opportunity to do something, to make something possible or feasible'. Empower is defined as 'to give somebody power or authority, to give someone a greater sense of confidence or self esteem' (*Encarta English Dictionary* 2008). These are the principles of the empowerment approach where the focus is on the development of community or individual confidence and development of the skills to enhance health and well-being. It is a 'bottom-up' approach which works on the community/client's agenda, rather than addressing needs identified by professionals. Empowerment is often separated out into community empowerment and individual empowerment (Naidoo and Wills 2000, Tones and Tilford 2001). Weare (2002: 106) suggests that 'free choice has to be at the centre of the concept, and the goals of empowerment must be self-determination and independence'. This takes away any coercion or persuasion. Individual empowerment is based on life skills teaching, building assertiveness, self-esteem, the development of social interaction skills and the opportunity to transfer theoretical aspects to practice (Weare 2002).

The principles of empowerment utilized when practising an empowerment approach are often poorly understood (Rodwell 1996, Tones and Tilford 2001). A concept analysis was undertaken by Rodwell and the following defining features were identified as being essential to empowerment: 'a helping process, a partnership which values self and others, mutual decision-making using resources, opportunities and authority and freedom to make choices and accept responsibility' (Rodwell 1996: 309). This brings to the forefront the importance of partnership working between the health promoter and individual or community and a power base that is equal between both parties. Naidoo and Wills (2000) point out that before an empowering approach can work, people need to accept responsibility, recognize and understand that they are able to make a difference to their health, be motivated to want to change things and feel that they are capable of influencing that change through the development of the appropriate skills. For some living in disadvantaged circumstances, beginning this way of thinking can be difficult and much effort may be required in working with people to build their confidence and self-esteem and influence their self-efficacy and internal locus of control. Self-efficacy refers to a belief in one's own ability to be able to influence and make decisions and actions and leads to increased self-esteem (Bandura 1997). Tones and Tilford (2001) comment that the higher one's self-efficacy, the more perseverance and persistence a person is likely to demonstrate. Perceived locus of control (PLC) is a term first referred to by Rotter (1966). The following extract provides an interpretation of locus of control:

> When a reinforcement is perceived by the subject as following some action of his own but not being entirely contingent upon his action, then, in our culture, it is typically perceived as the result of luck, chance, fate, as under the control of powerful others, or as unpredictable because of the great complexity of the forces surrounding him. When the event is interpreted in this way by an individual, we have labelled this an external locus of control. If the person perceives that the event is contingent upon his own behaviour or his relatively permanent characteristics, we have termed this a belief in internal control. (Rotter 1966: 1)

Possessing high self-efficacy and an internal locus of control has a direct and indirect relationship to health (Tones and Tilford 2001). If a person believes that they are able to influence their own health, then they are more likely to engage in health-enhancing activity. Those with an external locus of control would be less likely to do so, as their belief would be that their ill health was a matter of fate or chance. Self-efficacy is also likely to increase people's perseverance at making changes in their behaviour. For these reasons the empowerment approach can have far-reaching consequences in health promotion work and its success has been evaluated in relation to working with adolescent school children (Weare 2002) where children have been taught to resist peer pressure in relation to drug and alcohol misuse

and pressures to conform to adverse lifestyle behaviours.

Figure 7.2 demonstrates how use of an empowerment approach and building confidence through life skills teaching may increase people's self-efficacy – a belief in ones own ability to achieve, which in turn may influence personal perceived locus of control and possibly health-related behaviour. This becomes a 'feedback loop' in that once people have made positive lifestyle decisions, it leads to greater self-esteem and confidence in decision-making.

The advantages to using an empowering approach are that it is people centred and the focus is on issues important to the community or individual. For these reasons, then, success is more likely. It also acknowledges the context of people's lives and recognizes the social and environmental factors that influence health and health choices. Community empowerment would indeed perhaps help communities to focus on addressing external factors influencing their health. The disadvantages of the empowerment approach are that people need to recognize the need for change and feel they want to do something about their situation. They also require a belief in their own ability to be able to influence action. The outcomes may not be health orientated, making success sometimes difficult to measure. The other difficulty associated with using this approach is that issues raised by communities or individuals may conflict with the attitudes and beliefs of the health promoter, raising difficult ethical dilemmas.

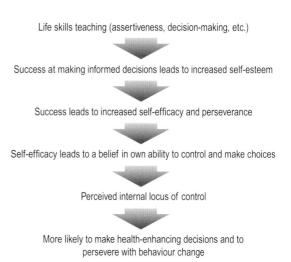

Life skills teaching (assertiveness, decision-making, etc.)

Success at making informed decisions leads to increased self-esteem

Success leads to increased self-efficacy and perseverance

Self-efficacy leads to a belief in own ability to control and make choices

Perceived internal locus of control

More likely to make health-enhancing decisions and to persevere with behaviour change

Figure 7.2 • Utilizing an empowering approach.

Social change approach

The social change approach aims to bring about change in the social, physical and economic environment. It is referred to as a 'radical approach' to health promotion (Naidoo and Wills 2000). It utilizes a top-down approach in that it sets out to work with governments, organizations, councillors, pressure groups, politicians, etc. Some examples of using a social change approach would be working to ban the use of mobile phones while driving or campaigning for green areas, parks, safe play areas and working conditions, or introducing no-smoking policies in public places. The focus is on societal change, rather than on working with individuals to influence behaviour change.

The opportunities for nurses to get involved in adopting a social change approach may be more limited for some and are dependent upon the environment and area of clinical practice in which they work. For example, specialist community public health nurses such as health visitors would be in a position to utilize a social change approach, while hospital-based nurses may have less opportunity (see Chapter 23 for more discussion regarding this issue).

Whatever approaches are used, the following principles are deemed important to include:

- client choice and participation
- recognition of the importance of wider determinants on the achievement of health and health choices
- equal power balance between professionals and clients/patients in all interactions
- the use of empowering strategies
- making links with other dimensions of public health activity where appropriate
- influencing political imperatives that seek to enhance and maintain health where possible
- utilizing a multidisciplinary, multiagency approach where appropriate.

Models of health promotion

There are various models of health promotion available which can offer a framework on which to base strategy and practice. Models act as a guide and allow for the theoretical basis of health promotion to be explored more fully. They also allow for analysis and synthesis of practice and are useful for planning and evaluation. Only two models will be presented in this chapter; Tannahill (1985) and Beattie (1993), although other models are available.

Tannahill's model of health promotion

The first model devised by Tannahill (1985) was later presented by Downie, Fyfe and Tannahill (1992). In this model health promotion is presented as three overlapping spheres in the form of a Venn diagram (Figure 7.3) and in some respects mirrors the dimensions of public health previously outlined in this chapter.

Figure 7.3 illustrates that there are three major overlapping dimensions of health education, prevention and health protection. Health education is any education based on promoting positive health and health-enhancing behaviour; prevention aims to prevent the occurrence of disease and this may be divided into primary, secondary and tertiary prevention, as previously outlined in this chapter; health protection is about protecting health through legislation, policy or procedures. This may be at a local, community or national level. Each of the spheres is then subdivided and there are seven areas in total, illustrating the overlapping nature of each part of the Venn diagram. These seven areas are outlined by Downie et al (1992) as:

1. Preventive services – this relates to any 'service' established which aims to promote health and prevent disease. This would include the many areas already discussed under primary,

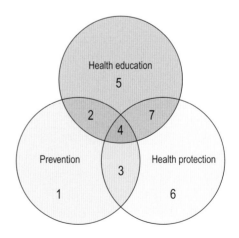

Figure 7.3 • Model of health promotion (Downie et al 1992).

secondary and tertiary prevention earlier in the chapter. Examples of primary preventive services include immunization and vaccination programmes, screening services, child health surveillance programmes. The emphasis here is on the provision of preventive services that aim to prevent or minimize the risks and outcomes of disease and ill health.

2. Preventive health education – this involves any 'education' that seeks to prevent disease or ill health from occurring. An example here would be the education required to inform people of the benefits of partaking in preventive programmes. For example, educating the elderly to take up influenza vaccination would fall into this category. It may involve educating people to take up preventive services such as cervical cytology.

3. Preventive health protection – relates to any service or intervention which brings about change for the benefit of the public's health, for example water fluoridation to reduce dental caries.

4. Health education for preventive health protection – this area brings together the three dimensions of health education, prevention and health protection. It illustrates how each dimension influences the others. An example of work within this area would be positive health education that aimed to educate people regarding adhering to relevant legislation to protect health, for example seat belt legislation. It may also involve empowering people to influence areas of health protection and prevention.

5. Positive health education – this area relates to the provision of education that seeks to empower individuals, for example the use of the empowerment approach previously discussed. The teaching of life skills, assertiveness and decision-making illustrates this area. It is also about trying to influence people to engage in positive lifestyle behaviour such as exercise, in an effort to promote positive well-being.

6. Positive health protection – would be the introduction and implementation of policies that protect health. Examples of this include no-smoking policies, seat belt legislation, health and safety policies in the workplace, infection control policies to protect staff and patients.

7. Health education aimed at positive health protection – includes education aimed at informing people about the benefits of adhering to policies or procedures or legislation and the positive effects it may have on their health.

Box 7.1

Tannahill's model of health promotion

Consider how you would apply Tannahill's model to one of the following areas:

- prevention of accidents in the home
- promotion of safe practice at work
- promotion of healthy eating
- prevention of suicide

Beattie's model of health promotion

Beattie's (1993) model of health promotion illustrates use of the approaches to health promotion previously discussed in this chapter. It presents health promotion as a continuum on a vertical and a horizontal axis. At one end of the vertical continuum is the mode of intervention which ranges from authoritarian with thought and decisions based on objective evidence, for example the outcomes of robust research. This is likely to demonstrate a top-down approach where experts set and lead the agenda for health promotion. On the other end of the continuum is a negotiated mode of intervention where thoughts and decisions would be based on more subjective information and gained through participatory processes. This is more likely to be a bottom-up approach where individuals and communities set the agenda and negotiate with professionals regarding what is important and how they would like change initiated. The horizontal continuum runs from individual health promotion through to working on a collective level. There are four dimensions to the health promotion activity which are health persuasion through to personal counselling which follows the continuum of authoritarian through to a more negotiated approach; and legislative action through to community development. Figure 7.4 illustrates the model.

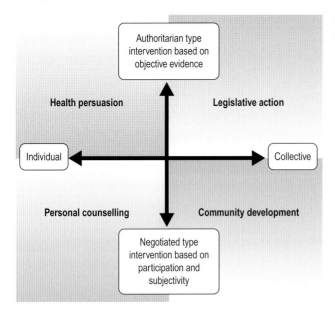

Figure 7.4 • Beattie's model of health promotion (Beattie 1993).

Beattie's model of health promotion provides a framework where all dimensions of health promotion are covered. It is important to note that in some circumstances an authoritarian top-down approach based on objective evidence may be justified, such as in an outbreak of salmonella, or meningitis within a local school. In these circumstances it is important that professionals take the lead to prevent further spread of infectious diseases. In other instances it would be appropriate to take a more negotiated approach which is client centred and based on personal counselling, where a more empowering approach could be utilized. Examples where this would be used may be promoting smoking cessation, helping someone to reduce their weight or to engage in exercise. The model includes legislative action and working at a community or an individual level. The approach used here may be a social change or socio-political one. All these areas have their place in trying to promote health and well-being.

This chapter would not be complete without reference to psychological theory and the role it plays in behaviour change. The following section will provide a very brief overview of selected behaviour change theories. However, the reader is advised to refer to other psychology literature to gain an in-depth understanding of the psychological theories that are so important to understand in working to promote health.

Psychological theories underpinning behaviour change

It is considered imperative that nurses are aware of the process people may pass through when making a change in their behaviour. As alluded to previously within this chapter, people rarely change their behaviour in relation to knowledge received. The majority weigh up the advantages and disadvantages of making a change in behaviour and usually it is not an immediate decision. There are a number of psychological theories available that try to explain this, and two of these will be discussed briefly:

- health belief model
- the stages of change model.

The health belief model

The health belief model (HBM) was originally devised by Rosenstock (1974) and later further developed by Becker (1978) and Janz and Becker (1984). It attempts to explain people's health behaviour by focusing on their attitudes and beliefs. The model suggests that factors may motivate people to consider a change in their behaviour; these are referred to as 'triggers for action'. The triggers may be in the form of health messages from the media or health professionals, illness of self, a close friend or relative. They motivate people to begin to look at their personal health and lifestyle and to question whether they may be at risk of ill health. Whether people decide to change will be influenced by a number of factors, and, within the process of considering whether they will make a change, a cost–benefit analysis takes place. Becker (1978) outlines the following stages, which may or may not be linear:

- *Perceived susceptibility* – a person questions how susceptible they are to a particular health risk or illness. They question – is it likely to happen to them? In some instances they will rationalize and go no further with their thinking, convincing themselves they are not at risk. Others will go on to consider how serious the risk would be.
- *Perceived severity* – the person begins to question how severe the health risk or illness would be – would they recover, or become disabled – would it inhibit their life if they were to become ill? Their analysis of the severity of the risk to health makes a difference as to whether people will, or will not, consider changing their behaviour to reduce risk.
- *Perceived benefits* – the person now moves into the cost–benefit stage and begins to weigh up the benefits of making a change and compares this with the barriers. They ask themselves whether the benefits outweigh the barriers or perceived difficulties in making a change.
- *Perceived barriers* – the person begins to identify the barriers to making a change. In this analysis they may identify more barriers than benefits. If this is the case, it is unlikely they will make a change. The barriers to change may come in a number of different guises; for example peer pressure to continue with adverse lifestyle behaviour; enjoyment of the habit such as smoking and losing its addictive properties; making the change and maintaining it, may all be seen as potential barriers.

The perceived benefits and barriers are 'weighed up' by the individual and should the barriers to change outweigh the perceived benefits, then it is unlikely the person will make the change. Becker indicates that the perceived severity may also influence action – the more vulnerable a person feels to a health risk causing a severe effect on their well-being, the more likely the person is to make a change.

There are obvious limitations to the use of this model in practice, in that a person must perceive themself to be at risk before embarking on a journey of considering a behaviour change. Fear is detrimental to people being able to perceive themselves at risk, and for this reason, victim blaming and fear tactics are unlikely to work. Self-efficacy (as previously discussed in this chapter) also plays a part in whether people perceive they will be successful in making a change. Low self-efficacy may exhibit itself as a perceived barrier to embarking on the change.

The HBM may be of particular use to nurses, as they are in close contact with those who may have experienced personal health problems, and/or ill health of family members, partners or close friends. These factors can act as a trigger to motivate people to consider their own health status, their susceptibility to further ill health may be increased and the severity may be highlighted by recent personal experiences. Utilizing the HBM in practice provides a framework on which nurses can base their practice. For example, providing health messages can act as a trigger and knowing that people will be undertaking a cost–benefit analysis associated with making a change allows the nurse opportunities to increase the patient/client's knowledge of the benefits and to help people to identify the barriers and plan strategies to overcome these. Part of this process is about increasing self-esteem and a person's belief in succeeding and gaining an understanding of the social and environmental constraints influencing health decisions. Working to help people make changes in their behaviour also requires an empowering approach which is led by the client (Whitehead 2001).

The stages of change model

The stages of change model was developed by Prochaska and DiClemente (1984) and is also referred to as the 'transtheoretical model' (for more detail and further reading, please refer to Millar and Rollnick 2002). It describes the course of action a person may pass through when making a change and consists of the following dimensions which are presented as a cyclical process (Figure 7.5).

Precontemplation

When someone is in the precontemplation stage they are not considering a change. Nurses can

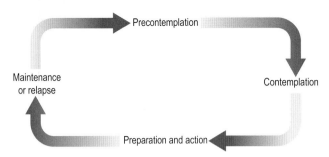

Figure 7.5 • Stages of change model (Prochaska and DiClemente 1984).

provide health promotion messages to people who are in this stage and it may trigger them to move into the next section of the wheel, which is the contemplation stage.

Contemplation

People may be contemplating change in this stage. They will weigh up the benefits and barriers as outlined previously in the HBM to help them make a decision. Again in this section, the nurse can provide information and support, helping people to identify strategies to overcome possible barriers. People in the contemplation stage may benefit from further discussion.

Preparing to change

Those who are preparing to make a change may begin to put strategies in place to make the change. An example here would be the person who may be considering taking up exercise; they may decide to buy trainers, or to join a gym. In this stage, people require help with strategies to put the change into place. It may be helpful for the nurse to negotiate with the client/patient small goals and action plans so that changes may be measured and act as motivators to continue with change.

Actioning the change

Here people activate the change. However, they will continue to require support and help to maintain the change. They are at risk of relapse at any time and re-entering the cycle.

Maintenance

Once the change has been maintained for a period of time, the person is less likely to relapse into old habits and behaviours.

This model can be of help to nurses in their everyday public health practice and it is possible to categorize people into the various stages through talking with them and ascertaining their thoughts and beliefs. It is important to note that people do not always go through the process of change in an orderly fashion (Prochaska et al 1992). It can be helpful if the nurse points out that 'relapse' is part of the normal course of events, and that if relapse takes place, it does not mean failure. It simply means re-entering the cycle and embarking on the journey of making the change again. The key to success is for the client to feel motivated to change (Naidoo and Wills 2000) and motivational interviewing may assist with increasing motivation (for further information relating to motivational interviewing see Millar and Rollnick 2002).

The use of social psychological theories must be viewed with caution, as they describe a 'possible' process people may pass through. They have their limitations and although they may present a 'pattern' for working to achieve health, each individual will be different and may not necessarily pass through the processes outlined. People are complex; the circumstances in which they live and work, and the experiences they have encountered will be unique. As nurses we cannot place ourselves in their shoes and tell people we 'know how they feel', because we cannot know what life is like for others. In any health promotion encounter, nurses should consider that people's individual experiences are as important as the expertise the nurse has to offer. These factors play an equal part in any health promotion intervention and are deserving of an equal power balance between the parties. Respecting this equality goes towards successful empowering public health work.

Conclusion

This chapter has discussed the emergence of health promotion and the inclusion of this within a true public health framework. It has defined health promotion and provided the theoretical basis to this concept. Approaches and models appropriate to the promotion of health have been discussed and their advantages and disadvantages analysed. A brief history of two psychological theories underpinning behaviour change have been outlined, although it is recognized that this is limited and readers are referred to further reading to increase their understanding of this area.

In conclusion, the author's opinion is that nurses should maximize on the potential opportunities available to them to promote health and to increase public health within their practice. Trying to differentiate between health education, health promotion and public health is not helpful. It leads to confusion and devalues nursing's contribution to the public health agenda. The way in which nurses can improve their practice is to underpin it by theory and an evidence base on effectiveness wherever possible, to adopt a non-persuasive and empowering approach, appreciate socio-economic issues that impact on health decisions and always take into account the client/patient's experiences.

Public health practice, whether it is termed health promotion, health education or public health, should move away from 'telling people what to do', to working in partnership, equal participation in the process and negotiation on goals and outcomes. This way of working can be in direct competition with the beliefs of health professionals whose goal is to change behaviour no matter what, in the interest of preventing further disease. The challenge to health professionals is to work in an empowering manner and in a way that regards the experiences of individuals and communities as essential to the success of health promotion, and as equal players in the move towards health improvement.

SUMMARY

- Public health is now seen as incorporating health promotion work fully into its remit.
- Approaches to promoting health should, wherever possible, be based around empowerment and take cognizance of the social determinants of health.
- Psychological theories form a useful basis for practice and can guide nurses in their interventions with patients based on promoting behaviour change.

DISCUSSION POINTS

1. How could nurses contribute further to taking forward the public health agenda in the United Kingdom?
2. Consider an issue that influences health and think about application of a health promotion model in the development of a public health strategy to address the issue identified.
3. In what way could health promotion practice undertaken by nurses on an individual level with clients/patients be adapted to include the principles of empowerment?

References

Acheson D 1998 Independent Inquiry into Inequalities in Health Report. Department of Health. The Stationery Office, London

Bandura A 1997 Self-efficacy: the exercise of control. WH Freeman, New York

Beattie A 1993 The changing boundaries of health. In: Beattie A, Gott M, Jones L, Sidell M (eds) Health and wellbeing: a reader. Macmillan–OU, Basingstoke

Becker MH 1978 The health belief model and personal health behavior. Health Education Monographs 2(4)

Bunton R, Macdonald G 2002 Health promotion: disciplines, diversity and developments. Routledge, London

Canadian Nurse Association 2005 Social determinants of health and nursing: a summary of the issues. Online: http://www.cna-nurses.ca/CNA/documents/pdf/publications/BG8_Social_Determinants_e.pdf

Catford J, Nutbeam D 1984 Towards a definition of health education and health promotion. Health Education Journal 43(2–3): 38

Cooper CL, Starbuck WH 2005 Work: contexts and consequences: three-volume set. Sage, London

Department of Health 2005 Delivering Choosing Health: making healthier choices easier. The Stationery Office, London

Downie RS, Fyfe C, Tannahill A 1992 Health promotion, models and values. Oxford University Press, Oxford

Drever F, Whitehead M 1997 Health inequalities: decennial supplement. ONS, London

Ewles L, Simnett L 2003 Promoting health: a practical guide. Baillière Tindall, London

Gillam S, Yates J, Badrinath P (eds) 2007 Essential public health. Cambridge University Press, Cambridge

Graham H 2000 Understanding health inequalities. Open University Press, Buckingham

Griffiths S, Jewell T, Donnelly P 2005 Public health in practice: the three domains of public health. Public Health 120: 1–7

Janz NK, Becker MH 1984 The health belief model: a decade later. Health Education Quarterly 11(1): 1–47

Lalonde M 1974 A new perspective on the health of Canadians. Government of Canada, Ottawa

Millar WR, Rollnick S 2002 Motivational interviewing: preparing people for change. Guilford Press, New York

Naidoo J, Wills J 2000 Heath promotion: foundations for practice, 2nd edn. Baillière Tindall, Edinburgh

Office for National Statistics 2002 The National Statistics Socio-economic Classification (NS-SEC). Online: http://www.statistics.gov.uk/methods_quality/ns_sec/

Prochaska JO, DiClemente C 1984 The transtheoretical approach: crossing traditional foundations of change. Irwin, Illinois

Prochaska JO, DiClemente CC, Norcross J 1992 In search of how people change. American Psychologist 47: 1102–1114

Rodwell CM 1996 An analysis of the concept of empowerment. Journal of Advanced Nursing 23: 305–313

Rosenstock I 1974 Historical origins of the health belief model. Health Education Monographs 2(4)

Rotter JB 1966 Generalised expectancies for internal versus external control of reinforcement. Psychological Monographs 80(1): 1–28

Smith P, Masterson A, Lloyd Smith S 1999 Health promotion versus disease and care: failure to establish 'blissful clarity' in British nurse education and practice. Social Science and Medicine 48: 227–239

Tannahill A 1985 What is health promotion? Health Education Journal 44: 167–168

Tones K, Tilford S 2001 Health promotion: effectiveness, efficiency and equity. Nelson Thornes, Cheltenham

Townsend P, Davidson N 1982 Inequalities in Health: The Black Report. Penguin, Middlesex

Tudor Hart J 1971 The inverse care law. Lancet 1: 405–412

Watkins D 2003 Health visiting/public health nursing. In: Watkins D, Edwards J, Gastrell P (eds) Community health nursing: frameworks for practice. Baillière Tindall, Edinburgh

Weare K 2002 The contribution of education to health promotion. In: Bunton R, Macdonald G Health promotion: disciplines, diversity and developments. Routledge, London

Whitehead 2001 Health education, behavioural change and social psychology; nursing's contribution to health promotion? Journal of Advanced Nursing 34(6): 822–832

Whitehead D 2003 Incorporating socio-political activities in nursing practice. Journal of Clinical Nursing 12(5): 668–677

Whitehead D 2004 Health promotion and health education: advancing the concepts. Journal of Advanced Nursing 47(4): 311–320

Wilkinson R, Marmot R (eds) 2003 Social determinants of health: the solid facts, 2nd edn. World Health Organization, Copenhagen

World Health Organization 1978 Report on the International Conference on Primary Care Alma Ata. WHO, Geneva

World Health Organization 1986 Ottawa Charter for Health Promotion, an international conference on health promotion. WHO, Copenhagen

Recommended reading

Millar WR, Rollnick S 2002 Motivational interviewing: preparing people for change. Guilford Press, New York

Naidoo J, Wills J 2005 Public health and health promotion: developing practice, 2nd edn. Baillière Tindall, London

Tones K, Tilford S 2001 Health promotion: effectiveness, efficiency and equity. Nelson Thornes, Cheltenham

Chapter Eight

8

Developments in promoting workplace health

Denis D'Auria

KEY ISSUES

- The meaning of work to the individual and to society
- The workplace as a setting for healthcare
- Employment of people with disabilities in the workforce
- Future opportunities

Introduction

This chapter is concerned with the relationship between healthcare and work. The United Kingdom has become a nation of workaholics. It has the lowest number of public holidays and the longest working week of any of its European partners. Unsurprisingly, British society has come to accept the central role of work in the life of the individual and the prosperity of the nation. This chapter will set the scene, by considering the meaning of work to the individual and to society. We consider such questions as: what benefits does a job confer on individuals? Second, we examine where we are in the economic cycle in order to place the changing demography of the workplace into perspective. The focus will then shift towards the workplace as a setting for healthcare, providing a framework for hazard assessment and consideration of appropriate counter measures. We will then examine the employment of people with disabilities in the workforce. Lastly, with an eye to the future, we will look at opportunities that may face us in the future and how these might be addressed in ways that may well change our future horizons.

The meaning of work to the individual and society

We consider 'meaningful occupation' rather than the more restrictive term 'work' in the sense of paid employment being central to human existence and the value of individuals in society. In a study of unemployment, the importance of work was expressed by Clarke (1982) in the following terms:

> Work is important because it provides us with a social arena in which a number of basic rights are met. (cited by Cantrell 1997: 115)

Clarke (1982) developed eight functions of work, which he hypothesizes are the reasons why people continue to work, most of which overlap with those of other writers (Cantrell 1997, Hayes and Nutman 1981). The functions of work are compared in Table 8.1 for all authors together with an indication of whether or not these values might apply to unpaid work such as hobbies, interests, or even work within the voluntary sector. One can infer therefore that there is a significant basis for regarding occupation as providing an individual with much more than just income. It is appreciated that these studies are dated but they are at the level more easily comparable with community health practice compared to the more modern meaning of the work research paradigm. Money is not the only result of work. Cantrell (1997: 115) cites Cox (1966) who states that a job is:

Table 8.1 The functions of work

After Clarke	After Hayes and Nutman	After Cantrell	Application to unpaid work
Income	Income	Income	No
Social honour	Status	Respect	Yes
Adulthood	Identity	Identity	Yes
Life script	Time structure	Time structure	Yes
Something for others	Activity	Usefulness	Yes
Sociability	Mastery	Company	Yes
Decision-making	Purpose	Group voice	Yes
Power		Being busy	Yes
		Achievement	Yes
		Ambition	Yes
		Choice	Yes

the key to the kingdom of consumption; it is the admission ticket by which the individual gains entrance to the goods and services that society produces.

From Table 8.1 it is obvious that income is a major component in the decision to continue in difficult and demanding jobs. Despite this, some paid employment may result in less income than would otherwise have been obtained from welfare benefit and workers affected by these factors are less well off than those out of work. The poverty trap may well apply to people with disabilities, who may obtain more from welfare benefits than from the jobs for which they usefully aspire. Clarke (1982) reviewed the history of the Calvinist work ethic as well as the stigmatization of the unemployed which took place in historical Roman, Elizabethan and Hebrew society. Those in regular employment seemed to be favoured by social standards and even public opinion. Job satisfaction is often derived from an individual's usefulness to other people, particularly if there is praise or gratitude. The gratitude of patients or colleagues is an obvious example for the healthcare professions.

Employment contributes identity to an individual. A new job for a young person is the reason to stop being a child. It is the sign of having a place in society, having gained the right to be an adult and gain the respect that goes with it. In the middle years, social introductions, say at a party, are frequently based on occupation rather than personal qualities. A professional or identifiable work label means more than whether the individual is doing a useful piece of work.

Status is accorded to those with a widely recognized label rather than to those who care for others. There is very little status in being unemployed, disabled or a housewife, as unjustifiable as that might be. A job can become overwhelming in our cash-limited society but nonetheless provides structure to one's day. Apart from the decision to go to work, each day, one deals with timetables, deadlines, expectations, work schedules and many forms of public or financial accountability that fill the day. For those not in an occupation, retired or severely disabled, the absence of this structure leads to apathy and boredom. Inability to continue in employment, having to rely on charity or needing physical help from other people becomes discouraging and even demotivating. Welfare may pay some of the bills but individuals may be denied any feeling of being valuable. On retirement, people lose their social contact at work, as they cease to be one of the crowd. They adapt by joining sports clubs, churches or interest groups. For many, premature retirement is very much worse, especially if combined with poor mobility, pain, speech defects or deafness.

The employed may belong to work-related groups that may have some influence on local or national decisions such as a union or employers' organization. Even if there are obvious power brokers in finance, politics or military systems, a place in a professional body or an industry or a union does allow participation in public debate. The unemployed have no such voice except perhaps associated with violence, emanating from boredom or the alcoholism of despair. Smith (1987) states how the loss of a job has been associated with apathy, depression and ill health and has been extensively studied. For instance, the effects of anticipated loss of work some two years ahead in a Calne factory affected sickness absence rates among employees (Beale and Nethercott 1985).

Activity is stimulating and prevents atrophy of body or mind. Inactivity rarely produces health. Many jobs produce challenges and results and if the work objectives are met, then success. The structure of work in some professions can lead to much greater energy if there are large or small achievements. Achievement is more difficult for those who have no work. Every day can be like the last – no results, no achievement. Hours spent in study, practice, research or skills training can be valuable, especially when they lead to qualification or an end result that gives public recognition. These are examples where behaviour is fired by specific goals, public acclaim or recognition as a driving force. For those unable to see such goals, each day can be grey pools of 'sameness', 'uniformity' and loss of self-respect.

Regular earners have more choice over what they can do or buy than do those in poverty. Purchasing power cannot be ignored in a society subject to great variations in finance, noticeable for those who have to live on pensions, welfare benefits or charity. Choice is reduced if financial reduction is associated with the expensive needs of being disabled and being short of transport, independence and lifestyle options. Isolation may be the only choice for those short of money. A wide range of health problems is associated with unemployment, particularly depression, high suicide rate, obesity, heart disease, smoking-related diseases and cancer (Beale and Nethercott 1985). However, studies need to resolve whether less healthy people are more likely to lose their jobs, or whether ill health is the result of loss of employment in otherwise fit people. The study in Calne is significant. Factory closure was the result of economic failure and affected a whole village population. Morbidity started to rise as soon as the closure

was announced even though the actual event was not to occur for two years (Jahoda 1982).

Stages of economic development

The impact of health in the workplace depends on the nature of work and society's economic development. The UK is termed a post-industrial society and to understand the relationship between health and work it is important to place this concept into context (Bell 1973).

Pre-industrial society

The living conditions of most of the world's population are described as subsistence level. The prime mover is work with muscle power and therefore health is a critical resource and a nation's most important asset. The workforce is engaged in the so-called primary and extractive industries – agriculture, mining and fishing. Life is conditioned by the elements – the weather, the quality of soil and, of course, the availability of water. Production is low and technology is not overwhelming. Farming, horticulture and forestry fit this model though mining in the UK has been mechanized considerably.

Industrial society

The predominant form of activity in the industrial society is the production of goods, seeking to make more with less. Energy and machines enhance the output per worker hour and structure the nature of work. Division of labour creates routine tasks, leading ultimately to the notion of the semi-skilled worker. People use machines to work in the artificial environment of the factory. Life is a game against the fabricated world of cities, factories and tenements. The rhythm of life is machine-paced, dominated by rigid working hours and time clocks. It is a world of schedules and an acute awareness of the value of time. The quantity of goods becomes an index of the standard of living. Production must be coordinated and goods distributed have resulted in the creation of large organizations, with impersonal operation and specific roles reserved for each member. The unrelenting pressure is subject to the countervailing effect of the trade unions.

Post-industrial society

Society today is different, being more concerned with the quality of life measured by the availability of services such as health, education and recreation. The key resource is information rather than energy or physical strength and the central figure, the professional. Bell (1973) suggests transformation resulted from three mechanisms. First, national development of services such as transport and utilities is needed to support industrial development. Engineering has provided more labour-saving devices incorporated into production. Therefore more workers engage in non-manufacturing activities such as maintenance and repair. Second, population growth and mass consumption increase the wholesale and retail trade along with banking, property and insurance. Third, as income increases, the proportion spent on the necessities of food and home decreases, and the remainder creates a demand for durables and then services (see Chapter 17 for further information on influences on health in the workplace).

Changing demography of the workforce

Throughout the last century, there have been a number of demographic changes in the workforce, all of which have important implications for both clinical practice and health service planning. Male activity rates have declined, counterbalanced by a large increase in female activity rates though men still predominate over women in all age groups. However, that position is slowly being eroded. The proportion of potentially economically active men and women actually in employment has declined in parallel with the rise in unemployment. The decline in male rates of economic activity is due to the increasing propensity to stay in full-time education as well as for early retirement.

Explanations for the increase in female economic activity rates have included a change in the perception of women working, an increase in the availability of part-time, key-time and flexible working arrangements, and an increase in the participation of married women and women with children in the labour force. The total population and that in employment has aged, suggesting that health-related issues such as functional capacity, age and ageing will become critical in the future. The patterns of employment have also changed and affected the demand for labour. There has been a dramatic fall in manufacturing, extractive and mining industries with an expansion in service sector employment. There has also been a move from manual to non-manual occupations as well as an increase in part-time working for both men and women. This has been accompanied by a rise in self-employment and an increase in shift working, the latter being due to growth in medical advances (for the NHS workforce in particular) and increased reliance on expensive plant requiring 24/7 operation in order to recoup costs.

So what have been the consequences of such demographic change? The loss of the mining, manufacturing and construction sectors, where accident and injury rates were highest, may produce a positive improvement in health and safety but this is unlikely in the short term. Many diseases have a long latent period between exposure to the cause of the disease and the development of the disease, e.g. cancer after exposure to a carcinogen. So the employee exposed to crocidolite asbestos has an increased chance of developing mesothelioma, a type of tumour, after a lapse of 10 to 20 years. As awareness of the link between health and occupation grows, reporting might also increase, thus further offsetting the downward trend. Diseases with shorter rather than longer latent periods are more likely to improve.

The profile and nature of the risk facing the workforce is evolving with changes in the configuration of industry and occupation because of growth in numbers of women and older people in the workforce. Slips, trips and falls, especially on the same level, affect both sexes and all types of industry and occupation. They are on the increase. The shift to non-manual occupations may bring with it new health-related problems arising from new technology, new types of working environment, such as computers, air conditioning units or increased stress, or the expansion of flexible working arrangements.

Hazard and risk: two definitions

In occupational health, the terms *hazard* and *risk* are commonly referred to and used in everyday practice. Unfortunately, the meanings attached to them do not correspond with the dictionary definitions. Nonetheless a clear understanding is essential to the integrity of clinical practice and decision-making. Hazard is to be understood as the potential to do harm whereas risk is to be perceived as the likelihood of such harm materializing. Any discussion of risk is usually carried out in defined circumstances and is often qualified by some statement of the severity of harm. If comparing risk between two groups of people, subject to all factors being equal, then the risk will be proportional to the hazard. However, relevant factors are very rarely equal and so it is important that they should not be considered as identical unless specifically proven satisfactorily.

Workplace hazards

There are various agents within the work environment which give rise to ill health arising from the fields of toxicology, medicine, biology, physics, engineering and chemistry. Space does not permit the coverage of all of them but instead a number of examples from each category of hazard will be reviewed from a principally public health perspective. Their effects on health will be dependent on the nature of the hazards and the degree of exposure. Hazards are commonly classified as:

- physical
- chemical
- biological
- ergonomic
- psychosocial.

Normally several hazards are involved, often against a background of psychosocial and ergonomic factors. It is therefore important to consider the combined effect of several hazards drawn from differing categories.

Physical hazards

Physical hazards are those hazards that arise from the physical aspects of the work environment including noise, vibration, temperature, light and radiation. They have a range of health effects depending on the physicochemical nature of the factor. Most effects, lacking the complexity of chemical exposure, are dependent on the absorbed energy and on the dose received. Together with chemical exposure, they occupy over 90% of the work of occupational health and safety professionals. This section will draw on noise and vibration as examples.

Noise: an example

Sound consists of waves of pressure which are passed through the air, received by the ear and interpreted by the brain. The key element is the sensing by the individual. Sound is therefore limited by the frequency response of the individual's ear. Above this range, it becomes ultrasound and below, it is known as infrasound. Neither can be heard. Acoustic pressure and frequency are the two parameters of noise emissions that are of interest (Ramsden and Saeed 2000). Frequency is defined as the number of times the pressure wave repeats within a given unit of time. Pressure is measured in newtons per square metre ($N\ m^{-2}$) or pascals, where one pascal is equivalent to one newton per square metre.

The changes in pressure perceptible by the human ear range from the minute to the extremely large and often by factors of several million. To compress this, a logarithmic decibel scale is used where a 3 dB increase in noise intensity is effectively a doubling of the exposure. As the human ear is frequency dependent, measurement must mimic it electronically using a specific circuit measuring 'A-weighted decibels' described as dB(A). Noise is described as unwanted sound and is therefore either a physiological or psychological response reflecting an individual consideration of incident sound energy. Listening to your chosen track on your iPod or MP3 player may be acceptable and probably pleasant. The same tracks coming from the apartment next door at 2.00 am in the morning are usually described as noise. The hum of the air conditioning unit or a neighbour on a train talking loudly into a mobile phone will often be perceived as annoyance, anger, frustration and stress. Otherwise, hearing is damaged by prolonged exposure to excessive high levels resulting in noise-induced hearing loss.

The perception of noise depends on the circumstances when the individual is exposed to the noise. There is wide individual variation. It may be possible to become accustomed to low-level continuous noise as might occur in an air conditioner. It is not possible with intermittent, infrequent, unexpected or simply loud noises. Noise can affect performance and is influenced by the degree of habituation. The largest reduction in performance arises from intermittent and unpredictable sounds as well as sudden increases in sound intensity. The likelihood of noise interfering with performance increases with the complexity of tasks, the degree of mental processing, vigilance and attention required (Piccone 1999). Noise also affects the ability to communicate, which is essential in most workplaces. Poor communication results in error and is a safety risk; it also causes annoyance, frustration and stress to both parties in attempts to communicate.

To be audible, speech must be 10 dB(A) higher than background. Keeping the background to less than 50 dB(A) limits speech to below 60 dB(A) and avoids strain on the vocal cords. Noise-induced hearing loss results from damage to the cochlea and can be either temporary or permanent. This is because the cilia lining the cochlea can recover from noise-related damage. Temporary hearing loss occurs following excessive noise exposure over a relatively short duration. For a short period after exposure ceases, auditory acuity is diminished but will usually recover within 24 hours. The degree of hearing loss and length of time taken to recover depends on the intensity and duration of initial exposure.

Permanent hearing loss is the result of cumulative damage over a long period of time. Hearing ability becomes increasingly poor over several years until there is a significant disability. This form of damage can sometimes be caused by a sudden loud sound such as gunfire or an explosion. Permanent hearing loss can nearly always be prevented. Health surveillance is required under the Management of Health and Safety at Work Regulations (1999). This relies on audiometry. However, for this to be valid, it is essential that appropriate and calibrated equipment is used for the performance of the test, by someone who is competent to perform the test and interpret the results.

Vibration: another example

Vibration is an oscillatory motion in an object, which is transmitted to the body in contact with it (Griffin 1990). It occurs along any axis but three principal directions are fore and aft motion (the x-axis); a sideways lateral motion (the y-axis); and vertical motion (the z-axis). It moves with velocity and acceleration in one direction and at its far point it returns. The number of times this happens is the frequency, measured in hertz. The velocity is measured in metres per second and the acceleration in metres per second/per second ($m\,s^{-2}$). Vibration is now known to cause two recognizable clinical enti-

ties: hand–arm vibration syndrome and whole body vibration.

Hand–arm vibration syndrome is also known as vibration-induced white finger (Gemme and Taylor 1983, Taylor and Pelmear 1975). It is a disorder of the blood vessels and nerves in the fingers that is caused by vibration transmitted directly to the hands (segmental vibration) by tools, parts or working surfaces. Reduced hand grip strength has also been noted in some groups of exposed workers. The condition is primarily characterized by numbness and tingling with blanching being a later sign, appearing first in the finger tips and eventually engulfing the entire finger. Symptoms usually appear suddenly and are often precipitated by exposure to cold and attacks last between 15 and 60 minutes but may stretch up to 1 or 2 hours in more severe cases. Recovery begins with a red flush, which normally starts in the wrist and moves down towards the fingers. With continuing exposure to vibrations, symptoms become definite and eventually irreversible, though this is questioned. In later stages, there is reduced sensitivity to heat and cold, with accompanying pain and impaired tactile sensitivity. Precise manual tasks become difficult because of joint stiffness. Fingers develop a dusty cyanotic appearance. None of the available objective tests is satisfactory. Peripheral vascular function, neurological function and radiographic appearances of the fingers and hands are useful but thermotactile aesthesiometry and vibration perception thresholds are higher in vibration-exposed workers with advanced neurological symptoms but not vascular symptoms.

The syndrome is caused by the direct physical transmission of vibration from the hand and arm through the use of vibrating tools or through other exposure to segmental vibration such as might be transmitted through a large goods vehicle or bus steering wheel or a part held to a grinding wheel. Exposure for 1 year is sufficient to initiate onset. Latency from first exposure to onset of symptoms is estimated to range from 1 to 17 years depending on the duration, frequency and intensity of the exposure and on work practices. The shorter the latent period the more severe will be the expected symptoms if exposure continues. Chronic exposure to low temperatures, especially during simultaneous vibration exposure, exacerbates the effects of vibration. These two exemplars illustrate the considerations in assessing risks from other hazards.

Chemical hazards

This category includes various materials including metals, solvents, pesticides, asbestos, carcinogens and drugs. The precise effects depend on the dose and duration as well as the nature of the substance concerned. Advances in technology result in exponential increases in chemical usage in industry that is so diverse that it is unlikely that common criteria can be elicited reflecting the relationship between their properties and health effects. Chemicals can be classified by customary chemical nomenclature or into organic and inorganic, contributing little to the debate. Physical state, such as gases, vapours, aerosols, liquids or solids, can be used with their specific dispersion and absorption properties.

Application of differences in chemical structure and biological effect might be useful. Solvents include alcohols, ethers, ketones and other compounds, as well as plasticizers, pesticides, organic dyes, etc. Some common characteristics become apparent, e.g. skin absorption and irritancy. Chemicals can be divided into reactants and non-reactants. Once absorbed, reactants undergo chemical reactions in yielding other entities. The toxic effect exerted may be due to direct action by the compound or its metabolites. Non-reactants are generally excreted unchanged.

Benzene is a reactant whose effect on the haematopoietic system is due to metabolites, e.g. phenol, pyrocatechol and hydroquinone. The aliphatic hydrocarbon series is a non-reactant. The effect of chemical substances on enzyme synthesis provides the basis for classification by principal target organ, e.g. hepatotoxic, nephrotoxic, cardiotoxic, etc., relating substances to their principal target organ. Chemicals can be classified by their specific adverse effect on the target organ, e.g. sensitizers, irritants, carcinogens or mutagens. Put succinctly, the Paracelsus principle states that the character of an adverse effect on an individual depends on the level of the exposure. Thus, the toxic effect following brief exposure to a high concentration is different from that of prolonged exposure to low concentration. Workplace-based epidemiological studies therefore are characterized by low intensity and long duration of exposure. The difference is believed to be due to repair processes which operate in the low-intensity exposure mode.

Many chemical substances possess a variety of toxic properties which vary with the concentration and duration of exposure, that is to say the dose. Classifying chemicals for toxicity appears reasonable, but no criterion is satisfactory and may yield serious limitations. Chemical hazards are best dealt with by individual assessment of toxicity and exposure. Attention needs to be paid to the raw materials and intermediates of the manufacturing process, their physical and chemical properties, possible transformation in the surrounding medium, sources of dispersion into the workplace, worker health effect, effects of the microclimate and other environmental factors. Concentrations of dusts, vapours and gases in the workplace are variable. Prediction of the response of an individual requires the proper quantitative estimate of exposure. Correlations between quantitative indicators of the effects of chemical agents and changes in workers' health must be determined. This might include data concerning:

- periodic medical examination
- health surveillance
- interval health history
- incapacity episodes such as sickness absence
- variations in functional state
- poisoning episodes following acute or chronic exposure
- mortality.

General non-specific effects must be distinguished from specific effects of a chemical agent upon the individual, related to pre-clinical and pre-pathological conditions occurring from time to time. Estimates of concentrations sit on the borderline between normal and abnormal or a pathological range of values, resulting from the dominant effects of chemical agents on the individual, produced by low levels of exposure. In workers exposed to low chemical concentrations, the distinction between specific and non-specific toxic effects is blurred. The toxic substance undergoes a change in its intrinsic specificity. A lengthy exposure to low concentrations of toxic substances causes the toxic effect to be demonstrated in a new form with the appearance of non-specific features.

A feature of prolonged low-level exposure is the ability of chemicals to modify the interaction between the individual and changing environmental conditions. These changes in the efficiency of adaptation mechanisms are caused by an unstable equilibrium between the individual and their environment and lead to a succession of stable and unstable conditions, accompanied by changes in the individual's adaptability. A reduction in adaptability caused by prolonged chemical exposure and the related instability determine intimately the ability of pre-morbid conditions to become transformed into pathological states.

Epidemiological studies have established causality between the appearance of several disease entities and exposure to such industrial chemical agents as carbon disulphide, hydrogen sulphide, hydrocarbons, amino compounds, organochlorines, phosphorus and heavy metals, corroborating the view that prolonged exposure has an effect on workers' health. Further complications arise from the fact that one agent at differing exposure intensities may cause different pathological or clinical pictures affecting one or more different target organs. High exposure to silica dust causes silicosis which is not as a rule associated with chronic bronchitis. Low concentrations lead to chronic bronchitis without evidence of silicosis. Different intensities cause qualitatively different pathological profiles, as a result of different target organ susceptibilities.

Absorption of a toxic agent is not critical in determining the adverse health effects of chemicals. Processes crucial to human risk assessment concern not only absorption but also distribution, metabolism and excretion. Metabolic transformation of the absorbed chemical is of interest, since many associated processes render absorbed toxic substances harmless. Information on intakes may be subject to considerable fluctuation, depending on:

- length of exposure
- interruptions during work
- character and level of intermittent concentrations
- intensity of work
- effect of other concomitant factors.

Epidemiological studies have achieved the dominant position for the reliable determination of occupational hygiene standards. It has been shown for example that:

- the thresholds for allergic effects of some chemicals are not unexpectedly much lower than those for toxic action
- the threshold for the gonadotropic effect may be drastically different from the toxic threshold for the same substance.

Establishing the occupational hygiene standards for benzene and aniline was based on an analysis of the specific actions of these compounds and their effects on each target organ. The standard for for-

maldehyde was corrected for its effect on the upper respiratory tract as a result of epidemiological study. Mercury and carbon disulphide affect the autonomic centres and limbic structures in the brain. The largest contributors are functional changes in the nervous system and mechanisms for regulation of arterial blood pressure. The prediction of safe concentrations of chemicals has also been based on the mathematical simulation of health effects compared to a control population. Setting out the exposure time relationship formally makes it possible to determine the threshold value that produces a health impairment.

Biological hazards

There are two broad categories:

- conditions producing adverse effects through infection
- conditions producing adverse effects in non-infective (allergic) ways.

Occupational infections are uncommon. They can be missed clinically unless a proper occupational history is coupled with knowledge of infections in occupational groups. Examples are drawn from the list of prescribed diseases under the Social Security Act 1975.

- *Streptococcus suis* from meat handling
- avian chlamydiosis from inhalation of dried excreta and feathers
- ovine chlamydiosis from sheep
- Newcastle disease from fowl
- histoplasmosis from chicken manure
- skin infections such as ringworm, orf or hydatid disease.

However, infections can be derived from other sources and some examples include:

- infective skin conditions in machine shop workers arising from reuse of cutting oils
- deep sea divers using saturation techniques who develop otitis externa due to *Pseudomonas*
- viral haemorrhagic fevers in those responsible for clearing crops, trees and forests
- Lassa fever in healthcare workers
- forestry workers at risk of Lyme disease due to infection with *Borrelia burgdorferi*.

Many allergens may cause attacks of hay fever or asthma (allergic rhinitis). High exposure in early life increases the risk of suffering from asthma later on. Increasing evidence suggests that air-borne chemical pollution acts synergistically with naturally occurring allergens and results in effects on lung function at concentrations lower than those at which either the allergen or chemical irritant on its own would have produced an adverse effect.

Ergonomic hazards

Ergonomics is the application of scientific information concerning human beings to the design of objects, system and environments for human use. Ergonomics in occupational health and safety overlaps with many other disciplines including occupational medicine, engineering, production management, etc. Ergonomics is about optimizing the interaction between work, productivity and comfort.

The same techniques, however, can be used to minimize health problems arising from application of force at the extremes of range of motion of joints, from constrained postures, etc. The advent of the video-display unit (VDU) has brought the value of ergonomics to the fore. It is of course regulated by the Health and Safety (Display Screen Equipment) Regulations (1992), which require application of ergonomic principles, as do the Manual Handling Operations Regulations (1992). Musculoskeletal problems associated with manual handling and constrained posture are intimately linked with society's performance culture. Without suitable rest pauses, muscle tends to build up lactic acid and fatigue results in eventual injury.

Psychosocial hazards

This group includes an eclectic mix of issues which cause problems in worker health, but the will to confront them is often absent and a knowledge base to place intervention on a firm footing is missing. Stress is the prime example. It is well known that moderate stress is a necessary stimulus, but when it becomes prolonged or excessive, then it can become pathogenic. Satisfactory measurement capability is unavailable and therefore it is impossible to determine an unacceptable level. Evidence in support of ill health arising from shift work is not yet completely convincing. It is regularly flouted by many workers because of personal preference. Excessive hours again are often condemned almost arbitrarily. However, many workers are happy to do long shifts because of the reduction in travel costs and interference with their social lives. It gives workers greater control over their free time. The list is endless. Some occupational groups such as pilots have their working hours strictly controlled by law. This does not apply to doctors or nurses.

Prevention of disease

Anticipating health hazards before they become manifest permits implementation of preventive measures before the onset of disease and injury. The best time to take preventive measures is when new facilities are being built or existing ones modified. Once operational, retrofit solutions are difficult to implement. The knowledge base concerning workplace hazard is large, but sadly seldom used in planning.

Beginning hazardous work should lead to medical evaluation. The incorporation of medical information with the detailed exposure inventory of the job can be used in satisfactory job placement. Comparison of pre-exposure health status to post-exposure changes can result in improved worker safety. In the workplace, surveillance means monitoring both exposures and health outcomes and it is desirable to link the two. Surveillance can be practised both at the individual workplace and within the primary care sector, as was carried out for many years with people who worked in the dyestuffs industry. Such surveillance assists with the detection of trends, clusters, associations and causal links between disease and injury. It provides guidance for preventive activities. Often the immediate consequence of surveillance and detection of an issue is the initiation of detailed investigations. Its ultimate purpose is to determine disease, so that resources can be allocated rationally for prevention.

Health-hazard surveillance requires an inventory of those hazards and a quantitative assessment of exposure. It may not be clear how the interest can be expressed in hazards that result in acute injury. Surveillance should include assessing the sources of energy, vehicles and circumstances. Sources of energy may be mechanical, electrical, thermal or chemical. They can be delivered to the victim through the medium of a vehicle, which may include stationary or moving machinery, work at heights or depths, work with electrical circuits, ovens, refrigerators, hot gases or chemicals. The circumstances may include the condition of walking, or working surfaces and the necessity of working with or near machinery, power tools, electrical circuits and sources of heat or acutely toxic chemicals. These are the type of issues which are important in maintaining an inventory of such hazards and the data which need to be recorded.

Quantitative assessment of exposure consists of measuring the concentration, the variation and the total duration of exposure, in addition to the total number of workers exposed. If exposure to hazards is excessive, it should be controlled irrespective of outcome and the health of exposed workers evaluated. Exposure is excessive if it approaches or exceeds established limits, some of which become legally enforceable. Within the UK, these can be found in a Health and Safety Executive publication known as EH40, which changes annually, and in relevant legislation. Measurement and evaluation of exposure may well be conducted by industrial occupational hygienists, ergonomists or safety practitioners, as well as non-specialists, including employees and managers.

Health is usually evaluated by physicians, nurses or other healthcare providers. Those who can identify occupationally-related conditions may well work within the NHS, but also work in independent occupational healthcare providers, as individual consultants, or as university academics. If seeking external help, the provider's credentials should be checked. Appropriate training and accreditation are the badges of competence. To identify whether or not a condition is work related, it is essential to identify occupational exposures, both quantitatively and qualitatively.

Medical surveillance may be passive or active. Passive surveillance requires the injured or ill employee to either register that fact or present themself at the occupational health centre for assessment. Medical certificates may assist in that process, but the true nature of the cause of the sickness absence is sometimes difficult to appreciate. It may be unclear to the general practitioner at initial presentation. The general practitioner may be deliberately vague in an effort to preserve confidentiality.

Active surveillance is more appropriate for workers who have higher risks of disease and injury than normal. These may take the form of periodic examinations or reviews for workers exposed to specific hazards, e.g. radiation, and screening and biological monitoring of groups of workers exposed to specific substances, e.g. lead and radionuclides. The precise form of medical monitoring depends on the

nature of the effects and the pattern of occupational exposure, involving a consideration of whether the effects are acute or chronic, whether screening tests are available, and whether a worker population is satisfactorily defined. If individuals are sick or injured or have pre-clinical signs or symptoms, or have other indicators of adverse effects, there are a range of options available for the healthcare staff to initiate:

- treat the sick or injured
- investigate their occupational history as an aid to diagnosis
- investigate the relevant workplace for possible causes and additional cases
- control exposure to prevent additional cases if a plausible source is found
- facilitate the recovery of the individual employee by appropriate rehabilitation and advice.

It may be necessary to remove the worker from the job, if there is a present, continuing and uncorrectable hazard. Injury surveillance is based on systematic investigation and recording of incidence resulting in injuries. These records can be used at individual workplaces to manage prevention activities, by safety representatives and committees to assure appropriate activity, and by regulators or others with a legitimate interest.

Epidemiology and occupational health have an intimate relationship. Since the 1990s, the relationship with public health has grown stronger. Standard methods and study designs are used in occupational epidemiology, but there are some important differences. Topics of analysis may be unique, e.g. silicosis, or adult lead poisoning. There are important logistical issues in studying disease and injury. Exposure must be carefully characterized and it is important to account for employee status as a carefully selected, healthier group than non-workers, often achieved by using non-exposed workers as a control group as a basis for comparison.

Analysis of occupational hazards is also conducted. Risk assessment utilizes controlled investigations by scientists from various disciplines, such as toxicology and biochemistry, by extrapolating results involving animal experiments and in vitro studies in human material. This type of analysis yields complex information that complements epidemiological data. On occasions, a primary source of information, such as structural similarity to chemicals of known toxicity, may be important, especially to establish the need for control. Primary prevention is the preferred means of disease control. In the workplace, this is largely an engineering activity. With very few exceptions, it is also likely to be the most cost-effective. There is a hierarchy of controls derived from a conceptual model, which places a hazard source at its centre, an environment into which the hazard may be released and the worker. From most to least effective, technical controls will include engineering activity, which prevents the generation of the hazard at its source, environmental controls that are implemented in the work environment and personal protective devices that individual workers can wear or use.

Examples of positive engineering include reducing the use of toxic materials, replacing toxic materials with less toxic alternatives and changing work design to eliminate or reduce hazards. Environmental controls might include the implementation of a ventilation system to reduce concentration of airborne pollutants, reduction of duration of exposure and shielding. Personal protective equipment includes masks, gloves, aprons and safety devices. Commonly, they include respiratory protection devices, which require a support programme of maintenance, training and fit testing for their effective use. They are less effective than the other two kinds of controls and should only be used as temporary measures, for example during maintenance or when positive engineering or environmental controls are impractical.

Prevention of disability

The Disability Discrimination Act (1996) represented a major shift in achieving, for people with disabilities, access to employment as of right. It represented a shift towards the social model of disability. In this model, disability is seen as a social construct, rather than a medical condition. Briefly, the Act defines a disability as 'a physical or mental impairment causing a substantial and long-term adverse effect on the ability to carry out normal day-to-day activities', which though obtuse, attempts to be pragmatic. Space does not permit a detailed analysis of the Act, though there is no doubt that it has made an impact on the practice of occupational health.

Once under the Act's protection, disabled employees acquire a right to expect reasonable adjustments, which may be considered alongside cost and resource information. Experience with the Americans with Disabilities Act, upon which the Disability Discrimination Act appears to be based, shows that significant expenditure is unnecessary. The UK Act was revised in 2005, restricting the defence of justification and widening the scope of application.

Current practice

The main obligations on employers are set out in the Health and Safety at Work etc Act (1974), where Section 2(1) requires employers to take reasonable care in the workplace as far as is reasonably practicable. Specific statutory duties are also set out here in this section as follows:

- to provide and maintain a safe system of work
- to ensure the safe use, transportation and storage of materials and substances
- to provide adequate information, instruction, training and supervision
- to provide adequate maintenance of buildings and premises
- to provide a safe working environment.

The Reporting of Injuries, Diseases and Dangerous Occurrences Regulations (1989) requires the reporting of death or major injury, an over-three-day injury, work-related disease or dangerous occurrences. This serves to furnish the surveillance action outlined above. Experience suggests that less than 30% of incidents are actually reported. Government policy now focuses on the positive promotion of health and well-being at work, on the understanding that those employees who are 'healthy, happy and here' are more likely to be productive, emulating the trend in the United States, forging links between health and productivity. The measure of the success is no longer sickness absence reduction, but the reduction of long-term incapacity and joblessness. Risk assessment is the process by which these workplace threats are identified and evaluated, allowing steps to be taken to implement appropriate countermeasures. Based on the premise that the workplace is a human construct, almost everything that takes place therein is potentially amenable to control and prevention. Risk assessment is a requirement of several statutory measures, including:

- Manual Handling Operations Regulations (1992)
- Control of Substances Hazardous to Health Regulations (2002)

- Control of Asbestos at Work Regulations (2002)
- Control of Lead at Work Regulations (2002)
- Noise at Work Regulations (1989)
- Health and Safety (Display Screen Equipment) Regulations (1992)
- Health and Safety (First Aid) Regulations (1981)
- Management of Health and Safety at Work Regulations (1999).

Known also as the Management Regulations, the last in the list is a 'catch-all' statutory measure, requiring assessment of risks not formally addressed in other regulations. It applies to thermal comfort, excessive working hours, stress, young people, pregnant women and susceptible groups. If work activity poses a significant health risk, the assessment should be written. This should be normal practice, since once identified, an employer is under a duty to reduce it. The discharge of this obligation can only be effected by those who are competent to do so. Unfortunately, there is no simple definition of competence, but involves consideration of skill, knowledge and experience.

Conclusion

Occupational health has evolved considerably in the last 30 years. Rarely do we hear the question 'occupational what?' any more and only a few people confuse us with occupational therapists. What has changed, however, has been the demand for and delivery of services. Britain has shifted away from the model of an in-house service to the buying-in of a service from a multi-client provider. This may be a private consultancy led probably by nurses or physicians or it may be an NHS trust often under the NHS Plus banner.

The future is unlikely to see universal provision via the NHS even in the presence of the new 'sick note' initiative and its associated rehabilitation projects. However, a reduction in the isolation of occupational health services might be feasible where patients can be referred from the primary care sector for opinions about fitness to work and prescription of rehabilitation plans. The introduction of rehabilitation plans to discharge planning for hospital inpatients might be another avenue for development. As more experience is gained with the Human Rights Act 1998, it is likely that it will begin to

---

Box 8.1

Recommendations of the Black Report

1. A robust cost–benefit model for investment in occupational health
2. Other disciplines should help promote investment
3. Government should initiate a health and well-being service for small and medium-sized enterprises
4. GPs/other professionals supported in efforts to help people enter, stay or return to work
5. Electronic 'fit for work' certificate to replace current paper incapacity certificate
6. Government to pilot a 'fit for work' service using multidisciplinary case-management principles
7. Occupational health and vocational rehabilitation should be integrated into mainstream healthcare
8. Clear professional leadership, standards of practice, formal accreditation, revitalized workforce, sound academic base, systematic collation and analysis of data

---

affect various aspects of employment. Although slow, this may well include action on various rights such as privacy to avoid employers accessing computer mailboxes or tracing calls; or the right to fair trial given that there is no legal aid for employment tribunals. Other challenges to inaction over such matters as right to health or work may well arise.

The future of the occupational health landscape in the UK was recently the subject of a major study by Dame Carol Black. The conclusions and recommendations of the report merit some study (Black 2008). The recommendations are set out in Box 8.1. However, we are still awaiting outcomes of the 10-year strategy of the Health and Safety Commission. We await government policy on the Black recommendations.

DISCUSSION POINTS

1. What will the world of occupational health look like in 5, 10 and 15 years' time?
2. What new emerging technologies are likely to cause health problems in a decade?
3. How can occupational professionals respond to the Black Report?
4. Is seamless care inclusive of occupational health desirable and achievable? If so, how?

SUMMARY

- The workplace is one area in today's society where healthcare in under-represented. The annual toll in terms of fatal and lost time accidents, avoidable disease and disability leaves no one in any serious doubt that working men and women are a vulnerable group in our society.
- Despite their contribution to the economic wealth of this country, the healthcare needs of this group have retained a low priority and have been effectively ignored over the last three to four decades by government health policy.
- Since the 1960s, each decade has seen attempts to fully integrate employee

healthcare into the NHS. All have resulted in inaction or tedious compromise. For these reasons, hopes are not high for the government response to Dame Carol Black's review.

- On the positive side, the care of employees is a thriving multidisciplinary subject, whose inherent satisfaction rests in keeping people with health problems economically active. There are firm roots in clinical practice, professionalism and a strong science base. The discipline is subject to rapid change buffeted both by changes in government and Health and Safety Executive policy and advances in scientific and medical research.

References

Beale MR, Nethercott S 1985 Job loss and family morbidity: a factory closure study. Journal of the Royal College of General Practitioners 35: 510–514

Bell D 1973 The coming of post-industrial society. Basic Books, New York

Black C 2008 Working for a healthier tomorrow: review of the health of Britain's working age population. TSO, London. Online: www.workingforhealth.gov.uk

Cantrell EC 1997 Work, occupation and disability. In: Wilson BA, McLellan DL (eds) Rehabilitation studies handbook. Cambridge University Press, London

Clarke R 1982 Work in crisis: dilemma of a nation. St Andrews Press, Edinburgh

Control of Asbestos at Work Regulations 2002 Statutory Instrument 2002 No. 2675. HMSO, London

Control of Lead at Work Regulations 2002 Online: http://www.opsi.gov.uk/si/si2002/20022676.htm

Control of Substances Hazardous to Health Regulations 2002 Online: http://www.opsi.gov.uk/si/si2002/20022677.htm

Cox H 1966 The secular city. SCM Press, London

Disability Discrimination Act 1996 Online: http://www.opsi.gov.uk/acts/acts1995/ukpga_19950050_en_1

Gemme G, Taylor W (eds) 1983 Foreword: Hand arm vibration syndrome and the nervous system. Journal of Low Frequency Noise Vibration XI

Griffin MJ (ed.) 1990 Handbook of human vibration. Academic Press, London: 571–575

Hayes J, Nutman P 1981 Understanding the unemployed. Tavistock, London

Health and Safety (Display Screen Equipment) Regulations 1992 Online: http://www.hse.gov.uk/foi/internalops/fod/oc/200-299/202_1.pdf

Health and Safety (First Aid) Regulations 1981 Approved code of practice and guidance. HSE Books, London

Health and Safety at Work etc Act 1974 Online: http://www.hse.gov.uk/legislation/hswa.htm

Human Rights Act 1998 Online: http://www.opsi.gov.uk/ACTS/acts1998/ukpga_19980042_en_1

Jahoda M 1982 Employment and unemployment. Cambridge University Press, Cambridge

Management of Health and Safety at Work Regulations 1999 Online:http://www.opsi.gov.uk/si/si1999/19993242.htm

Manual Handling Operations Regulations 1992 Online: http://www.opsi.gov.uk/SI/si1992/Uksi_19922793_en_1.htm

Noise at Work Regulations 1989 Online:http://www.opsi.gov.uk/si/si1989/Uksi_19891790_en_1.htm

Piccone P 1999 Environmental design. In: Jacobs K (ed.) Ergonomics for therapists. Butterworth Heinemann, Boston

Ramsden RT, Saeed SR 2000 Sound, noise and the ear. In: Hunter's diseases of occupation, 9th edn. Arnold, London: 285–305

Reporting of Injuries, Diseases and Dangerous Occurrences Regulations 1989 Online: http://www.opsi.gov.uk/si/si1989/Uksi_19891457_en_1.htm

Smith R 1987 Unemployment and health. Oxford University Press, Oxford

Social Security Act 1975 HMSO, London

Taylor W, Pelmear PL 1975 Introduction. In: Vibration white finger in industry. Academic Press, London: XVII–XXII

Recommended reading

Adams PH, Baxter PJ, Aw TC,
Cockcroft A, Harrington JM
(eds) 2000 Hunter's diseases of
occupation, 9th edn. Arnold, London
*This book addresses diseases caused
by occupations and the assessment,
management and treatment of the*
*individual patient. This is an ideal
text for clinicians, as well as for
occupational physicians and other
occupational health professionals.*

Agius R, Seaton A 2001 Practical
occupational medicine, 2nd edn.
Edward Arnold, London
*This is a key text which covers all
aspects of the clinician's role from
occupational history taking to
rehabilitation and health promotion.*

Section **Three**

The family as a framework for practice

The third section continues to develop important themes for public health and community nursing by focusing on the family and the particular perspective of family nursing. Both sociological and psychological perspectives are adopted to explore the diversity of experiences in family life, aspects of continuity and change and perhaps more importantly the impact of external influences mentioned in previous chapters. Given the emphasis placed on quality assessment and the identification of risk factors as the basis for decision-making and intervention, the family is usefully examined both as a potential source of ill health as well as a resource for enhancing health and quality of life. Particular importance is given to the potential for violence within intimate family relationships and to child protection issues, as well as those to do with older people. Current theory and research are explored in detail as the basis for the public health nursing role in child protection.

The concept of 'family' is explored in depth in the first chapter, adopting a sociological perspective to consider changing patterns of family living and the diversity of experiences across time. Special reference is made to the demographic aspects of marriage and cohabitation, to the changing and unchanging roles of women and to current expectations for personal fulfilment. The impact of divorce and the rise in one-parent family households are two

issues of particular significance for community nurses given established links with poverty, child and women's health.

The psychological perspective adopted in the second chapter alerts the public health and community nurse to the costs and benefits to the individual of family life, to the styles of interaction and life events which can predict positive mental health, or a risk of breakdown in family relationships. The concept of a dysfunctional family is mentioned because of the special challenge this presents for healthcare professionals.

The next chapter addresses the difficult problem of violence within the family, exploring explanations for abuse to women, children and older people and highlighting the size and extent of the problem and its links with overall physical and emotional ill health. The final chapter in this section focuses particularly on the theory and research which underpins public health nursing intervention in the prevention of physical abuse of children. It looks specifically at sociological, structural and environmental factors which seek to offer explanatory models; but of greater interest for a public health nursing assessment is the discussion of interacting variables within the family which predict increased risk. In conclusion, different models of prevention are clearly presented emphasizing the importance of the social context in which abuse occurs.

The family: a sociological perspective

Graham Allan and Graham Crow

KEY ISSUES

- Continuities and changes in households and families
- Diversity in people's experiences of families
- New forms of family are emerging

Introduction

While we all talk about 'the family' as though it were obvious and unproblematic, in a very real sense 'the family' as such does not exist. Rather what we have are many different forms of family, each of which gets modified and changed, over time, generally slowly, but sometimes more radically. This point is not as banal as it might seem. Indeed arguably the key to understanding the nature of family life lies in recognizing the interplay between continuity and change which characterizes all aspects of family relationships. It is this notion of the family as dynamic rather than static, variable rather than uniform, which will provide the framework for much of what follows in this chapter.

We can recognize that change occurs within families at a variety of levels. Clearly individual relationships within families change over time. Think here about your relationships with your parents. Whether or not they are still together, the ways they have treated you, their expectations about your behaviour, and the forms of control they have exercised over you, have all altered as you have grown older. In adulthood, your relationship with them is likely to continue but not in anything like the same form as when you were a child. So too relationships

Activity box 9.1

Consider the nature of parent–child dependencies and how these alter over time. In particular, write down a list of the different ways that you are still dependent on your parent(s). How does this differ from the list you might have written five years ago? How different do you think the list will be in five years' time? As you do this, think about the ways you feel obligated or indebted to your parent(s). What do you 'owe' them? What demands can they make of you? Think too about what you consider their obligations to you to be. How will these change over time?

between husbands and wives, between brothers and sisters, or any other family members also alter as people age and take on different responsibilities. Most of the time this change is considered routine and normal, though there are occasions, such as divorce or the onset of severe infirmity, when it is more traumatic and requires more rapid adjustment.

But just as relationships between family members alter over time, so too the patterns of family living within a society are liable to change as wider social and economic conditions alter. Traditionally within sociology, a great deal of attention has been paid to the impact that industrialization had on family relationships. For example, there has been much debate around whether industrialization led to the decline of extended family relationships or, in contrast, actually generated the conditions necessary for greater solidarity between extended family members.

Such debates are echoed in much popular discourse, though this tends to emphasize the pathological character of contemporary family life and the decline of family values. Thus, we often hear claims that family life has become more insular and less community oriented, or that elderly people do not receive sufficient support from their families. Recently too there has been much emphasis placed on shifts occurring within marriage, though here there are more conflicting views as to how this should be interpreted. Some argue that in comparison to the past – though exactly how far back in the past is often left unspecified – marriage is now a much more equal relationship, a far more genuine partnership than it used to be. Others point to the rising levels of divorce and cohabitation as indicators that many no longer regard marriage with the sanctity it deserves.

So what has been happening to family life and family relationships? How different are our experiences from those of our grandparents? How much change has there been and how much continuity? In order to examine these issues, this chapter will focus on key aspects of the social organization of family and domestic life pertinent to community nursing. These include marriage, cohabitation, divorce, lone-parent households, lesbian and gay partnerships, and the family circumstances of older people. We will begin by examining the contemporary patterning and social organization of marriage and cohabitation.

Marriage and cohabitation

Throughout most of the 20th century marriage became a more common experience. By the early 1970s approximately 95% of men and women were or had been married by the time they were in their mid 40s. Marriage age also decreased over this period, with the average age of first marriage for men being 23 and for women 21 in the late 1960s. Since the mid 1970s, though, demographic aspects of marriage and partnership formation have altered markedly. To begin with, age at first marriage has shown a steady increase. By 2004 the average age had risen to 30.4 for men and 28.3 for women (Office for National Statistics (ONS) 2007a) (Table 9.1). In part this reflects the massively increased levels of cohabitation now occurring (Kiernan 2004, Seltzer 2004). In this regard, marriage is becoming less normative as a mode of household and family formation. Until the 1970s, very few couples cohab-

Table 9.1 Selected family changes 1971–2004 (England and Wales)

	1971	2004
Number of first marriages	320 347	163 007
Women's median age at first marriage	21.4	28.3
Rate of divorce per 1000 marriages	5.9	14.0
Number of lone-parent households[a]	570 000	1 750 000[b]
Number of single-person households[a]	3 350 000	6 990 000
Percentage of births to unmarried mothers	9.2	42.2
Percentage of unmarried women aged 16–59 cohabiting[a]	13[c]	27

Sources: Haskey (1998, 2002), ONS (2001, 2005a, 2006a, 2007a, 2007b).
[a]These figures are for Great Britain.
[b]This figure is for the year 2000.
[c]This figure is for 1986. Data on this were not gathered before the mid 1980s.

Activity box 9.2

- Consider why there has been such a rapid growth in cohabitation since the 1970s.
- Why has marriage declined and cohabitation increased?
- Is this just a matter of personal choice? What social factors have fostered the growth of cohabitation?
- To what degree do cohabitation and marriage represent different forms of commitment?
- Are there different forms of cohabitation? How important are the differences between these different forms?

ited prior to marriage, with most of those who did being separated or divorced. At the beginning of the 21st century, some 80% of all marrying couples had previously cohabited (ONS 2007a). Importantly too, many couples now live together without marriage being an explicit project. Indeed, in 2004 over a quarter of all unmarried women aged 18–59 were cohabiting (ONS 2005a). Thus, while religious and ethnic variations persist, behaviour that was censured a generation ago is now accepted by most as an uncontentious and morally appropriate way of developing romantic/sexual relationships.

Along with these changes in the demography of marriage and partnership formation, there is also a widely held belief that the basis of these relationships has been altering. Contemporary visions perceive marriage as being much more of a partnership between equals than it was in the past. It is now seen as an emotionally closer relationship, based on developing conceptions of personal compatibility, commitment and love. It consequently carries with it a heightened range of expectations, including a greater belief that personal expression and mutual satisfaction provide the central rationale for the relationship. It is this which people forming partnerships and getting married seek. More than their grandparents or even their parents, they want their unions to encompass a mutual sharing, a partnership between equals, premised on contemporary images of romantic love as a means to personal fulfilment. In this light, changing terminology is also important. The increased use of the term 'partnership' reflects these changing aspirations, as well as solving the 'dilemma' of what status to give cohabitation.

However, despite these ideologies, the basic organization of marriage and 'coupledom' has remained relatively constant. While cohabitation appears sometimes to entail a more symmetrical and equal relationship, once married, couples usually develop a more traditional pattern. Moreover, the division of labour and domestic responsibilities between a couple, and consequently the division of opportunities and constraints affecting each partner, become most marked when (and if) the couple have children. Generally, men are still seen as having a primary commitment to the job market and the main responsibility for securing household finances, while women take on the principal responsibility for domestic labour, childcare and household management (Oates and McDonald 2006).

The patterns here of course are not identical to those occurring in the past. There have undoubtedly been important changes, particularly with respect to wives' employment. For example, in 1961 fewer than 40% of wives aged 16–59 were in employment. In 2005 70% of married and cohabiting women in this age range were employed, with 30% in full-time employment (ONS 2007c). Equally mothers return

to employment much sooner after childbirth than they did even 20 years ago. Yet while most couples now depend on two incomes for their household's standard of living, men's earnings are still seen as 'primary' in a way in which women's are not. In turn, even when employed full time, wives/mothers are still taken to be the person with primary responsibility for the smooth functioning of household and family matters. (For a fuller discussion of these issues, see Allan and Crow 2001.)

As children grow older, as mothers return to employment and as the couple develop different commitments outside the home, we might expect that some aspects of their division of work are renegotiated. Yet, while there are modifications over time, rarely does such renegotiation appear to lead to radical change (Crompton and Harris 1999). Husbands and older children may help somewhat more in household tasks, but the primary responsibilities for domestic management and familial care usually continue as before. Even following major changes in household circumstances, as for example with male unemployment, the renegotiation of responsibilities appears to be limited. In general, the household division of labour continues to be patterned in the gendered ways established earlier.

The continuation of a high division of labour within marriage and other committed relationships is linked very strongly to the inequalities which flourish within the job market. Notwithstanding British and European Equal Opportunities legislation, occupations still tend to be highly gendered. For example, many women employees work in a few female-dominated service occupations, e.g. as secretaries, healthcare workers, teachers, sales staff and cleaners. Importantly too, the jobs women are in typically pay significantly less than male occupations. For the last three decades, and with very little variation between years, full-time women employees have received approximately 70% of the wages male employees receive, with this relationship being broadly consistent across different skill levels. Part-time employees, the vast majority of whom are married women, usually receive even lower proportional pay (Crompton 1997).

Overall, it is not really surprising that a conventional division of labour continues to be 'negotiated' by most couples. As well as husbands earning more than wives, women are socialized into being more accomplished at domestic activities than men and tend to have childcare and other relationship responsibilities built more into the construction of their personal and social identities. Of course, in principle a division of labour need not be associated with an unequal distribution of resources within a marriage or other partnership, nor with the dominance of one spouse over the other. Yet research has regularly shown that within most marriages, though not all, this is the outcome. Despite the prevalence of ideologies of coupledom, men have greater control of financial resources, more freedom for leisure and more control over key decisions than their wives do (Allan and Crow 2001). So notwithstanding modifications in employment patterns, in marital ideology, in domestic standards, in childcare practices and the like, the point remains that individual couples construct their marriages within an economic and social context which remains structurally unequal and usually provides men with more options and a greater access to resources than women.

Divorce

Divorce is another aspect of family life where there has been a clear change in the last 30 years. Whereas in the late 1960s there were only 45 000 divorces each year, over the last decade there have been between 140 000 and 150 000. This is a rise in the annual rate from 4 per 1000 marriages to 14 per 1000 in 2004. Each year approximately 150 000 children under the age of 16 experience their parents' divorce, almost a doubling since 1971. Alongside this there has been an expansion in the number of lone-parent families, not all of which arise through divorce of course, and a large increase in the number of step-families. This has resulted in much more diversity in family patterns compared to even a short while ago. It also means that many individuals now experience different forms of family life at first hand, moving, say, from a two-parent family to a lone-parent one, and then later forming a step-family.

It is difficult to be precise about the reasons for the rise in divorce. Divorce, like marriage, is a legal procedure, so at one level the heightened rate of divorce merely reflects changes in the law, with the 1969 Divorce Reform Act having been especially important. However, the law itself reflects changed marital ideologies; moreover the fact that divorce is made more available does not of itself explain why people have increasingly chosen it as an option. Three factors seem particularly important. First, as we have already noted, there have been changes in marital ideologies. Increasingly people are expecting continued personal satisfaction from marriage and not just a convenient domestic, sexual and economic arrangement. Indeed, the 1969 Divorce Reform Act – which is still the basis of current divorce law – itself symbolized this. Instead of viewing marriage as essentially a legal contract between two people which could be terminated only if broken by a specific action of one of the spouses, for example adultery or desertion, under the 1969 Act, marriage was understood more as a personal arrangement which could be terminated if it had 'irretrievably broken down', irrespective of what led up to this or of the behaviour of either spouse.

Second, increasing divorce rates are feasible only if both spouses normally have access to sufficient material resources to sustain themselves. Of particular importance here are the changes there have been over the last 50 years allowing separated women to maintain a sufficient standard of living independently of their (ex-)husbands. The creation of increased employment opportunities for married women has been significant in this, as has the availability of social security payments and the protection given in divorce settlements to the housing needs of those caring for children. Third, divorce is now far less stigmatized than it once was. It is seen as personally undesirable, but is no longer treated as a moral issue in the way it was, nor as indicative of questionable character. As divorce becomes accepted as an unfortunate but not unusual occurrence, so it comes also to be seen as a solution to marital difficulties that in a previous era would have been tolerated. It is this 'normalization' of divorce in both legal and social terms which lies at the heart of the currently high levels of divorce.

In understanding the impact which divorce has on those involved, it is crucial that it is viewed as a process occurring over time, rather than as a specific event. While divorce is the legal ending of a marriage and in that sense takes place at a particular moment in time, it is also the result of a (usually quite drawn out) process of relational disharmony and conflict. The factors that lead up to the separation and ending of the marriage, and the understandings each spouse has of these, will have a significant influence on the way in which the divorce and its aftermath are managed. This is particularly important when there are children, for as is now better recognized, divorce represents the ending of a marriage but not the ending of parenting. Legislation since the 1990s has highlighted the continuing financial responsibilities parents have to their children, irrespective of their household arrangements, but increasingly there is also social and legal recognition of the importance of the non-residential parent–child relationship continuing after separation and divorce. Research, particularly in the US, has demonstrated that children usually cope better with the experience of divorce if they are able to maintain an active and positive relationship with both parents (see Richards 1999).

Of course, separation and divorce are generally traumatic for all those involved, whether adults or children. As a consequence, the negative impact of divorce on children is always a concern for parents and others involved in a child's life. Much research has focused on the negative outcomes of divorce, showing for example that children whose parents divorced tended to do less well at school, to form committed relationships earlier and do less well occupationally. However, the differences here between children whose parents did or did not divorce are relatively small. Moreover there is a good deal of variation among those whose parents have separated. Increasingly research on the impact of divorce on children has examined the diversity of their experiences. Often parental separation is just one of a series of changes. As we will discuss, separation and divorce may result in household poverty. It may also result in housing change and geographical mobility, with consequences for the child's friendship networks as well as their schooling. Moreover, in the longer term parental separation and divorce may be followed by further domestic changes, such as the formation of a step-family when a parent re-partners. The cumulative consequences of these various changes, and how they are managed, will shape the outcomes of the parental separation for the child, rather than the simple fact of divorce itself.

A key issue within this is how the parents manage their conflict both prior to the separation and after it. As noted above, it is best for the child to maintain positive relationships with both parents following their separation. Indeed, it is in the child's interests that the two parents develop a consistent and cooperative relationship with one another with respect to parenting. However, this is rarely easy, given the history of hostility and conflict characterizing much pre- and post-divorce behaviour (Smart and Neale 1999). When parents continue to be in conflict over, say, financial arrangements or childcare responsibilities, or indeed when recrimination, jealousy and other strong emotions are still being experienced, it

Activity box 9.3

- Discuss the reasons why some non-residential fathers have a limited relationship with their children.
- Consider here personal, social, economic and legal factors.
- What policies might be developed to encourage continued relationships between non-residential fathers and their children? What difficulties are there with the policies you are suggesting?

is difficult to develop a mutually consistent and supportive stance in relation to children. Given the tensions and problems which can be generated, it is perhaps not surprising that a third of non-residential fathers appear to see their children less than once a month (Bradshaw et al 1999).

Lone-parent households

Over the last 30 years, the number of lone-parent households has increased quite dramatically, both as a result of high levels of divorce and because more children are being born outside marriage. As the numbers have grown, the range and diversity of experiences of those living in such households have also increased. Undoubtedly the majority of lone-parent households have much in common, especially with respect to their poverty and material deprivation. Yet variations in the living conditions, family histories and economic opportunities of different lone-parent households should not be ignored. Just as the routes into, and indeed out of, lone-parenthood have become more complex, so too the social, economic and domestic circumstances of those involved have become more diverse (Crow and Hardey 1999).

By the beginning of the 21st century there were 1.75 million lone-parent households in Britain, containing approximately 2.9 million children – nearly 1 in 4 of all dependent children (Haskey 2002). Of these lone-parent households, a little over 200 000 were headed by men. While this is not an insignificant number in itself, the predominance of female-headed lone-parent households warrants emphasizing as it plays a major part in shaping the experience of lone-parenthood. Of the one and a half million female-headed lone-parent households there were in 2000, over 50% were the consequence of divorce or separation, with only 90 000 being the result of widowhood. Over a third are headed by single (i.e. never married) women (Haskey 2002). This represents a quite remarkable demographic change since the mid 1970s. Then, fewer than 10% of children were born 'out of wedlock'. By 2005, the figure was over 40%, with over 90% of teenage mothers being unmarried (ONS 2006a, Office of Population Censuses and Surveys (OPCS)). However, it is worth noting that in 2005 nearly two-thirds of all mothers recorded as being unmarried on their child's birth certificate were cohabiting with the father of the child when the birth was registered.

The great majority of lone-parent households live in poverty (Rowlingson and McKay 2002). In 2002 nearly 50% of all lone mothers had a gross income of less than £10 000 a year, compared to 8% of married couples (ONS 2004). Many lone mothers rely on state benefits for their standard of living. However, the route into lone-parenthood has some bearing on this. In general, lone fathers and widowed mothers tend to be somewhat better off than other lone parents (though not as well off as two-parent households). These groups usually have older children than other lone parents, and as a result fewer problems with the coordination and costs of childcare. They are also more likely to have employment or pensions which make them less dependent on state benefits. In contrast, divorced, separated and single mothers – collectively nearly 85% of all lone parents – frequently experience high levels of poverty for long periods.

The reasons for this are various. Women's disadvantaged position in employment is one factor. The relatively low pay of many female jobs, especially for women without significant qualifications, means that many lone mothers have little prospect of enhancing their financial position. In addition, the need for flexibility over childcare often makes it difficult to coordinate employment and parenting responsibilities. When children are at school, part-time employment may become feasible though the financial benefits of this, as distinct from its social and personal advantages, are generally quite limited. In recent years, state policies have been attempting to reduce the numbers of lone mothers in poverty through more generous employment allowances, enhanced provision of childcare facilities, and through ensuring that non-residential fathers pay higher levels of maintenance for their children. However, despite these initiatives, the great majority of lone-mother households continue to experience poverty (Rowlingson and McKay 2002, 2005).

As well as being poor, lone mothers tend to be disadvantaged in other ways. For example, they have worse than average housing conditions, with a disproportionate number being in rented accommodation, or sharing their home with other adults. Only about a third of lone-parent families are in owner-occupation compared to 80% of all other households with dependent children living in them. So too, lone-parent households are three times as likely to live in flats compared to other households with children in them (ONS 2004). Equally there is evidence that lone parents, but especially lone mothers, suffer more health problems than other families (Shouls et al 1999). This is not altogether surprising, given the relationship between material well-being and good health. Families in poverty and in poor housing, as so many lone-parent families are, generally experience worse health than those who have adequate resources (see Chapter 1 and Chapter 5 for further information on the association between poverty and health).

Overall, there is no doubt that a majority of lone-parent families are disadvantaged, especially those that are female-headed. Yet while poverty and material deprivation is the norm, various aspects of lone-parenthood come to be valued by many. Simply in financial terms, some lone mothers are, in Hilary Graham's telling phrase, 'better off poorer' (1987: 59), because they now control all the household resources, whereas previously they received only a proportion of the overall larger 'household' income, with their husbands or partners retaining the rest. Equally, while many lone parents experience social isolation and a sense of having to cope with a wide range of demands alone, others value the freedom and autonomy over their use of time, domestic organization and social activities which lone-parenthood offers. For some too, the curtailment of disharmony and marital violence more than compensates for poverty. The point here is not that these more positive aspects of lone-parenthood necessarily counter its negative features, but rather that lone-parenthood is often an ambiguous and diverse experience.

Lesbian and gay couples

With the increases in divorce, cohabitation and step-families, it is evident that family life is now characterized by a greater degree of diversity than in the recent past. One further indication of this greater

Activity box 9.4

Write out in some detail the principles you think should apply to determine the financial contribution that a non-residential parent should pay for his or her child(ren).

Now go to the Child Maintenance and Enforcement Commission (CMEC) website at http://www.dwp.gov.uk/childmaintenance/csa_report.pdf and compare the principles you have specified with those recommended by the CMEC.

If there are differences, consider the benefits and disadvantages of your proposals and the CMEC scheme.

In your view, should non-residential parents who make an appropriate financial contribution to their child(ren)'s care have more rights to involvement in their child(ren)'s life than parents who don't make such a contribution? Why and who would benefit?

diversity can be seen in the increased acceptance of lesbian and gay sexualities and the growth in the number of openly lesbian and gay couples. Although Britain has not followed the lead of countries like Canada in accepting that the legal right to marriage should be available to all couples whether heterosexual or non-heterosexual, from 2005 it created the option of 'civil registration'. Although not termed 'marriage', effectively this allowed non-heterosexual partners the same legal rights and obligations as marriage did heterosexual couples. Some 18 000 civil registrations were celebrated in the first year of this legislation (ONS 2006b). Of course, many gay and lesbian couples prefer to cohabit rather than having their partnerships formalized through civil registration.

Lesbian and gay couples face many of the same issues of sustaining intimacy and managing long-term commitment that cohabiting and married heterosexual couples face (Kurdek 2004, Patterson 2000). Equally though many of those involved in gay and lesbian partnerships seek to develop forms of relationship that do not directly mirror the organization of heterosexual marriage. In particular, they wish to create more equal relationships in which the negotiated division of labour does not represent a power imbalance within their relationship. In any partnership a division of labour is likely to emerge over time. However, in the absence of the structural gender inequalities that pattern heterosexual relationships, gay and lesbian couples are more likely to

be able to construct relationships in which differentials in power and access to resources are more equitably managed (Heaphy et al 1999).

Despite the changes there have been in general attitudes, gay and lesbian individuals are still frequently confronted with hostility and stigma as a result of their sexual preferences. For some, this has significant consequences for their involvement in wider family networks, especially where genealogical family members are intolerant of their sexuality. In a major British study, Weeks et al (2001) have emphasized the importance of 'families of choice'. This refers to the pattern by which some gay and lesbian individuals (and couples) create strong ties with specific friends who come to be seen as 'family'. These are the people who form their intimate circle and who can be relied on for practical and emotional support. Their unconditional acceptance of the individual's gay or lesbian identity and lifestyle results in their developing the forms of committed solidarity that are more commonly associated with conventional family ties.

Step-families

There has been a significant growth in the number of step-families, with cohabitation and marriage representing major routes out of lone-parenthood. According to official estimates, more than 10% of families with dependent children were step-families in 2005, with many other children having a non-residential step-parent (ONS 2007c). As might be expected, some lone parents are more likely to repartner than others. Generally, single mothers form new unions quicker than those who have been married previously, with age, educational attainment and family size affecting the chances of remarriage for those who have divorced (Rowlingson and McKay 2002). Given the number of step-families there now are, it is surprising how little research there has been in Britain on their organization and functioning. Similarly it is surprising how little official concern there is about them. The assumption has tended to be that step-families are essentially similar to other two-parent families.

However the diversity and complexity of step-families make this an oversimplified view (Ribbens McCarthy et al 2003). Aside from factors like the age of the children and how long they have known their step-parent, the social roles of step-father and step-mother are ill-defined. There are few guidelines about just how much of a parent a step-parent should be. For example, the extent of the step-parent's involvement, their rights to impose discipline, and the commitment expected between step-parent and step-child, are all much more open to negotiation than in 'natural' families, so that the potential for disagreement and conflict is that much greater.

Equally the 'boundaries' around step-families tend to be more permeable than in 'natural' families, especially where contact is maintained with the non-residential parent and his or her kin. In addition, the different members of a step-family have different family and kinship networks to each other, often resulting in different kinship loyalties. In essence, the symbolic 'unity' of a step-family cannot be assumed in the way it is in 'natural' families. Given these structural dilemmas, it is hardly surprising that step-families appear particularly prone to friction, notwithstanding their members' frequent efforts to present themselves as just 'ordinary' families (Ganong and Coleman 2004).

Table 9.2 The population over 65	
Female population over 65[a]	6.9 million
Male population over 65[a]	3.9 million
Female population over 75[a]	2.8 million
Male population over 75[a]	1.6 million
Percentage of women over 75 who live alone[b]	59%
Percentage of men over 75 who live alone[b]	28%
Percentage of people over 65 with incomes less than 60% of the UK median[a]	25%
Percentage of men aged 75–84 with limiting long-term illness[c]	56%
Percentage of women aged 75–84 with limiting long-term illness[c]	59%

Sources: ONS (2005a, 2005b).
[a]UK 2001.
[b]Great Britain 2005.
[c]England and Wales 2001.

Old age

There is a strong belief that kinship ties outside the household have become less significant than they once were. In particular, the solidarities that exist across the generations are now seen to be weaker than in the past, with the result that many elderly people are left isolated, leading lonely and largely unfulfilling lives. This picture of contemporary old age is highly questionable, though there have been many changes in the circumstances of older people.

There are now for example nearly four and a half million people over the age of 75 compared to half a million in 1901, a rate of increase which is over 15 times that of the general population. Moreover nearly 60% of all women over 75 live alone, though only a little over a quarter of men of this age live alone (ONS 2005a) (Table 9.2). Along with these demographic shifts, there have been important changes in elderly people's social and economic circumstances. In particular, it is becoming increasingly inappropriate to treat the elderly population as homogeneous. The divisions between them are as important as the similarities. For example, the rise of private pension plans and of owner-occupation since the mid 20th century have exacerbated differences in income and wealth among those aged 65 and over. These factors, together with variations in

life expectancy, have also led to very important gender differences in the experience of old age (Arber et al 2003, Phillipson 1998).

On the surface, the fact that so many elderly women especially live alone appears to give credence to the claim that elderly people no longer receive the support they deserve and need. Undoubtedly some of these people are very isolated and receive inadequate social support; some will never have married, or have no surviving children to whom they might turn. Yet there are other factors at work here too, which give a rather different picture. In particular, culturally a high priority is often given to maintaining household independence, though there are important ethnic variations in this (Phillipson et al 2001). That is, while there is strong value placed on relationships between genealogically close adult kin being generally supportive, there is also much weight given to the idea that in adulthood, personal and household autonomy takes priority. Kin, including parents and children, should not interfere too much in each other's lives. Here there can be a fine line between supporting and interfering, between assuming some responsibility and maintaining independence. Indeed, rather than neglecting their elderly parent(s), it would seem many adult children play a major role in helping them to sustain independent lives as infirmity encroaches (Connidis 2001, Phillipson et al 2001).

Of course the nature of the relationship which elderly people have with their children varies a good deal. In part, this will be shaped by the past development of their bond, but it will also be influenced by a range of other personal factors, such as geographical location, employment, other familial and domestic responsibilities, material resources and health. It is important to recognize here that older age of itself does not have any necessary impact on family relationships. The great majority of older people are relatively fit and active, well able to manage their own lives, and have no reason for fuller involvement with their children than in preceding life stages. As in earlier times, the relationships are likely to be characterized by a degree of reciprocity with both sides providing support of different forms for one another, but without either being in a position of dependence.

It is not old age per se which alters the nature of these exchanges, but rather changes – sometimes gradual, sometimes radical – in older people's circumstances. However, such changes as reduced income, widowhood and poor health have a differential impact on the older population. Expressed simply, those with most resources, in particular those who have higher levels of private or occupational pensions and significant investments, are in a better position to sustain their lifestyle and independence through purchasing services privately. Those with fewer resources, a position in which many older women find themselves, especially after their husband's death, are likely to become more quickly dependent on kin for support. In nearly all cases though there is a desire to maintain some semblance of balance and reciprocity in these ties. This can often require careful and quite subtle 'negotiation' if the older individual's sense of self-worth is not to be undermined.

When extensive care is required, it tends to be provided by family members, though usually the responsibility falls most heavily on one particular person. This is typically the spouse where there is one, or another adult living in the same household. Otherwise it is usually daughters or daughters-in-law who are most active in providing informal care. While this has now been much discussed in the research literature on caring (see, for example, ONS 2005b, Ungerson and Kember 1997), it is still easy for health professionals and others to underestimate the actual level of work which such caring entails and its impact on the lifestyles and well-being of those who do it.

Conclusion

There has been little explicit focus in this chapter on issues directly concerned with health behaviour or practice. Other chapters discuss these matters more directly. Its aim has been to provide a broad framework through analysing key aspects of contemporary family experience. However, the arguments made in this chapter certainly have relevance for healthcare provision and the work of community nurses. Three particular issues are worth highlighting in conclusion. First, there is growing diversity in household and family patterns, both demographically and materially, with recent increases in cohabitation, divorce and remarriage. In delivering healthcare, advice and support, the particular circumstances of individual families need to be recognized. Second, the family itself is not a single entity or social unity. It comprises sets of relationships which change over time but which also typically entail marked divisions of labour, resources and power. Recognizing these divisions and the impact they have on the experiences of different household members can be important in providing appropriate health services. Finally, it is important that all health workers recognize the extent to which healthcare continues to be delivered informally, principally by family members and predominantly by females responsible for the household's domestic organization. Despite the changes which are imagined to have occurred, most non-specialized nursing and healthcare is carried out by wives, mothers and daughters. At times the burden of such care can be extremely heavy, a fact which should not be downplayed even when those involved give the impression of 'coping'.

SUMMARY

- The structure of families is constantly changing; these changes may be sudden or gradual, and although families can be categorized into different family types, differences between different families in the same grouping can be marked.
- The numbers of couples not marrying but cohabiting have increased dramatically over the past 30 years. However, the roles men and women have, no matter the legal relationship, still tend to be patterned by gender, with men having more options and access to resources.
- The divorce rate has escalated over recent decades due to its 'normalization'; however, to understand the implications of divorce on family members, separation and divorce must be seen as a long-term process rather than a single event for the family.

- Lone-parenting, usually with women at the head of the family, has increased over the past two generations; the large majority of female-headed, lone-parent households experience poverty.
- There has been a growth in the number of lesbian and gay couples; for some, 'families of choice' are more central in their lives than family ties based on conventional genealogical principles.
- Step-families are more complex than 'natural' families, especially in terms of family unity and belonging.
- Older people's experiences are not uniform; they have diverse individual and family biographies, differing levels of financial security, different levels of family support, different health experiences and different needs.

DISCUSSION POINTS

1. Why might it be useful for community nurses to profile family diversity in the neighbour-hood served by the practice team?

2. How would you record family differences in a way which would account for variation in community nursing intervention?

3. Why would it be important to assess in detail the impact that caring for frail older people has on different family members?

References

Allan G, Crow G 2001 Families, households and society. Palgrave, Basingstoke

Arber S, Davidson K, Ginn J (eds) 2003 Gender and ageing: changing roles and relationships. Open University Press, Maidenhead

Bradshaw J, Stimson C, Skinner C, Williams J 1999 Absent fathers? Routledge, London

Connidis I 2001 Family ties and aging, 2nd edn. Sage, Thousand Oaks, CA

Crompton R 1997 Women and work in modern Britain. Oxford University Press, Oxford

Crompton R, Harris F 1999 Attitudes, women's employment and the changing domestic division of

labour: a cross-national analysis. In: Crompton R (ed.) Restructuring gender relations and employment. Oxford University Press, Oxford

Crow G, Hardey M 1999 Diversity and ambiguity among lone-parent households in modern Britain. In: Allan G (ed.) The sociology of the family: a reader. Blackwell, Oxford

Ganong L, Coleman M 2004 Stepfamily relationships: Development, dynamics, and interventions. Kluwer/Plenum, London

Graham H 1987 Being poor: perceptions and coping strategies of lone mothers. In: Brannen J, Wilson

G (eds) Give and take in families: studies in resource distribution. Allen & Unwin, London

Haskey J 1998 One-parent families and their dependent children in Great Britain. Population Trends 91: 5–14

Haskey J 2002 One-parent families, and the dependent children living in them, in Great Britain. Population Trends 109: 46–57. Online: http://www.statistics.gov.uk/downloads/theme_population/PT109.pdf

Heaphy B, Donovan C, Weeks J 1999 Sex, money and the kitchen sink: power in same sex couple relationships. In: Seymour J, Bagguley P (eds) Relating intimacies:

power and resistance. Macmillan, London

Kiernan K 2004 Redrawing the boundaries of marriage. Journal of Marriage and Family 66: 980–987

Kurdek L 2004 Are gay and lesbian cohabiting couples really different from heterosexual married couples? Journal of Marriage and Family 66: 880–900

Oates C, McDonald S 2006 Recycling and the domestic division of labour: is green pink or blue? Sociology 40: 417–433

ONS 2001 Population trends 103. Office for National Statistics, London. Online: http://www.statistics.gov.uk/downloads/theme_population/PT103book_v3.pdf

ONS 2004 Living in Britain No 31: Results from the 2002 General Household Survey. Office for National Statistics. Stationery Office, London. Online: http://www.statistics.gov.uk/downloads/theme_compendia/lib2002.pdf

ONS 2005a Social trends No. 35. Office for National Statistics. Stationery Office, London. Online: http://www.statistics.gov.uk/StatBase/Product.asp?vlnk=5748

ONS 2005b Focus on older people, 2005 edition. Office for National Statistics. Palgrave Macmillan, Basingstoke. Online: http://www.statistics.gov.uk/downloads/theme_compendia/foop05/Olderpeople2005.pdf

ONS 2006a Birth statistics 2005, Series FM1, No. 34. Office for National Statistics, London. Online: http://www.statistics.gov.uk/downloads/theme_population/FM1_34/FM1_no34_2005.pdf

ONS 2006b In brief. Population Trends 126: 3. Online: http://www.statistics.gov.uk/downloads/theme_population/PopTrends126.pdf

ONS 2007a Marriage, divorce and adoption statistics, Series FM2, No. 32. Office for National Statistics, London. Online:http://www.statistics.gov.uk/downloads/theme_population/FM2no32/FM2_32.pdf

ONS 2007b Population trends 128. Office for National Statistics, London.Online: http://www.statistics.gov.uk/downloads/theme_population/PopulationTrends128.pdf

ONS 2007c Social trends No. 37. Office for National Statistics. Palgrave Macmillan, Basingstoke. Online: http://www.statistics.gov.uk/downloads/theme_social/Social_Trends37/Social_Trends_37.pdf

OPCS 1978 Birth statistics 1976, Series FM1, No. 3. HMSO, London

Patterson C 2000 Family relationships of lesbians and gay men. Journal of Marriage and the Family 62: 1052–1069

Phillipson C 1998 Reconstructing old age. Sage, London

Phillipson C, Bernard M, Phillips J, Ogg J 2001 The family and community life of older people. Routledge, London

Ribbens McCarthy J, Edwards R, Gillies V 2003 Making families: moral tales of parenting and step-parenting. Sociologypress, Durham

Richards M 1999 The interests of children at divorce. In: Allan G (ed.) The sociology of the family: a reader. Blackwell, Oxford

Rowlingson K, McKay S 2002 Lone parent families: gender, class and state, Pearson Education, Harlow

Rowlingson K, McKay S 2005 Lone motherhood and socio-economic disadvantage: insights from quantitative and qualitative evidence. Sociological Review 53: 30–49

Seltzer J 2004 Cohabitation in the United States and Britain: demography, kinship, and the future. Journal of Marriage and Family 66: 921–928

Shouls S, Whitehead M, Burström B, Diderichsen F 1999 The health and socio-economic circumstances of lone mothers over the last two decades. Population Trends 95: 41–46

Smart C, Neale B 1999 Family fragments? Polity, Cambridge

Ungerson C, Kember M 1997 Women and social policy: a reader. Macmillan, Basingstoke

Weeks J, Heaphy B, Donovan C 2001 Same sex intimacies: families of choice and other life experiments. Routledge London

Recommended reading

Allan G 1999 The sociology of the family: a reader. Blackwell, Oxford
The essays in this collection cover a wide range of topics relevant to this chapter. It includes sections on changing families; marriage intimacy and power; domestic organization; divorce and lone-parenthood; and family, kinship and care.

Allan G, Crow G 2001 Families, households and society. Palgrave, Basingstoke
This book provides an introduction to the sociology of the family, reviewing recent research and highlighting the changes there have been in domestic life. Written principally for sociology students, it develops some of the arguments made in this chapter.

Ganong L, Coleman, M 2004 Stepfamily relationships: development, dynamics, and interventions. Kluwer/Plenum, London
This book reports on a wide variety of mainly American studies examining different aspects of step-family life. It provides a very thorough introduction to many of the key issues.

McRae S 1999 Changing Britain: families and households in the 1990s. Oxford University Press, Oxford
This is a very useful collection of specially commissioned papers, all based on recent research into different aspects of family life. It is particularly useful for understanding patterns of change and continuity in family relationships over the last generation.

Phillipson C, Bernard M, Phillips J, Ogg J 2001 The family and community life of older people. Routledge, London
This fascinating study of the family and community relationships of older people in contemporary Britain

contains much of interest to community nurses. It is particularly interesting because it compares the current and past circumstances of elderly people in three different urban locations.

Smart C, Neale B 1999 Family fragments? Polity, Cambridge

This book reports on research into post-divorce family arrangements. In doing so, it engages with recent theorizing about changing family relationships and highlights key aspects of family organization. By focusing on the consequences of marital breakdown, it reveals much about the patterning of contemporary marriage and domestic organization.

Weeks J, Heaphy B, Donovan C 2001 Same sex intimacies: families of choice and other life experiments. Routledge, London

This is a major empirical study of gay and lesbian individuals in England. It focuses on the personal networks respondents sustained. Among other topics, it examines partnerships, intimate ties and family relationships.

The family: a psychological perspective

Neil Frude

KEY ISSUES

- The family as a system whose benefits and costs impact on health
- Relationships and life events
- Interactional styles
- Intimacy, well-being and health
- Family types and coping mechanisms

Introduction

The individual person was traditionally the principal unit of examination, diagnosis and treatment in medicine. Indeed, in many cases attention was focused on a narrower 'subsystem' such as the respiratory system or the cardiovascular system. In recent decades it has been recognized as appropriate to adopt a more holistic approach in which biological, psychological and social factors are all acknowledged to be important contributors to physical and emotional health. This focus now extends beyond the 'whole person' to include wider systems such as the family and the community. Thus 'family medicine', 'family nursing', 'family therapy', 'community medicine' and 'community nursing' have all become well-established disciplines.

This chapter will examine some of the ways in which psychologists think about families. Of course, there are other ways of looking at family issues, including those offered by the political, ethical, legal and sociological perspectives (see Chapter 9 for examples). The various perspectives can often be seen as complementary although they tend to focus on different issues and employ different concepts and methods of analysis. Thus while a sociologist is likely to be concerned with the family as an institution within society, and might therefore emphasize the relationship between the family unit and wider systems such as the health service or the taxation system, psychologists are typically more concerned with the interactions and relationships within particular families and how these change as a result of the impact of events such as illness, death or the birth of a child.

The aim of this chapter is to provide a basic framework for thinking, psychologically, about families rather than to summarize knowledge about the effects of particular illnesses or treatments on families. Extensive reviews of the impact of illness, handicap, divorce, bereavement, etc. on family life are available elsewhere (Frude 1991, Power and Del Orto 2004). The first part of this chapter examines the family as the background or context for understanding the individual and demonstrates that family relationships have a substantial impact on individuals' physical health and psychological well-being. The second half of the chapter focuses on the family group, discusses the nature of 'healthy' and 'dysfunctional' families and considers how different families respond when an individual member becomes ill.

The family as the context for the individual

The value of family relationships

Being part of a family brings a number of costs and benefits to an individual. If a person decides that the costs of family membership outweigh the benefits (so that family membership has a negative value), then he or she may decide to withdraw from the family. According to one influential psychological theory ('social exchange theory'), the decisions that people make about their lives, including their family life, reflect their own cost–benefit analyses (Nye 1982, Ruben 1998). This kind of analysis has been used, for example, to explain why people choose to have (or not to have) children, why they may choose to separate, and why older children choose to leave home or to continue living with their parents (Rigazio-DiGilio and Cramer 2000, Veevers and Mitchell 1998). A good deal of research has been aimed at discovering what people want (i.e. the benefits they hope for) from relationships, and what they wish to avoid (i.e. the costs). Some adults who have ended an unsatisfactory marital relationship feel that the risks associated with any close relationship are too high, and avoid such relationships. On the other hand, the majority of people who have experienced a divorce hope for a better relationship in the future and exert considerable effort to find 'the right person'. When interviewed, such people are often able to identify what they are looking for in a relationship – they are able to provide a list of hoped-for benefits.

It is clear that many marriages and long-term cohabiting relationships eventually end (according to some estimates, around 50% of all those who are currently entering into a marriage will eventually divorce). There is also a good deal of conflict and violence within families. Few families, indeed, could be described as completely harmonious. In view of these facts, it might be tempting to conclude that the family is a disaster area and that people would be better off without family ties. However, such a conclusion would be unjustified. We have to consider the benefits as well as the costs, and the love and support as well as the conflict and violence. On average, people value their relationships positively and there is strong evidence that, on the whole, close relationships benefit individuals.

When people are asked what makes them happy, what provides them with satisfaction, and what gives meaning to their lives, they emphasize their close relationships much more than any other aspect of their life, including their occupation, hobbies, health or money (Carr 2003). This is not to deny that many people blame a key relationship for their unhappiness, or that intimate relationships often provoke the most intense anger, anxiety and sadness, but, on the whole, people do assess the impact of their closest relationships in positive rather than in negative terms. Furthermore, in support of such subjective assessments, there is objective evidence suggesting that, overall, the effects of close relationships are more often favourable than unfavourable.

Relationships and life events

It is now well established that psychological and physical health is profoundly affected by life events such as divorce, the birth of a child, bereavement or moving house. Several lists (or 'inventories') of commonly experienced life events have been compiled, with each item being assigned a weighting to reflect the likely impact of an event of that nature. These inventories can be used to assess how much 'life change' an individual has experienced in the past 6 months, or the past year. Individuals' total life change scores have been found to predict many health outcomes, including susceptibility to infection, the risk of being involved in a serious accident and the risk of cardiovascular disease (Richter and Guthke 1993). Generally speaking, those who have experienced several recent major changes are more vulnerable to physical and psychological illness than those who have not experienced such changes.

A high proportion of the events listed in inventories compiled to assess major life changes (e.g. Gray et al 2004, Holmes and Rahe 1967) are directly related to family life. Such events include the illness of a family member, a bereavement, a child leaving home, marital separation and sexual problems. Lists of major positive events in people's lives also show a preponderance of family-related items (Argyle and Henderson 1985), and the same is true of minor positive and negative events (sometimes referred to as 'uplifts' and 'hassles' respectively). Compared with those who live in isolation, people who live in a family setting have lives which are relatively full of incident. They experience more 'entrances' (such as the birth of a child) and more 'exits' (the death of a family member, marital separation or a young adult leaving home). They experience more 'uplifts' (such as birthdays, anniversaries and school successes), but they also experience more 'hassles' (such as minor illnesses of family members, or family rows) (Harper et al 2000, Maybery and Graham 2001). Many of those who live in isolation are lonely and feel that their life lacks interest, excitement or involvement. Whereas many early studies stressed the potential danger of exposure to 'excess life change', it is now appreciated that a modest degree of incident and transition promotes healthiness and well-being.

Intimacy, well-being and health

Studies that have asked people to report how happy they are, how lonely they feel and how stressed they feel, have revealed a number of interesting findings. For example, Wood et al (1989) conducted a 'meta-analysis' whereby they re-analysed the findings from 93 previously published studies that had addressed the issue of happiness and positive well-being. They showed that, overall, women reported greater happiness and life satisfaction than men (despite the fact that women are twice as likely to be clinically depressed as men). They also showed that marriage was associated with higher levels of well-being both for women and for men, a finding that has been demonstrated repeatedly in other research (Wilson and Oswald 2005). Similarly, studies comparing the reported happiness, loneliness and stress experienced by married people, single people, the widowed and the divorced also indicate that those who are currently married have fewer problems and have a greater sense of positive well-being than those in any of the other groups (Cohen 2004).

Objective indicators point in the same direction. Overall, married people have better physical health than those who have never married or are divorced or widowed. They are less likely, for example, to suffer from asthma, diabetes, ulcers, tuberculosis, cancer of the mouth and throat, hypertension, strokes and heart attacks (Cohen 2004). The association between health and being married is even apparent in mortality data. Married people are at significantly less risk of dying at a young age, compared to those who are single, widowed or divorced (Wilson and Oswald 2005).

A broadly similar pattern emerges when the statistics for mental health are considered. When groups of people matched for age, sex and social class are compared in terms of their psychiatric history, morbidity rates are lowest for the married population (Bebbington et al 2000). General community surveys also reveal that married people experience the fewest psychological symptoms, with an intermediate rate among widowed and never-married adults, and the highest rates among those who are divorced or separated.

Before we conclude that 'marriage is good for you', however, it does need to be stressed that the statistics merely show an average advantage for those who are married. It must be remembered that for many people the marital relationship is oppressive or violent, and that conflict and aggression can jeopardize both physical and psychological health. There can be little doubt that many people would be much healthier if they were to opt out of an unhealthy relationship. Although divorce is often a major stressor, many divorced people adjust to a new lifestyle and end up healthier and better adjusted than many of those who opt to remain in a conflictual or violent marital relationship (Kim and McKenry 2002).

Why do good relationships promote health?

How can we explain the association between a stable, intimate relationship and relatively good health? One explanation is that people who are in a secure relationship are likely to have a greater sense of well-being than those who lack a partner, and that as a result they may be less vulnerable to stress. Another suggestion is that it might be especially useful to have access to a partner and confidant(e) during critical periods, for example when the individual faces a major life change. One way in which a partner may help is by listening to the person's worries and providing informal therapy. In their classic study of the social origins of depression among women, Brown and Harris (1978) found that the presence of an intimate partner and confidant was associated with a relatively low impact of stressful events.

People often 'consult' their partners when they are under emotional strain, and many report that they derive great comfort from their partner's counsel and that it helps them to survive a crisis. Health and counselling professionals are often a 'last resort' for those who seek help for psychological problems. Relatives, friends, work colleagues, neighbours, volunteer helpers (e.g. the Samaritans) and other professionals (e.g. religious leaders) are frequently used as counsellors, advisers and 'sounding boards'. However, when people are asked whom they 'really depend on' when personal problems arise, they are more likely to cite their partner than anyone else (Griffith 1985). Informal psychotherapy is a feature of the majority of marriages and it has been found that those who are satisfied with their partner's 'therapeutic' efforts are likely to be satisfied with the marriage as a whole (Nye and McLaughlin 1982).

The presence of a partner may also contribute to health because one partner acts as a 'guardian' of the other, monitoring behaviours and providing encouragement and guidance. Thus partners, relatives and close friends often encourage a person to comply with certain 'rules' and help them to refrain from dangerous activities (Tucker and Mueller 2000). A partner will often keep a watchful eye on an individual's smoking and drinking, encouraging them to eat well, to exercise regularly, to attend for medical check-ups and to comply with medical advice. People who are socially isolated do not receive the mixture of encouragement and censure that helps others to check any excessive or dangerous behaviour. Although it may not be experienced as pleasant or useful to be on the receiving end of such frequent 'nagging' about the need to maintain a healthy lifestyle, it is undoubtedly beneficial for many people. Those who do not have a partner to support them in this way are more likely to lead disordered lives and to expose themselves to danger. Thus many of those who are newly divorced eat and sleep irregularly, smoke and drink to excess.

The family unit

So far, family relationships (especially marital relationships) have been considered in terms of their costs and benefits to the individual. We have focused exclusively on adults and the costs and benefits they derive from their relationship with their partner, but we could also examine the costs and benefits that an adult or a child may derive from the relationship with any other family member. But we might also consider what any individual gains (or loses) overall by being a member of the family and we can go beyond this and focus on the whole family as a unit.

Families are not merely 'backdrops for individuals' or simply collections of individual people. A family is a unit in which 'the whole is greater than the sum of the parts'. A family unit, indeed, can be viewed as if it were an organism in which the individual family members are constituent elements. The organism metaphor can be a fruitful one, for it leads to a number of interesting questions. What are the anatomical features of this type of organism? What is known of its physiology? What is known of the life cycle? What variations are there between different organisms (families)? And what forms of pathology are found?

Like organisms, families pass through a developmental sequence or 'career'. They are 'formed', they undergo changes, and in the end they 'die'. Some analysts divide the 'family life cycle' into a number of stages. In one classic formulation, for example, Duvall (1977) distinguished eight stages, starting with a 'newly formed' couple who have no children and ending with the ageing family – a stage that lasts from retirement until death. Such models are clearly oversimplified, but they can be useful in mapping broad patterns of change and identifying common problems at particular stages of development. Thus the pressures typically experienced by 'young families' are somewhat different from those faced by families with adolescent children.

Families (like organisms) must adapt in response to both internal and external changes. The birth of a first child, for example, presents the couple with many new tasks and gives them new roles as parents. The family boundary becomes extended to include the infant, and there are marked changes in the nature of the couple's interactions. The original two-person ('dyadic') relationship (i.e. the couple) is replaced by three dyadic relationships (mother–father, mother–infant and father–infant) and one 'triadic' relationship. Even with this simple arrangement we can begin to get some idea of the 'reverberations' that occur within families. For example, a change in an infant's behaviour or health is likely to bring changes to the mother–infant relationship. These changes may then affect the relationship between the parents, and the changed interparental relationship is then likely to affect the infant. This provides an example of the reverberations that occur constantly throughout the family system.

The elements within a family system are not just the individual family members but also the relationships between them, and any change in one individual or one relationship will be likely to have effects on all other elements and on the 'tone' or 'atmosphere' of the family as a whole. Another metaphor which may be useful at this point is that of the family as a 'hanging mobile'. Such a mobile consists of a frame, the various suspended items (or 'elements'), and the strings by which these elements are suspended from the frame. Any change in one element will affect every other element as well as the position and movement of the mobile as a whole. It is impossible to move any element without having a global effect on the mobile. Furthermore, it is impossible to move any one element without affecting all of the other elements and the resulting movements will reverberate back to affect the element that was originally moved.

Within a family system, any change such as an 'entrance' (a child being born; an elderly relative coming to live in the home) or an 'exit' (the death of a family member; an adolescent leaving) will have profound effects on individual family members. It will also affect the relationships between them and may completely transform the family interaction patterns. Thus in a family in which there is normally a good deal of hostility and open conflict, the knowledge that one family member is seriously ill may bring a period of apparent harmony and a cessation of hostilities. A family member who has previously appeared selfish and unhelpful may suddenly change to become cooperative and helpful. Such changes will affect the overall 'family atmosphere'. A crisis, such as that precipitated by a serious illness, inevitably brings many changes to the family. Some families become stronger, more united, and function better than ever before, whereas others become disorganized and lose their ability to function effectively. Any family can be expected to experience several 'entrances' and 'exits' throughout a lifetime, and many other changes will also alter the pattern of family relationships. Over a 30–40-year span there may be a complete reversal in roles, as the once-helpless infants grow towards middle age and perhaps eventually take on the care of their aged parents. The normal processes of family development demand major changes in interaction patterns. But in addition to such expected, or 'normative' changes, many families also experience exceptional circumstances such as the birth of a disabled child or the sudden death of a young parent that require extraordinary adaptations.

Structural differences between families

There are many different ways of classifying families. One obvious variation is that of structure. Some families are single-parent units while others are two-parent families. Some families are childless, some have a single child, some have two children, etc. Families also differ in terms of their stage of development. Thus there are new partnerships without children, families with young children, families with adolescent children, and 'empty nest' families in which all of the children have grown to adulthood and left home. Working out a comprehensive system for classifying families, even in such concrete structural terms, is not easy because we would have to include families that include three or even four generations, step-families (sometimes known as 'reconstituted families') and same sex partnerships (including formalized civil partnerships) with and without children living in the home. There has been a notable broadening of 'family configurations' in recent decades, and only a minority of families now fit into the traditional 'married couple with their children' category.

Differences in family interaction styles

There are many contexts in which it is useful to group families in terms of their structural characteristics (for example, when addressing social policy issues). However, families that share a common structural characteristic may differ markedly in terms of the interactions between family members. Psychologists are typically less interested in structural aspects than in interactional and relationship characteristics and therefore tend to differentiate families in terms of their 'character' or 'interactive style'. Thus psychologists may differentiate between 'harmonious' and 'conflictual' families or between 'depressed families' and 'non-depressed families'.

There are of course many thousands of characteristics such as these that might be used to distinguish families, although it is likely that some of them will be far more useful than others. Thankfully, a wealth of research evidence, as well as clinical experience, points to two dimensions that are particularly useful in differentiating family interaction styles. The two dimensions that emerge consistently as providing a useful basis for classification are 'adaptability' and 'cohesion'. 'Adaptability' refers to the family's ability to change its structure, roles and rules when adjustment is called for. 'Cohesion' relates to the degree of emotional bonding between family members and to their independence and autonomy.

According to the 'circumplex model' devised by Olson and his colleagues (Olson 2000, Olson et al 1979), families can be classified into one of four 'types' on each of the two key dimensions. On the 'adaptability' dimension, the classification proceeds from one extreme – 'rigid' – through 'structured' and then 'flexible' to the other extreme – 'chaotic'. On the 'cohesion' dimension, the classification proceeds from one extreme – 'enmeshed' – through 'connected' and then 'separated' to the other extreme – 'disengaged'. The labels used for the extremes of each dimension were chosen to convey the belief that all extreme positions are relatively 'unhealthy'. Thus families at either end of the adaptability dimension (i.e. either rigid or chaotic) are likely to experience special problems, particularly when they face a need to change. Families classified in terms of the middle positions on the adaptability dimension (i.e. structured and flexible families) would be expected to respond to change more effectively.

In 'rigid' families each member maintains fixed roles and rarely strays into another person's allocated role. The family has set ways of doing things. The power structure within such families is inflexible, leadership is authoritarian, and discipline is managed in an autocratic way. 'Rules are rules' and compromise is rare. At the other extreme, chaotic families have few clear rules. Lacking established patterns of action and interaction, they are constantly having to work out how to do things. Because there is no clear allocation of special roles or responsibilities between members, for example, discussion will be needed (and conflict may result) whenever a chore needs to be done. The power structure within such families is unstable, and there is no reliable mutual support between family members. The lack of rules is likely to lead to frequent confusion and, in the face of erratic and inconsistent parental discipline, children are likely to lack guidance.

The other dimension in the circumplex model is 'cohesion'. Families that are very low in terms of cohesion are said to be 'disengaged' while those that have extremely high cohesion are described as 'enmeshed'. Families classified in positions between these extremes are described either as 'separated' or

as 'connected'. The two mid positions on the cohesion dimension are associated with relatively good family functioning. Connected and separated families, in their different ways, avoid the lack of family unity and family feeling typical of disengaged families, while also avoiding the suffocating closeness found in enmeshed families. Members of enmeshed families identify with the family so closely, and the bonds between members are so tight, that individuals have little sense of personal identity (Davies et al 2004).

Extreme families

Many families can be identified as occupying an extreme position on one of the two dimensions of adaptability and cohesion. Some families, indeed, occupy extreme positions on both dimensions (they may be rigid–disengaged, rigid–enmeshed, chaotic–disengaged or chaotic–enmeshed). A family placed at an extreme on one or both dimensions is likely to have difficulty in maintaining a good level of functioning and in providing for the needs and personal growth of family members. Extreme families may well develop problems even without external pressures, and they are certainly unlikely to function well in the face of severe stress. Such families are likely to experience a crisis when they are under pressure and the health of family members may suffer as a result (Jacobvitz et al 2004).

Extreme families provide a major challenge for the health professional. Enmeshed families tend to be 'closed' to the outside world and are so used to keeping themselves to themselves that they are likely to regard all agencies and professionals with suspicion and disdain. The tight-knit nature of enmeshed families may mean that when one person becomes seriously ill, every other family member feels personally stricken. At the other extreme, in a disengaged family, there is little family feeling. When one member becomes ill, the others may resent the inconvenience and may attempt to carry on their own lives regardless of their relative's illness or disability. The professional cannot rely on such families to offer significant emotional and practical support to the patient. If a child or adult from a disengaged family is hospitalized, for example, the other family members may prefer the patient to remain in hospital until completely recovered.

The two extremes on the adaptability dimension are labelled 'rigid' and 'chaotic'. Faced with the illness of one family member, a rigid family will find it difficult, or even impossible, to make appropriate adaptations. If the father is incapacitated, for example, his routine tasks will be left undone. No-one will attempt, temporarily, to 'step into his shoes'. The family will find it very difficult to make allowances for the new situation and to evolve ways of dealing with new demands. Eventually, family life may become untenable. The challenge for the health professional is to help such a family to modify its rules and interactional patterns so that the patient is protected from undue pressure to 'carry on as normal'. At the other extreme, chaotic families present a different kind of challenge. The fact that they have very few established patterns of interaction, or problem solving, means that they are unlikely to be effective in dealing with a crisis such as that arising from a serious illness. Such families are unable to 'get their act together' even in normal circumstances and are likely to be completely thrown when a threatening situation arises. There may be a willingness to help the patient, but because family members hardly ever consult one another or engage in forward planning, their attempts to adapt to a changed situation are unlikely to be effective (Seligman and Benjamin Darling 2007). To assist such families in providing care for their relative, it may be necessary for professionals to make highly specific suggestions concerning the timetabling and allocation of tasks. The normal assumption that a family will work out its own routines and devise strategies for handing over responsibility, etc. does not apply to families that are extremely chaotic in their organization.

Some families that manage to adapt fairly well to a patient's illness have difficulty in readjusting when the patient is recovering. Thus a patient from this type of family may be maintained in the sick role long after he or she has returned to health. In some cases an individual's recovery from a physical or psychiatric illness threatens to disturb a precarious and convenient equilibrium within the family, and the family as a whole may then have a 'vested interest' in the patient remaining unwell. Family therapists have long recognized the fact that an illness may be 'useful' to a family (for example, by postponing serious long-term arguments that threaten to destroy the family). Family therapy addresses such issues by dealing with the family system as a whole (Carr 2000, Dallos and Draper 2000). All families maintain certain 'myths', most of which are harmless and some of which are constructive. When a family member is seriously ill, for example, many families develop positive myths about the quality of service they are receiving. They may regard their general practitioner as a leading authority in a highly specialized field, for instance, or believe that their local clinic has an international reputation for treating the relevant condition. For the most part, such myths instil hope, alleviate anxiety and contribute to good relations between the family and professionals. However, some families evolve a 'rescue myth' which can encourage passivity. Families that subscribe to this myth may believe that they only have to wait and maintain a 'helpless' stance and someone will come to provide all the help necessary to rescue them from their predicament and to solve all of their problems. Any professional who comes into contact with the family may therefore be considered as a candidate for the role of 'saviour'. Family members may believe that there is little point in actively seeking to improve the current situation before the 'saviour' arrives on the scene and takes over (Gayer and Ganong 2006).

Other families develop more hostile myths about the professionals involved in the patient's care and the quality of service being provided. Services and professionals are sometimes 'demonized' and blamed for any problems or deterioration in the patient's health. Such myths may jeopardize the patient's recovery in a number of ways, for example by lowering family morale, or reducing compliance with medical advice. It is important to recognize that some families have well-established suspicions about all aspects of healthcare and that these may lead to one or more professionals being unfairly 'scapegoated' by the family.

Healthy families

Well-functioning, or 'healthy', families occupy the middle ground in terms of both adaptability and cohesion. They are neither rigid nor chaotic, neither disengaged nor enmeshed. Family members have reasonably warm and close relationships with one another, each identifying with the family as a whole and having some sense of 'family pride'. Within such families, members share common goals. There is a general air of solidarity, but each person is also allowed to be an individual. Healthy families act as 'open' systems and are willing to accept help and advice from external sources. They interact with neighbours and feel integrated within the wider social community. They welcome professional help but are appropriately assertive when they feel that the level of service being provided falls short of the ideal. They do not regard professionals as 'saviours' and maintain an active role in the patient's care.

Healthy families share power fairly, and everyone is encouraged to share their opinions and feelings. Such a sharing of power, however, does not mean that all members are treated as equals. The parents work together as a unit in the care and control of their children. Roles within the family are clearly differentiated and are complementary. Tasks are assigned fairly and appropriately to particular individuals, but some degree of flexibility is maintained so that when one person is unavailable another person is able to take on some of his or her responsibilities. Family 'rules' are understood and supported by all family members, and infringements of these rules are confronted openly. Appropriate sanctions are applied firmly but without hostility or vindictiveness. Family rules are changed when necessary (e.g. as children get older) and such changes are brought about through a process of negotiation (Carr 2000).

Communication within healthy families is open and effective. Questions are clearly asked and plainly answered, and all transactions have a clear beginning, middle and end (in that order!). Family members are able to disclose their opinions, hopes and fears without anxiety and there is also a healthy respect for an individual's (or the couple's) privacy. Any conflicts that arise are usually resolved by negotiation and compromise. Healthy families are able to deal effectively with a wide range of challenges, for they have at their disposal a wide repertoire of effective coping strategies and are able to respond flexibly.

Conclusion

Although many families are devastated by serious troubles, in many cases both individuals and family units manage to endure the most formidable upsets and tragedies. Families often adapt to severe misfortune with remarkable resilience and resourcefulness. Thus, despite the fact that family life often produces extreme anxiety, fear or depression, and despite the fact that many families break down in disarray, the majority display an impressive range of strategies for coping with changing circumstances. But when a family faces a sudden major change, or significant adversity, the inner resources of the system may not be sufficient to maintain the equi-

librium, and support from other sources – from relatives, neighbours, community organizations and from professionals – can make a substantial contribution to the well-being of the family system and of the individuals who constitute the family group.

SUMMARY

- Family relationships are important determinants of an individual's physical health and psychological well-being.
- Families bring costs and benefits to the individual, but, on the whole, close relationships are seen as beneficial.
- There is a correlation between major adverse life changes and physical or psychological illness.
- The family should not be seen merely as a group of individuals, but as a unit in its own right, with events 'reverberating' around family members rather than affecting them on an individual basis.
- Families should be identified less by their structure and more by their 'adaptability' and 'cohesion'.

DISCUSSION POINTS

1. How does nursing practice (as you have experienced it) involve a consideration of family interactions, family influences and family styles?
2. Consider two women aged in their 30s. One is single (never married, with no children). The other is married with two young children. Discuss how their lifestyles might compare in terms of such factors as stress and social support.
3. Discuss the possible reasons why (as research has shown) a good relationship with an adult partner promotes an individual's physical and psychological health.
4. Using an (anonymized) example of a family known to you personally or professionally, use the metaphor of 'the family as an organism' to explore some key aspects of family life.
5. Compare the interactional styles (and 'family atmospheres') of two contrasting families that you know reasonably well (either professionally or personally). Try to make use of the concepts from the 'circumplex model' in your account.

References

Argyle M, Henderson M 1985 The anatomy of relationships. Penguin, Harmondsworth

Bebbington P, Brugha T, Meltzer H, et al 2000 Psychiatric disorder and dysfunction in the UK National Survey of Psychiatric Morbidity. Social Psychiatry and Psychiatric Epidemiology 35: 191–197

Brown GW, Harris T 1978 The social origins of depression. Tavistock, London

Carr A 2000 Family therapy. Wiley, Chichester

Carr A 2003 Positive psychology: the science of happiness and human strengths. Routledge Brunner, London

Cohen S 2004 Social relationships and health. American Psychologist 59: 676–684

Dallos R, Draper R 2000 An introduction to family therapy. Open University Press, Milton Keynes

Davies PT, Cummings EM, Winter MA 2004 Pathways between profiles of family functioning, child security in the interparental subsystem, and child psychological problems. Development and Psychopathology 16: 525–550

Duvall E 1977 Marriage and family development. JB Lippincott, Philadelphia

Frude NJ 1991 Understanding family problems: a psychological approach. Wiley, Chichester

Gayer D, Ganong L 2006 Family structure and mothers' caregiving of children with cystic fibrosis. Journal of Family Nursing 12: 390–412

Gray MJ, Litz BT, Hsu JL, Lombardo TW 2004 Psychometric properties of the Life Events Checklist. Assessment 11: 330–341

Griffith J 1985 Social support providers: Who are they? Where are they met? And the relationship of network characteristics to psychological distress. Basic and Applied Social Psychology 6: 41–49

Harper JM, Schaalje BG, Sandberg JG 2000 Daily hassles, intimacy, and marital quality in later life marriages. American Journal of Family Therapy 28: 1–18

Holmes TH, Rahe RH 1967 The social readjustment rating scales. Journal of Psychosomatic Research 11: 213–218

Jacobvitz D, Hazen N, Curran M, Hitchens K 2004 Observations of early triadic family interactions: boundary disturbances in the family predict symptoms of depression, anxiety, and attention-deficit/ hyperactivity disorder in middle childhood. Development and Psychopathology 16: 577–592

Kim HK, McKenry PC 2002 The relationship between marriage and psychological well-being: a longitudinal analysis. Journal of Family Issues 23: 885–911

Maybery DJ, Graham D 2001 Hassles and uplifts: including interpersonal events. Stress and Health 17: 91–104

Nye FI 1982 Family relationships: rewards and costs. Sage, Beverly Hills, CA

Nye FI, McLaughlin S 1982 Role competence and marital satisfaction. In: Nye FI (ed.) Family relationships: rewards and costs. Sage, Beverly Hills, CA

Olson DH 2000 Circumplex model of marital and family systems. Journal of Family Therapy 22: 144–167

Olson DH, Russell CS, Sprenkle DH 1979 Circumplex model of marital and family systems II: Empirical studies and clinical intervention. In: Vincent J (ed.) Advances in family intervention, assessment and theory. JAI, Greenwich, CT

Power PW, Dell Orto AE 2004 Families living with chronic illness and disability: Interventions, challenges, and opportunities (Springer series on rehabilitation). Springer Publishing, New York

Richter V, Guthke J 1993 Life events as indicator of change in life and as risk factor for cardiovascular heart disease. In: Schroeder H, Reschke K (eds) Health psychology: potential in diversity. Roderer Verlag, Regensburg

Rigazio-DiGilio SA, Cramer BD 2000 Families with learning disabilities, physical disabilities, and other childhood challenges. In: Nichols WC, Pace-Nichols MA (eds) Handbook of family development and intervention. Wiley, New York

Ruben DH 1998 Social exchange theory: dynamics of a system governing the dysfunctional family and guide to assessment. Journal of Contemporary Psychotherapy 28: 307–325

Seligman M, Benjamin Darling R 2007 Ordinary families, special children: a systems approach to childhood disability, 3rd edn. Guilford, New York

Tucker JS, Mueller JS 2000 Spouses' social control of health behaviors: use and effectiveness of specific strategies. Personality and Social Psychology Bulletin 26: 1120–1130

Veevers JE, Mitchell BA 1998 Intergenerational exchanges and perceptions of support within 'boomerang kid' family environments. International Journal of Aging and Human Development 46: 91–108

Wilson CM, Oswald AJ 2005 How does marriage affect physical and psychological health? A survey of the longitudinal evidence. Discussion Paper No. 1619, The Institute for the Study of Labor, Bonn

Wood W, Rhodes N, Whelan M 1989 Sex differences in positive wellbeing: a consideration of emotional style and marital status. Psychological Bulletin 106: 249–264

Recommended reading

Power PW, Dell Orto AE 2004 Families living with chronic illness and disability: Interventions, challenges, and opportunities (Springer series on rehabilitation). Springer Publishing, New York

Violence within the family

Neil Frude

Introduction

Although families commonly provide invaluable support, protection, nurturance and guidance for family members, the family is also frequently the context for many forms of abuse including physical (injurious) abuse, sexual abuse, emotional abuse and neglect. Abuse may take place between members of the same generation (marital abuse or sibling abuse) or between different generations (e.g. child abuse by parents, or elder abuse).

Table 11.1 provides an overview of some forms of family-based abuse. The columns specify particular forms of abuse and the rows specify the relationship between the victim and the perpetrator. It would not be difficult to quote cases which illustrate each of the 16 boxes in the grid in Table 11.1. Box 10 for example, would include marital rape, and Box 16 would include cases in which the needs of elderly people are neglected by other family members. This chapter will begin with a general discussion of violence within the family and will then consider four specific types of family violence: marital violence, the physical and sexual abuse of children and abuse of older people.

Violence within the family

The family is the setting for a substantial proportion of the violence that occurs within society. Most estimates agree that in any average week at least two children in the UK die as a result of a violent attack by a parent or caregiver; many more women are seriously injured as a result of marital battering than as a result of road accidents and street violence; and violence is a significant cause of bruising and more severe injuries among older people living with relatives. Estimates of the prevalence of the various forms of family violence depend to a great extent on the definitions used, and on diagnostic criteria, but it is clear from the available evidence that many forms of family violence are all too common.

Explanations of family violence

The issue of how family violence is best explained is somewhat controversial. Some authorities consider violence in families to be a 'natural' effect of the kind of society in which we live, and a reflection of the attitudes that adults generally have towards children and that men generally have towards women. Others, while not denying the relevance of the cultural climate, suggest that acts of domestic violence are 'deviant' behaviours that are best explained as aggressive responses to interpersonal conflict. Such 'interactional' explanations account for physical abuse by focusing on the relationships and interactions between the assailant and the victim, particularly in conflict and disciplinary situations, and attribute the violence to the assailant's

Table 11.1 An overview of some forms of family-based abuse

	Physical	Sexual	Emotional	Neglect
Parent to child	1	2	3	4
Sibling	5	6	7	8
Partner	9	10	11	12
Elderly	13	14	15	16

high level of anger and low level of inhibition regarding the aggressive assault.

In trying to understand particular incidents of family violence it is useful to bear in mind the distinction between hostile and instrumental violence. Hostile violence is driven by anger and the principal motive for the action is that of hurting the victim. Instrumental violence is driven principally by a desire for certain 'gains', with aggression being used merely as a means to this end. Thus the 'mugger' is aggressive not because he wishes to hurt his victim but because he believes that his attack will enable him to steal money. Some incidents of family violence are best explained as examples of instrumental aggression. A husband may be violent towards his wife, for example, because he believes that if he can make his wife fearful of him then he will be able to totally dominate her. Instrumental violence may also be used strategically to 'teach' the wife that a beating will follow if she dares to criticize or to refuse any demand.

On the other hand, most incidents of marital violence, physical child abuse and elder abuse are probably best understood as examples of hostile aggression. Typically, one person does something which makes another person very angry and, in the absence of sufficient inhibitions, the angry person then assaults the victim. This simple model suggests that in order to understand the nature of family violence we need to understand what triggers anger, how people judge (or 'appraise') other people's behaviour, the dynamics of anger, and inhibitions against physical violence. The model also suggests that effective interventions might involve strategies for reducing anger, for increasing inhibitions, and for maintaining self-control (Frude 1991).

The interactional model will form the basis for much of the analysis provided in this chapter, and

the discussion will focus, for the most part, on hostile rather than on instrumental violence. Four types of family violence will be examined – marital violence, physical child abuse, child sexual abuse and elder abuse. But first we will consider the general issue of why violent assaults occur so frequently in so many families.

Why is there so much violence within the family?

One reason why family violence may be considerably more common than street violence, or violence towards neighbours, friends and work colleagues, is that contact between family members is prolonged and is often intense. People who live together, eat together, sleep together and play together will be in close proximity for so much of the time that strong emotions, including anger, are likely to be generated at least occasionally. In addition, family members are locked into the family situation. It is possible to avoid or to walk away from an annoying stranger, but a crying baby or a dependent older relative cannot be avoided or ignored.

Irritating behaviours such as constant 'complaints' or 'nags' by one partner about the other, a child's persistent attention seeking, or a baby's continual 'grizzling' are likely to lead to extreme annoyance. Family members are interdependent, and the behaviour of one person will affect everyone else. A parent, partner or carer who invests a lot of time and energy in helping or caring for others is likely to feel aggrieved if there is no appreciation of the effort involved. Babies, children and the elderly infirm, especially, demand a great deal of attention and their care involves considerable 'costs' to carers in terms of time, effort and money. In such circumstances it is not difficult to appreciate that a carer might become angry in response to an apparent lack of gratitude or when additional demands are made. Thus a parent who is finding it difficult to cope with a demanding child may become angry if an infant soils a nappy immediately following a change, or if a child refuses to eat food that has taken a long time to prepare.

Anger may also result when there is a conflict over the allocation of space, money or other resources, and such disputes may be especially bitter if the relevant resources are very limited (for example, if the family is poor). Thus some marital fights concern money, with one partner being accused of wasting money (for example, on drink or gambling). Other conflicts focus on the allocation of duties, responsibilities and household chores. Those who feel that they are being exploited or 'taken for granted' are likely to object, and their complaint will often generate an angry response. Conflicts on such matters may escalate, with accusations being made and insults thrown, until one person becomes physically violent and attacks the other.

Anger is often preceded by the judgement that someone has behaved badly or has 'broken a rule'. Family life is governed by so many unwritten 'rules' that these are likely to be broken frequently even in families that function well. Thus accusations of rule breaking (or 'transgressions') are likely to feature prominently in family interactions. Such accusations are usually expressed in terms of what a person 'should' or 'should not' have done. The person being accused in this way is likely to defend himself or herself and may make a protestation of innocence or a counter-accusation. Real or supposed transgressions frequently initiate an episode that ultimately results in violence. Some parents even judge that very young babies are guilty of rule breaking and regard certain aspects of the infant's behaviour as 'naughty' and 'blameworthy'.

Family violence is not simply a reflection of the fact that family situations frequently generate anger, but also reflects the fact that people have relatively few inhibitions in the home situation. In most other contexts expressions of anger are regularly inhibited, or at least 'toned down', but people often have few reservations about expressing their disagreement with other members of the family, making complaints to them, or even threatening them. In contrast to a disagreement arising in a work situation, for example, or a dispute with a neighbour, family conflicts may involve little verbal sparring before a rapid onslaught of insults and disparagements focuses on particularly sensitive areas. Family members know about each other's vulnerabilities and therefore have the 'advantage' of being able to inflict maximum hurt.

Furthermore, inhibitions against physical aggression are often particularly low in family situations, and many people feel justified in behaving aggressively towards family members within the home. Parents may believe that it is their right to physically discipline children by smacking them, and some men maintain that they have a right to physically abuse a wife who has 'misbehaved'. If pushing, pulling or slapping a relative is regarded as accept-able, and becomes habitual, then regular low-level physical aggression may occasionally escalate to a dangerous level to include punches, kicks and the use of weapons. In addition, the constraints that normally inhibit violence towards strangers are often absent in the family situation. For example, a man may assume that, if he were to attack his wife, his child or his aged mother, his actions would not come to the attention of the police. In addition, his physical size and strength may eliminate any fear of physical reprisal by his victim. If previous assaults have passed without serious repercussions, then inhibitions about a further assault may be particularly low. Thus it appears that family aggression is relatively common because a good deal of anger is generated in family situations and because there are relatively few inhibitions that prevent this anger from being expressed in the form of physical aggression.

Domestic (partner) violence

The term 'domestic violence' is generally confined to partner violence, while 'family violence' is a broader term that generally includes physical child abuse, elder abuse and other violent acts between family members. Traditionally, domestic violence tended to remain hidden because this form of abuse occurred 'behind closed doors'. However, violence against women by their partners became a major focus of social concern as a result of pressure from the women's movement in the 1970s and since that time it has had a much higher profile. Despite this, it is still only a minority of cases that get reported. Thus in the study based on the British Crime Survey (BCS) of 2001, 31% of female victims of domestic violence and 63% of male victims had not told anyone about the abuse that they had suffered during the past year (Walby and Allen 2004).

The 2001 BCS asked a sample of more than 22 000 women and men about their experiences in order to ascertain the most accurate estimates of the extent and nature of domestic violence for England and Wales. The BCS estimated that 4% of women and 2% of men were subject to domestic violence in the 12 months prior to interview. Among women subjected to domestic violence, the average number of incidents during the year was 20, while 28% experienced only one incident. For men who were victims of domestic violence, the average number of incidents during the

12-month period was seven, although almost half of these men (47%) had experienced a single incident. These figures allowed the number of incidents of domestic violence in England and Wales in the year prior to interview to be estimated as 12.9 million incidents against women and 2.5 million against men (Walby and Allen 2004).

These are figures for domestic violence experienced during 'the past 12 months', and the lifetime (adult) prevalence figures will clearly be higher. The BCS estimated that one in five (21%) women and one in ten (10%) men had experienced at least one incident of non-sexual domestic threat or force since they were 16. These figures reveal that men, as well as women, are often victims of domestic violence. The principal focus of domestic violence has always been on women victims, and this is certainly justified because many more women than men are abused in this way and the injuries they sustain are often more severe. In the BCS, of those who were subjected to four or more incidents of domestic violence by the same perpetrator, the overwhelming majority (89%) were women (Walby and Allen 2004). However, it is clear that men can also be victims of domestic violence, and that some men are brutally beaten up by their wives (Archer 2000, Carney et al 2007, Dutton and Nicholls 2005). The rise of the men's movement, and an increasing focus on men's rights, has led to a call for men, as well as women, to be offered protection from domestic violence.

Domestic violence in same-sex partnerships

There has recently been a good deal of interest in violence within same-sex relationships, and the research has generally indicated that there are many similarities between the partner abuse that occurs among same-sex couples and that which occurs in heterosexual relationships. Thus Lehman (1997) suggested that the rates of violence are similar, that violence in gay or lesbian couples, as with heterosexual couples, is associated with such conditions as unemployment, substance abuse and low self-esteem, that the victims' reactions are similar (fear and feelings of helplessness) and that the reasons for staying with an abusive partner are also similar ('love', 'we can work it out', 'things will change' and psychological denial). At the same time, Lehman

pointed to certain differences, including a less understanding or sympathetic approach by police to violence in same-sex relationships, and a lack of support from peers who may be reluctant to reinforce negative attitudes to gay people.

A typology of domestic violence

Various analysts and commentators have focused on specific factors to distinguish between different types of domestic violence. Thus one typology (Johnson 2005) focuses on the power relationship between the couple and distinguishes between the following types of domestic violence:

- *'Situational couple violence'*: here, ordinary conflicts and disputes between partners escalate to violence. Violence reflects a flare-up of anger and does not mark a strategic assertion of power. This kind of episodic violence is probably the most common type of violence between partners.
- *'Intimate terrorism'*: here, one partner uses violence systematically to dominate and control the other partner. Intimate terrorism is a characteristic of the relationship as a whole. The level of violence involved often escalates over time and may eventually result in extreme threats and serious injuries.
- *'Violent resistance'*: this is violence perpetrated, usually by a woman, as a form of self-defence against an abusive partner.
- *'Mutual violent control'*: here, both partners engage in a battle for dominance and control. This type of intimate partner violence is relatively rare.

Explanations of domestic violence

Two principal models are used to explain domestic violence. Psychological theories focus on the personality, beliefs and habitual behaviour patterns of the perpetrator as well as on the nature of the relationship and interactions between the offender and the victim. Social theories focus largely on external factors in the perpetrator's environment, such as cultural attitudes to gender and power. One sociological model suggests that wife battering is a socially approved strategy that reflects patriarchy and is used to maintain women in an inferior position in society (Dobash and Dobash 1979). The psychological interaction model regards marital abuse as a hostile aggressive attack by an assailant on a victim, usually following a conflictual encounter between the two (Frude 1994). It is important to recognize that although the interactional model attempts to explain violent attacks as the outcome of the behaviour of both the aggressor and the victim, the blame for the violence is attributed solely to the assailant.

The interactional explanation

Psychological accounts suggest that the majority of cases of domestic violence arise out of partner conflict and that most violent marriages are generally difficult and quarrelsome. Many men who beat their wives have extreme and objectionable views about how a wife should behave and judge many of the woman's actions as 'out of order'. If a man judges his wife to be unsupportive, or believes that she is failing to provide him with due attention, consideration, power or privileges, then the extreme hostility that he feels may lead to physical aggression. The issue of power is clearly central to this analysis, and a wide status difference between the partners is associated with a higher frequency of violence, particularly if the man has lower status than his wife (Holtzworth-Munroe et al 1997).

The marriages of assailant–victim couples are generally tense and conflict ridden, and aggressive attacks usually arise out of conflicts and arguments (Goldsmith 1990). There is generally little power sharing within such relationships, and little discussion or negotiation. Studies have shown that even in those arguments that do not end in violence, physically abusive husbands are likely to be hostile and offensive in their manner and to accuse their wives of many misdemeanours. Conflicts between at-risk couples tend to escalate rapidly, and both partners may fight 'unfairly', each attacking their partner's self-esteem and making serious assertions about the other person's conduct or personality. Many abusive husbands are aggressive not only to their wives but also to their children, to neighbours and to relatives and strangers (Hamel 2005). They are likely to be jealous (sexual jealousy often features in dangerous conflicts), and they are typically low in self-esteem. Such men also have a high 'need for power' and they usually hold strong traditional ('sexist') attitudes regarding women and marriage (Frieze and McHugh 1992).

The violent incident

Gelles (1987) maintains that an assailant's attack is almost always 'spontaneous' (i.e. not planned), 'justified' from the abuser's perspective and 'interactional' (a reaction to some aspect of the victim's behaviour). (This last characteristic, which suggests that the victim's behaviour plays a key role in precipitating the attack, does *not* mean that the victim is responsible for the violence.) Marital abuse frequently results from conflicts over such issues as child discipline, meals, chores, alcohol, sexual conduct or performance and money (Hamel 2005, Pahl 1985).

Gelles found that physical attacks were often precipitated by some aspect of the victim's verbal behaviour (including criticizing, name-calling or gibes about sexual performance) and that these usually reflected the victim's own extreme anger. Partners become experts at identifying each other's weaknesses, and when one decides to 'go for the jugular' or to 'hit below the belt', then the other is likely to regard the allegations as outrageous and highly offensive. A man who feels that his wife's verbal attacks against him are vicious will often, in his rage, feel that he is fully justified in beating her.

Alcohol is often implicated in marital violence. Drunkenness may be a cause for complaint, and alcohol tends to reduce inhibitions, so that a person who is both angry and intoxicated is likely to attack in a violent and uncontrolled way. The abuse of alcohol is often a key factor in marital abuse and efforts to control the drink problem may be highly effective in preventing further attacks on the partner (O'Farrell and Murphy 1995).

Intervention

The physical and psychological effects of marital abuse are often extremely severe, and once a relationship has become violent there is a high probability of recurrent attacks. However, victims of domestic abuse are often reluctant to come forward for medical treatment or to seek legal help. One UK study found that, on average, women experienced 35 incidents of domestic violence before seeking treatment (Bowen et al 2002). In the study based on the British Crime Survey of 2002, only 27% of women and 14% of men who suffered injuries as a result of domestic violence sought medical assistance. Of the women who sought medical assistance,

94% were asked about the cause of their injuries by the attending doctor or nurse and 74% disclosed a cause. However, only 26% were referred on to a potential source of help (Walby and Allen 2004).

The availability of shelters or refuges has been a major contribution to the safety of women and children, but around half of those who enter a shelter eventually return to live with the man who attacked them. Various forms of 'treatment' have been developed, some of which focus principally on a violent husband (e.g. anger control training) and some of which focus on the victim's need to develop an effective 'personal safety plan'. A number of extensive couple-based intervention programmes aim to modify the couple's conflict interactions, to teach the assaultive husband anger-control techniques, and to help the victim to promote her own safety (Hamel 2005). Changes in social policy and law enforcement practices in recent decades (for example, the setting up of police domestic violence units and the adoption of a 'zero tolerance' philosophy) may have gone some way to reducing the extreme danger that so many women face within their own home, but their effect has clearly been limited.

A great deal more needs to be done, and it is clear that there will never be a universal solution to the problem of domestic violence. Some cases require incarceration of the perpetrator, some require one partner to acquire anger management skills, many cases require the partners to separate, while in some cases the best solution may be family therapy (Cooper and Vetere 2005, Hamel 2005).

Physical child abuse

Definition and prevalence

The 'physical abuse of children' refers to aggressive attacks made on children. Most estimates of the prevalence of this form of child abuse are based on extrapolations from injuries that are known to have been deliberately inflicted. Such methods, however, may lead to a serious underestimation, since only a proportion of injuries to children are ever reported, and many injuries that are attributed to accidents may be the results of parental attack. Some people maintain that any assault on a child which leaves a bruise should count as a case of physical child abuse, while others go further and insist that any form of physical disciplining constitutes physical abuse (in

which case over 90% of parents in the UK might be described as 'abusive' – Nobes and Smith 1997, Nobes et al 1999). Physical methods of discipline are used in the majority of homes and the average child is subjected to hundreds or maybe thousands of slaps before he or she reaches adolescence. The definition of physical child abuse is therefore a matter of some controversy. Some people equate abuse with any physical disciplining method while others maintain a sharp distinction between such 'ordinary' behaviours and those which cause injury to a child (see Chapter 12 for further information on associations between physical punishment and physical abuse).

Demographic patterns

Focusing on serious assaults (those which result in some degree of injury to a child), roughly equal numbers of boys and girls are victims of attacks made by a parent or caregiver, and the attacker is equally likely to be a man or a woman. Babies and young children are much more likely to be injured by their parents than older children (hence the term 'baby battering' originally used to describe physical child abuse), partly because the very young are physically more vulnerable, but also because babies are very demanding and need continuous care. They cry a lot, the reason for their crying is not always easy to judge, and it is impossible to 'reason' with them or to cajole, beg or threaten them in order to gain compliance. Factors associated with a relatively high risk of physical abuse include poor accommodation, poverty, marital instability and social isolation. At one stage it was hoped that information about such correlates (or 'risk identifiers') would permit the 'high-risk' families to be recognized before any damage had been done to the child, but attempts to formulate a useful 'risk index' in this way have not succeeded because, typically, they result in far too many 'false positives' – that is, many families that have many of the presumed 'hallmarks' of potential abuse do not in fact become physically abusive.

An explanation of physical child abuse

According to the interactional model (Frude 1980, 1991, Mammen et al 2002), physical abuse is best understood as a form of aggression, a hostile attack made by an angry parent who has been intensely annoyed, usually by some action of the child victim. The child's behaviour triggers a high degree of parental anger so that, in the absence of effective inhibitions against attacking the child, an assault will occur. The suggestion that the victim's behaviour plays an important role in the events leading up to an attack does not mean, of course, that children are to be held responsible for the injuries that they suffer. Certain children, however, are more vulnerable to attack than others by virtue of their physical characteristics, their behavioural style and their response to the parents' attempts at discipline (Mammen et al 2002). Parents who are at high risk of abusing a child include those with an aggressive personality, those who have poor childcare and disciplining skills, those whose beliefs about children are inappropriate and those who generally lack self-control (Frude 1991).

Briefly, the interactional model of physical child abuse suggests that a poor parent–child relationship is likely to lead to disciplinary problems, and that frequent and badly handled disciplinary encounters are likely to escalate in seriousness and may lead to habitual low-level aggression. Against such a background, it is suggested, it is likely that on one or more occasions the aggressive parent will lose control and attack the child so severely that the child is injured.

The effects of physical abuse on the victim

Some physically abused children die as a result of a parental attack, others are permanently scarred and some sustain serious brain damage. Even where there are no external injuries, an action such as the parent shaking the child severely may lead to neurological damage (Coles and Collins 2007). Blows to the head can also result in permanent visual impairments, and intraocular bleeding can lead to retinal scarring, squints and a loss in visual acuity (Cirovic et al 2005).

Abused children show a higher incidence of various types of behavioural disturbance, although some of these may predate the abuse (a child's high level of aggressiveness, for example, may be the result of abuse or may have been a contributing factor leading up to the abusive incident). Compared to non-abused children, abused children show relatively high rates of bed wetting, tantrums, aggression, 'oppositional behaviour', social withdrawal, disturbed attachment to parents, depression, low self-esteem, self-destructive behaviour and suicide attempts (Cicchetti and Toth 1995).

However, no psychological symptom or syndrome inevitably follows abuse, and some children who are abused, including some who suffer serious injuries, appear not to show any significant psychological effects. As Wolfe (1987) notes: 'a remarkable number of children seem capable of adapting successfully to extremely traumatic and stressful situations'. The degree of disturbance caused by physical abuse depends on such factors as the number and severity of attacks, the age of the child and the quality of the everyday relationship between the parents and the child. Protracted legal proceedings and a history of frequent placement changes are associated with a relatively poor outcome while factors associated with a positive outcome include the child's retention of a basic sense of 'trust' in adults and the presence of supportive relatives (Wolfe 1987).

Many victims of physical child abuse show evidence of delinquency during adolescence and, in adulthood, victims as a group have a relatively high rate of convictions for violent crimes (including murder and rape). Springer et al (2007) also showed that adults who were subjected to physical abuse in childhood had higher rates of depression, anxiety, anger, physical symptoms and various medical diagnoses. However, although victims are over-represented in these troubled and troublesome groups, it needs to be stressed that only a minority of abused children go on to lead a life of crime or violence. It is therefore very important to avoid the suggestion that an abused child is somehow destined to lead a life of assaultive lawbreaking. Although victims may be at greater risk than non-victims of becoming perpetrators of family assaults, most abused children do not grow up to become abusive parents or abusive partners.

Therapy for abusive families

Some parents confide to a professional that they are under considerable stress and that their child may be at risk, and many different types of treatment can be offered to such high-risk families. Parents who frequently use severe and dangerous methods of disciplining, for example, can be guided towards the use of more refined techniques that are not only more appropriate but also much more effective. Parents may also be helped to develop effective childcare skills, to manage their anger and to formulate a range of 'escape tactics' for emergency use when they feel that they might attack the child (Browne and Herbert 1997, Stevenson 1999, Veltkamp and Miller 1994). Some parents have strong pro-punishment attitudes and these may need to be challenged directly by parent education programmes (Cowen 2001).

Various techniques, including behavioural, cognitive, counselling and family therapy techniques, have been incorporated into intervention programmes. Although such programmes are often successful in bringing about positive change, it is often considered necessary for the child to be removed from the home, at least temporarily. While it is judged that there is a continuing risk of injury, the child may need to be accommodated elsewhere until it is judged that it is safe for the parents to resume their role as the principal caregivers (Dale et al 1986). The issue of removal is not easy, however, for there is evidence that this carries its own risk of adverse psychosocial effects on the child (Drach and Devoe 2000).

Child sexual abuse

Whatever criteria are employed to define sexual abuse, it is clear from prevalence estimates that sexual abuse is much more common than was imagined until recent times. It is also clear that inappropriate sexual attention leads to enormous suffering both during childhood and in the longer term (Haugaard and Repucci 1988, Oddone-Paolucci et al 2001, Stevenson 1999).

Most victims of sexual abuse are aged between 8 and 14 years, and girls are at somewhat greater risk than boys. It was always assumed that the vast majority of perpetrators of sexual abuse were male, but it is now recognized that sexual abuse by females is by no means rare (Elliot 1996, Saradjian and Hanks 1996). Whereas physical abuse is an aggressive act carried out in anger and intended to hurt the victim, sexual abuse is essentially motivated by sexual feelings rather than by feelings of hostility. Sexual abuse is sometimes, but by no means always, perpetrated by a member of the victim's family (in which case it is referred to as 'intrafamilial abuse'). The victim's older brothers are the relatives most likely to be perpetrators of intrafamilial sexual abuse, but other perpetrators include the father, an uncle, a grandfather or a female relative.

Most cases of sexual abuse do not involve sexual intercourse. Most involve other abusive actions including oral–genital contact, masturbation, fondling, exposure to pornography and indecent exposure. The term 'incest' is best used in the legal sense (in which case it refers to intercourse between two people who have a close blood relationship – neither need be a child). Once a child has become a victim of intrafamilial sexual abuse, the victimization is likely to continue for some time; incidents may be numbered in hundreds, and the abuse may extend over several years (Frude 1985). Abusive adults use a variety of strategies to overcome their own inhibitions and those of their victims. They may insist that the victim is 'old for her years' or play upon the positive and loving nature of their relationship. The sexual approach will typically be very gradual, and may begin with the perpetrator conversing on sexual topics with the child, or indulging in various kissing, touching or tickling games.

Explaining sexually abusive behaviour

Why do adults interfere sexually with children? The idea that those who sexually abuse children are all 'psychopathic', 'psychotic' or 'criminal types' can safely be dismissed. Evidence has shown that the vast majority of perpetrators of sexual abuse do not engage in other forms of serious crime and are not suffering from any psychiatric condition.

Neither is it true that all or most sexual abusers are 'paedophiles' in the true sense of that term. Paedophilia is a well-defined psychiatric disorder in which the person's sexual interests are focused exclusively on young children. Although it is true that active paedophiles abuse children, and are thus responsible for a proportion of cases of sexual abuse, the majority of those who commit sexual offences (especially perpetrators of intrafamilial abuse) are not paedophiles. Typically, their sexual desires are not restricted to children.

One model portrays sexual abuse as a variation of a 'normal' seduction pattern in which the age of the seduction 'target', the victim's inability to give informed consent and the relationship between the victim and the 'seducer' make the behaviour aberrant and unacceptable (Frude 1982, 1989). The model suggests that, either because they develop an inappropriate romantic passion for a particular child, or because they have unmet sexual urges, certain adults come to find a child sexually attractive. Some of these adults attempt to engage the child in sexual practices, usually through persuasion and the subtle exertion of power rather than through physical force. Power is a central feature of the model, since the adult is seen to misuse his power (his adult status, his 'rights' as a trusted family member, and his greater sophistication) to gain sexual access to the child. However, power is regarded as a means rather than an end, and the principal motive for sexual abuse, it is suggested, is not the acquisition of power but the pursuit of sexual gratification.

In an earlier section of this chapter we considered the issue of why the family context is the setting for so much violence. We can ask a similar question about sexual abuse, and suggest a number of reasons why sexual abuse is so often perpetrated against young family members. A child is likely to be trusting and compliant with a close relative, and some adults take advantage of their loving relationship with the child and regard the child as a legitimate target for a sexual advance. Family members generally have little suspicion that a child might be at risk from one of their number, and a potential perpetrator is therefore likely to have many opportunities to be alone with the child. Such opportunities can be used initially to implement gradual and subtle strategies that initiate the seduction process (these are labelled 'grooming strategies'). A child who has been initiated into abusive activities may then be especially susceptible to threats and bribes and may thus continue to comply with the perpetrator's wishes. The adult's position and power within the family may persuade him that even if the child were to disclose to other family members, his denials would be believed and that, even if his protestations of innocence were not accepted, his secret would remain safely hidden within the family.

Although some victims do protest and struggle when they are approached sexually, most behave in a compliant way, either because they feel threatened or because the approach by the perpetrator has confused the child about the nature of the interaction (Kaufman et al 2001, Meiselman 1978). The victim's acquiescence may encourage the perpetrator in the belief that 'she is enjoying it', 'she doesn't mind' or 'she won't be harmed'. Perpetrators generally act as 'careful seducers' rather than as 'rapists', partly because they have no desire to hurt the victim and partly because they realize that an aggressive attack would be much more likely to lead to disclosure.

Consequences for the victim

Sexual abuse may lead to physical injury. Attempts at intercourse with young children (or anal intercourse with a child at any age) may lead to bruising or to more severe injuries. Some victims contract a sexually transmitted disease and older girls who are subjected to intercourse run the additional risk of pregnancy. In the majority of cases, however, the abuse takes the form of masturbation, fondling or indecent exposure and does not lead to any physical damage or leave any forensic evidence. In terms of psychological effects, there is no 'post-sexual abuse syndrome' and symptom patterns vary greatly in nature and degree. Immediate effects are sometimes, but not always, traumatic and may include extreme anxiety, depression, various forms of behaviour disturbance and an abnormal interest in sexual matters (Haugaard and Repucci 1988, Oddone-Paolucci et al 2001). Some abused children continue to show symptoms into adulthood, and some victims who appear to be relatively unscathed during childhood develop symptoms much later in life.

It is unfortunate that many people believe psychological trauma to be an inevitable consequence of sexual abuse, for the relevant research has consistently shown that a significant proportion of abused children are resilient and cope relatively well following sexual abuse (Himelein and McElrath 1996, Putnam 2003). There is a danger that professionals who simply assume a traumatic consequence of abuse will communicate this assumption to the children in their care. Hunting for 'latent trauma' in children who present as healthy and well-adjusted is rarely helpful and may do considerable harm. The resilience shown by many children following sexual interference should be appreciated and enhanced rather than disregarded or undermined. In many cases, of course, the child *will* be in need of specialist psychological help, and any child who has been sexually abused needs to be carefully assessed. Following this, appropriate forms of intervention may be used, for example, to alleviate any feelings of guilt or depression, to promote self-esteem, to deal with any outstanding sexual issues and to foster relationship-building skills (Edgeworth and Carr 2000). Traumatic effects are more likely when the child is young at the time of abuse and in the relatively rare cases in which force is used. Needless to say, sexual abuse is an appalling infringement of a child's rights and any such interference runs the risk that the child victim may suffer severe acute and chronic psychological problems. Even when such effects are not apparent, however, the grievous nature of such abuse is clear.

Difficulties of adult survivors of childhood sexual abuse include mood disturbances (feelings of guilt, low self-esteem and depression), interpersonal difficulties (isolation, insecurity, discord and inadequacy) and sexual difficulties (sexual phobias and aversion, and sexual dissatisfaction) (Jehu 1988). Again, some survivors adjust very well in adulthood so that it would be a mistake to simply assume that a person who has been victimized in this way will experience adverse effects as an adult (O'Dougherty Wright et al 2007).

In recent years various therapeutic strategies have been developed to help survivors, and these are offered both by professional agencies and through voluntary and self-help groups (Ainscough and Toon 2000). Unfortunately, the sexual abuse of children is by no means rare, and any professional who comes into regular contact with families should be vigilant for evidence of such abuse. Child protection policies and practices are now very specific and there are well-articulated guidelines for all professionals who come into contact with children specifying what they must do if they suspect that a child may have been subjected to sexual victimization or other forms of abuse (see Chapter 12).

Abuse of older members of the family

Elder abuse is increasingly recognized as a common problem with serious consequences for the health and well-being of older people. It takes many forms including neglect (for example, failure to provide help with personal care), financial abuse, psychological abuse, physical abuse and sexual abuse. As older people become increasingly dependent on others, including family members and professional carers, they become more vulnerable to abuse. An older person's deteriorating health may mean that he or she can no longer live independently and if this places a high 'burden of care' on relatives then the resulting stress, resentment and anger may in some cases lead to physical abuse. Physical attacks on elderly people by their younger relatives are almost always driven by anger, with very few assaults being 'cold-blooded' (Gordon and Brill 2001, Zdorkowski and Galbraith 1985).

The UK Study of Abuse and Neglect of Older People (O'Keeffe et al 2007) surveyed 2100 people aged 66 and over living in private households. Overall, 4% reported having experienced some form of abuse within the past 12 months. Approximately one-third of this abuse was by partners, one-third by other family members and one-third by acquaintances and neighbours. The majority of those who had been abused said that this had had serious effects on them. In general, only a minority of cases of elder abuse ever come to light because both the perpetrators and the victims may be reluctant to report or admit such abuse. Perpetrators may be profoundly ashamed of the way they have treated their elderly relative and fear possible legal consequences. Victims may be unable or reluctant to report incidents because of their isolation, their sense of shame, fear of possible reprisal and the fact that, even if they have been seriously assaulted within the home, they may dread the thought of being admitted to a residential institution.

Certain characteristics of caregivers are recognized as risk factors for elder abuse (Levine 2003), including stress and physical or emotional exhaustion as a result of providing care over an extended period. Many of those who abuse elder relatives are clinically depressed and alcoholism is also frequently a contributing factor. Relatives who are financially dependent on the older person, or dependent on the person for housing, are at increased risk of becoming abusive (Lachs and Pillimer 2004). Factors associated with increased risk of elder abuse include poor health, increased frailty, sensory impairment (deafness and blindness), high physical dependency and disruptive behaviours, such as the wandering, confusion, agitation and anger that are often found in cases of Alzheimer's disorder and other forms of dementia. Many studies have suggested that older women are more likely to be abused than older men and that those who are over 75 years old are at especially high risk.

Health professionals and family violence

Health professionals are likely to come into contact with abuse victims through their work and have an important role to play in helping victims of family violence. For example, many cases of domestic abuse and physical child abuse are brought into A&E and many nurses working in the community will be confronted with situations that indicate child mistreatment or elder abuse.

In the traditional biomedical model of healthcare, injuries were diagnosed and treated without enquiring into possible social causes, but practitioners today operate in a more holistic or 'biosocial' way. As well as sometimes identifying the fact that abuse has been perpetrated, health professionals are often in a special position to empower victims, to offer guidance and to refer victims to appropriate services. However, they are sometimes very reluctant to take on this role, preferring not to 'interfere in people's private lives'. Abbott and Williamson (1999) found that health professionals' knowledge and understanding of domestic violence was limited and that they did not regard themselves as major players in helping women victims of domestic violence.

Reporting abuse in the UK

All professionals who work with children, including teachers and health professionals, are required to report any concern that they have regarding a child's welfare if they feel that there is danger of 'significant harm' (neglect, physical, sexual or emotional abuse). Social Services work closely with the police in cases of possible abuse.

Social Services departments are required to investigate reports of possible abuse, to keep an 'at risk' register and to take appropriate action to protect children. Such action can range from giving advice and support to families through to immediate removal of the child under an Emergency Protection Order. If, as the result of care proceedings, a court believes that the child is in danger of significant harm then it may order that the child be placed temporarily or permanently outside the family. In care proceedings the welfare of the child is paramount and all professionals must disclose any information affecting the welfare of a child regardless of the interests of their own clients.

Conclusion

Family violence takes many different forms and is alarmingly common. Partner violence occurs in a relatively high proportion of relationships and many children and older people are mistreated by those on whom they depend for support and safety. Some explanations of family violence focus on anger and conflict arising within the context of family life while other explanations focus on widespread societal attitudes to women, children and older adults. The physical abuse of children is probably best understood as an act of aggression by an angry parent, while child sexual abuse may be seen as a form of exploitation in which a sexually motivated adult engages in various strategies to gain sexual access to a child. Some cases of elder abuse reflect extreme stress precipitated by a chronic burden of care, while other cases reflect a deliberate attempt to take advantage of the older person's frailty or limited cognitive powers. The evidence suggests that interventions targeted at reducing family violence are sometimes effective, but a great deal of family abuse remains hidden. Health professionals need to be aware of the full range of family violence and to maintain vigilance. They are mandated by the agencies they work for, their professional bodies and by the legal framework, to follow set procedures when they believe that they come across a case of abuse.

SUMMARY

- Abuse within the family comes in many forms including marital, child and elder abuse.
- Estimates of the prevalence of the various forms of family violence differ widely. This is partly because a good deal of family violence remains undisclosed and hidden and partly because definitions differ substantially. Thus, in the case of physical child abuse, some authorities include any physical disciplining of children as 'abuse', whereas others only include attacks that result in injury.
- The majority of assaults, especially those involving marital and child sexual abuse, are carried out by men. However, some women also act as perpetrators across all forms of abuse.
- A significant proportion of older adults are subjected to abuse. The most common form of such abuse is neglect, but other types of abuse are also commonly found.

DISCUSSION POINTS

1. Why is there so much violence within the family?
2. Consider the immediate and longer-term psychological effects of child physical abuse.
3. Do you think that any form of physical punishment (e.g. slapping) is acceptable in the context of a parent disciplining a young child?
4. Why do you think so many women stay in relationships in which they are subjected to physical abuse by their partner?
5. Why do many carers neglect the needs of older people or physically abuse them?

References

Abbott P, Williamson E 1999 Women, health and domestic violence. Journal of Gender Studies 8: 83–102

Ainscough C, Toon K 2000 Breaking free. Sheldon Press, London

Archer J 2000 Sex differences in aggression between heterosexual partners: a meta-analytic review. Psychological Bulletin 126: 651–680

Bowen E, Brown L, Gilchrist E 2002 Evaluating probation based offender programmes for domestic violence perpetrators: a pro-feminist approach. The Howard Journal of Criminal Justice 41: 221–236

Browne K, Herbert M 1997 Preventing family violence. Wiley, Chichester

Carney M, Buttell F, Dutton D 2007 Women who perpetrate intimate partner violence: a review of the literature with recommendations for treatment. Aggression and Violent Behavior: A Review Journal 12: 108–115

Cicchetti D, Toth J 1995 A developmental psychopathology perspective on child abuse and neglect. Journal of the American Academy of Child and Adolescent Psychiatry 34: 451–565

Cirovic S, Bhola RM, Hose DR, Howard IC, Lawford PV, Parsons MA 2005 Mechanistic hypothesis for eye injury in infant shaking: an experimental and computational study. Forensic Science, Medicine, and Pathology 1: 53–60

Coles L, Collins L 2007 Barriers to and facilitators for preventing shaking and head injuries in babies. Community Practitioner 80: 20–24

Cooper J, Vetere A 2005 Domestic violence and family safety: a systemic approach to working with violence in families. Whurr/Wiley, London

Cowen PS 2001 Effectiveness of a parent education intervention for at-risk families. Journal of Social Pediatric Nursing 6: 73–82

Dale P, Davies M, Morrison A, Waters J 1986 Dangerous families: assessment and treatment of child abuse. Tavistock, London

Dobash RE, Dobash R 1979 Violence against wives. Free Press, New York

Drach KM, Devoe L 2000 Initial psychosocial treatment of the physically abused child: the issue of removal. In: Reece RM (ed.) Treatment of child abuse: common ground for mental health, medical, and legal practitioners. The Johns Hopkins University Press, Baltimore, MD

Dutton DG, Nicholls TL 2005 The gender paradigm in domestic violence research and theory: Part 1 – The conflict of theory and data. Aggression and Violent Behavior: A Review Journal 10: 680–714

Edgeworth J, Carr A 2000 Child abuse. In: Carr A (ed.) What works with children and adolescents? A critical review of psychological interventions with children, adolescents and their families. Routledge, London

Elliot M 1996 Female sexual abuse of children. Wiley, Chichester

Frieze IH, McHugh MC 1992 Power and influence strategies in violent and nonviolent marriages. Psychology of Women Quarterly 16: 449–465

Frude NJ 1980 Child abuse as aggression. In: Frude N (ed.) Psychological approaches to child abuse. Batsford Academic, London

Frude NJ 1982 The sexual nature of sexual abuse: a review of the literature. Child Abuse and Neglect 6: 211–215

Frude NJ 1985 The sexual abuse of children within the family. Medicine and Law 4: 463–469

Frude NJ 1989 Sexual abuse: an overview. Educational and Child Psychology 6: 34–41

Frude NJ 1991 Understanding family problems: a psychological approach. Wiley, Chichester

Frude NJ 1994 Marital violence. In: Archer J (ed.) Male violence. Routledge, London

Gelles RJ 1987 The violent home: updated edition. Sage, Beverly Hills, CA

Goldsmith HR 1990 Men who abuse their spouses: an approach to assessing future risk. Journal of Offender Counseling, Services and Rehabilitation 15: 45–57

Gordon RM, Brill D 2001 The abuse and neglect of the elderly. International Journal of Law and Psychiatry 24: 183–197

Hamel J 2005 Gender-inclusive treatment of intimate partner abuse: a comprehensive approach. Springer Publishing, New York

Haugaard JJ, Repucci ND 1988 The sexual abuse of children. Jossey-Bass, San Francisco

Himelein MJ, McElrath JV 1996 Resilient child sexual abuse survivors: coping and illusion. Child Abuse and Neglect 20: 747–758

Holtzworth-Munroe A, Smutzler N, Bates L, Sandin E 1997 Husband violence: basic facts and clinical implications. In: Halford WK, Markman HJ (eds) Clinical handbook of marriage and couples intervention. Wiley, Chichester

Jehu D 1988 Beyond sexual abuse: therapy with women who were childhood victims. Wiley, Chichester

Johnson MP 2005 Domestic violence: it's not about gender – or is it? Journal of Marriage and Family 67: 1126–1130

Kaufman KL, Hilliker DR, Dalieden EL 2001 Subgroup differences in the modus operandi of adolescent sexual offenders. Child Maltreatment 1: 17–24

Lachs M, Pillimer K 2004 Elder abuse. Lancet 364: 1192–1263

Lehman M 1997 At the end of the rainbow: a report on gay male domestic violence and abuse. Minnesota Center Against Violence and Abuse, Minnesota

Levine JM 2003 Elder neglect and abuse. Geriatrics 10: 37–44

Mammen OK, Kolko DJ, Pilkonis PA 2002 Negative affect and parental aggression in child physical abuse. Child Abuse and Neglect 26: 407–424

Meiselman K 1978 Incest: a psychological study of causes and effects. Jossey-Bass, San Francisco

Nobes G, Smith M 1997 Physical punishment of children in two-parent families. Clinical Child Psychology and Psychiatry 2: 271–281

Nobes G, Smith M, Upton P, Heverin A 1999 Physical punishment by mothers and fathers in British

homes. Journal of Interpersonal Violence 14: 887–902

Oddone-Paolucci E, Genuis ML, Violata C 2001 A meta-analysis of the published research on the effects of child sexual abuse. Journal of Psychology 135: 17–36

O'Dougherty Wright M, Crawford E, Sebastian K 2007 Positive resolution of childhood sexual abuse experiences: the role of coping, benefit-finding and meaning-making. Journal of Family Violence 22: 597–608

O'Farrell TJ, Murphy CM 1995 Marital violence before and after alcoholism treatment. Journal of Consulting and Clinical Psychology 63: 256–262

O'Keeffe M, Hills A, Doyle M, et al 2007 UK study of abuse and neglect of older people. Prevalence survey report. National Centre for Social Research, London

Pahl J (ed.) 1985 Private violence and public policy: the needs of battered women and the response of the public services. Routledge and Kegan Paul, London

Putnam FW 2003 Ten-year research update review: child sexual abuse. Journal of the American Academy of Child and Adolescent Psychiatry 42: 269–278

Saradjian J, Hanks H 1996 Women who sexually abuse children. Wiley, Chichester

Springer KW, Sheridan J, Kuo D, Carnes M 2007 Long-term physical and mental health consequences of childhood physical abuse: results from a large population-based sample of men and women. Child Abuse and Neglect 31: 517–530

Stevenson J 1999 The treatment of the long-term sequelae of child abuse. Journal of Child Psychology and Psychiatry and Allied Disciplines 40: 89–111

Veltkamp LJ, Miller TW 1994 Clinical handbook of child abuse and neglect. International Universities Press, Madison, CT

Walby A, Allen J 2004 Domestic violence, sexual assault and stalking: findings from the British Crime Survey (Home Office Research Study 276). Home Office Research, Development and Statistics Directorate, London

Wolfe DA 1987 Child abuse: implications for child development and psychopathology. Sage, Beverly Hills, CA

Zdorkowski RT, Galbraith MW 1985 An inductive approach to the investigation of elder abuse. Ageing and Society 5: 413–423

Recommended reading

Ainscough C, Toon K 2000 Breaking free. Sheldon Press, London

A practical self-help guide for adult survivors of child sexual abuse based on many years of experience in helping survivors. It investigates the persistent effects of child sexual abuse including guilt and shame, depression, fear of relationships and sexual problems. The book draws on accounts of survivors and offers a

positive and optimistic approach to help survivors break free from the past.

Browne K, Herbert M 1997 Preventing family violence. Wiley, Chichester

An evidence-based review of the facts, theories and intervention strategies relating to spouse abuse, child abuse and maltreatment of the elderly within the family setting. Discusses the nature and causes of abuse as

well as treatment and prevention measures.

Carr A 1999 The handbook of child and adolescent clinical psychology. Routledge, London

Covers a wide range of concerns within the field of child psychology, including emotional problems, learning disabilities, child protection, depression, drug abuse, divorce, foster care and bereavement.

12

Safeguarding children from physical abuse

Dianne Watkins and Judy Cousins

KEY ISSUES

- Defining child physical abuse
- Macrotheoretical perspectives on the causation of child physical abuse
- Microtheoretical perspectives on the causation of child physical abuse
- A framework for prevention

Introduction

There is an explicit expectation in contemporary British healthcare systems that all healthcare professionals, regardless of their expertise or the context of their practice, should possess the knowledge and skills to enable them to recognize and respond appropriately to concerns about a child's safety. Roles and competencies for healthcare staff have been jointly developed by the Royal Colleges of nursing, midwifery and medicine with advice from 'Skills for Health'. These have been published by the Royal College of Paediatrics and Child Health (2006) and are in accordance with statutory government recommendations outlined in *Working Together to Safeguard Children* (Department for Education and Skills (DfES) 2006). These roles and competencies are aimed at all healthcare professionals who come into contact with children and young people, reiterating how all have a duty to safeguard and promote child welfare. This chapter specifically focuses on safeguarding children at risk of physical abuse. For those who wish for more comprehensive information on all categories of child abuse, guidance on further reading is provided at the end of the chapter.

This chapter will define child physical abuse and explore macrotheoretical and microtheoretical perspectives, which attempt to explain the possible contributing factors associated with the physical abuse of children. Macrotheory includes reference to cultural and sociological factors, structural characteristics of the family and stress attributed to the environment. Microtheory incorporates parental biological and lifestyle factors, biological differences in the child and the socialization experience of parents. The chapter will conclude by presenting a framework to inform primary preventive nursing practice in the field of child maltreatment.

Background

Society's focus on child abuse as a uniquely contemporary issue, both in terms of numerical prevalence and social/moral intolerance, is an erroneous one. Awareness of this issue was initiated by an American, Henry Kempe, who first diagnosed the 'battered baby syndrome' in the 1960s (Kempe et al 1962). Since this time there has been a growing realization that children are meaningfully abused by their parents and others in society. Although many of the studies which attempt to explain the reasons why child abuse occurs are retrospective and lack the rigour associated with randomized control studies, there is agreement that the causes of child abuse are multifaceted, and in most instances cannot be isolated to one determinant (Browne and Hamilton-Giachritsis 2007). Studies in the 1980s tended to focus on a positivist approach which blamed the perpetrator, placing child abuse within a medical framework (Parton 1985). However, more recent literature reflects a paradigm shift away from a 'cause and effect' model towards an 'ecological' model, which incorporates a complexity of interactions between the individual, family, community and society (Belsky and Stratton 2002).

Physical abuse: definitions, effects and prevalence

Definitions currently used in England and Wales for children recorded on child protection registers can be found in the categories outlined in *Working Together to Safeguard Children* (DfES 2006: 37). These include physical abuse, emotional abuse, sexual abuse and neglect. Physical abuse is defined as:

> *Hitting, shaking, throwing, poisoning, burning or scalding, drowning, suffocating, or otherwise causing physical harm to a child. Physical harm may also be caused when a parent or carer fabricates the symptoms of, or deliberately induces, illness in a child.*

The National Society for the Prevention of Cruelty to Children (NSPCC; 2008), and Hanks and Stratton (2007) inform on the type of injuries that physically abused children present with. The most common external injuries include bruises from beatings and kicks, cuts, torn frenulum from rough feeding practices, black eyes and broken bones. Common internal injuries consist of brain injuries, retinal haemorrhages and internal injuries of the abdomen. Signs which the NSPCC (2008) state are a cause for concern include:

- injuries that the child cannot give an explanation for or the explanation provided is unconvincing
- untreated or poorly treated injuries
- injuries where accidents are unlikely, such as the abdomen, back and thighs
- bruising that looks to incorporate hand or finger marks
- human bite marks and cigarette burns
- burn and scald injuries.

Behavioural signs exhibited by children experiencing physical abuse may include:

- being sad, withdrawn or depressed
- having difficulty sleeping

- behaving aggressively or becoming disruptive
- showing fear towards certain adults
- lacking confidence and having low self-esteem
- using drugs or alcohol.

Creighton (2007) explains how child abuse statistics are obtained from the numbers of children placed on child protection registers in England and Wales. Each social service department in the United Kingdom holds a central 'child protection register' and children's names are placed on the register as the result of a child protection conference, where a decision is made that the child is at risk of significant harm and therefore in need of an interagency child protection plan. The primary purpose of the child protection register is to assist in the protection of children, and the statistics it generates are of a secondary benefit. Figures collated from the register should be viewed with caution, as under-reporting is a constant feature discussed in literature pertaining to child abuse (Creighton 2007). In 2007 there were 27 900 children in England who were the subject of a child protection plan (registered), representing 25 children per 10 000 of the population aged under 18 years. This rate has increased from 26 400 in 2006 and 25 900 in 2005 (Department for Children, Schools and Families 2007). Of the children registered in 2007, 44% were included under the category of neglect, 25% under the category of emotional abuse and 15% under the category of physical abuse.

This distribution is very different from that of 20 years ago. Of the children included on child protection registers between 1980 and 1990, those who had experienced physical abuse formed the largest group, followed by sexual abuse, neglect and finally emotional abuse. However, by 2004 children registered for emotional abuse nearly equalled those registered for physical abuse and registrations for neglect far exceeded any other of the three categories. Changes in child characteristics are also evident; the average age of a child on a child protection register for physical abuse rose from just over three and a half years of age in 1975 to seven years in 1990. Other characteristics remain static, such as the persistent over-representation of boys versus girls registered for physical abuse (Creighton 2007).

The Welsh Child Protection Systematic Review Group at Cardiff University, the NSPCC and the Department for Children, Schools and Families have produced a range of evidence-based information leaflets on physical child abuse that health professionals will find invaluable (Box 12.1).

Box 12.1

Information resources for professionals

Oral injuries and bites on children (2007)

http://www.nspcc.org.uk/Inform/publications/
Downloads/oralinjuriesandbites_wdf48007.pdf

Thermal injuries on children (2006)

http://www.nspcc.org.uk/Inform/
trainingandconsultancy/learningresources/coreinfo/
ThermalInjuriesOnChildren_wdf54671.pdf

Fractures in children (2005)

http://www.nspcc.org.uk/Inform/publications/
Downloads/fracturesinchildren_wdf48020.pdf

Bruises on children (2005)

http://www.nspcc.org.uk/Inform/research/Findings/
bruisesonchildren_wda48277.html

Safeguarding children in whom illness is fabricated or induced (2008)

http://www.everychildmatters.gov.uk/_files/7582-
DCSF-Safeguarding%20Children%20WEB.pdf

Safeguarding children who may have been trafficked (2007)

http://publications.everychildmatters.gov.uk/
eOrderingDownload/DCSF_Child%20Trafficking.
pdf

A macrotheoretical perspective on child physical abuse

A macrotheoretical perspective allows a broad approach to examining contributing factors associated with the physical abuse of children, one that moves away from a focus on blaming the perpetrator. It includes reference to cultural and sociological reasons and stress attributed to the environment (Watkins and Cousins 2005).

The influence of culture on child physical abuse

Authors discuss cultural norms as a possible theory to explain violence in families and punitive patterns of discipline (Browne and Hamilton-Giachritsis 2007, Korbin 2007). Intertwined with this is the 'privacy' of the family regarded as a cultural value in Britain, which often inhibits society from becoming involved in family affairs (Lyon 2007). However, while much discipline may not be regarded as a deliberate act of cruelty, it becomes difficult to differentiate between that which is considered 'tolerable' and that which is 'abusive' (Frude 1991: 176).

Historically, the physical punishment of children has been an accepted cultural norm in British society and continues to influence child-rearing patterns in many families in the 21st century. Smith et al's (1995) findings confirmed this where, of 403 socially diverse families with children, 97% of 4-year-olds had experienced physical punishment, 16% had experienced a blow that would have fitted the criteria for physical abuse and 75% of infants aged under 1 year of age had been smacked, with 38% being smacked more than once a week. More mothers than fathers smack their child at 79% versus 58% respectively, probably reflecting the greater time mothers spend with children (Cawson et al 2000). More recently, Ghate et al (2003) found that nearly 60% of parents reported slapping or smacking their child during the previous 12 months and 9% stated they had used severe physical punishment. Hobbs (2003) estimates that 150000 children a year experience physical punishment of a degree likely to cause them physical harm. This supports Cousins and Watkins' (2005) belief in a continuum between child physical punishment and child physical abuse.

Escalation theory offers one explanation for the association between physical punishment and physical injury. Quite simply, as children grow, parents are invariably required to increase the force they use when administering physical punishment. What starts as little 'taps' may escalate into smacks or even worse, and where this occurs, so does the risk of injury (Phillips 2007). Indeed, many parents prosecuted for physically injuring their child state how their intention was never to injure, just to discipline. Intentionality is discussed by Krug et al (2002), highlighting how an individual's violent behaviour against another, such as a parent shaking a crying baby to quieten it or smacking an infant for perceived bad behaviour, can have unintended consequences. Force is used, not necessarily with an intention to cause harm. However, such actions can result in serious injuries or even death; especially where parental perception of the fragility of infants and children is underestimated.

For those children who experience frequent, intentional and harsh physical punishment the associated outcomes are the poorest. Worst case scenarios involve the death of a child and the younger the child the greater the risk of death (Krug et al 2002). As a measure or indicator of children's life experience, homicide rates may be considered the absolute tip of the iceberg, or at one end of a continuum where 'taps' used to instil discipline are at the other. Bridging the two are behaviours ranging from smacks, slaps, shakes, scaldings, burns, kicks, thumps and beatings and at any one time an infant or child may experience one, some or all of these reactions from a caregiver. The morbidity associated with physical punishment and violence experienced behind the closed door of the home must never be underestimated. Frequent harsh physical punishment is also associated with a range of psychological effects including evoking feelings of rejection, provoking feelings of anger towards the perpetrator, engendering low self-esteem and inhibiting the development of self-worth, as well as socializing children in the use of physical force against others, and perpetuating long-term aggressive and delinquent behaviours (Gershoff 2002, Ghate et al 2003).

As well as the risk of injury from physical punishment, evidence suggests that children living in violent environments also face increased risk of physical abuse (Hester et al 2007). The Royal College of Psychiatrists (2004) report that in families where there exists domestic violence, approximately three-quarters of children witness the event and about half experience being badly hit or beaten themselves. At least one-third of children are injured when trying to protect their mothers, and in a quarter of cases, abusive men also exhibit violence towards children (Mullender 2004, Royal College of Psychiatrists 2004, NCH Action for Children 1994). Apart from the obvious risk of physical injury, witnessing violence in these situations can result in anxiety, tummy-aches, temper tantrums, sleep difficulties and bedwetting in younger children. In older children, boys may exhibit aggressive and disobedient behaviour and girls exhibit tendencies to become withdrawn and depressed (Royal College of Psychiatrists 2004).

The influence from living in violent conditions appears to influence disciplinary choices. Kanoy et al's (2003) longitudinal study found an association between high rates of hostility and marital conflict and more frequent and severe use of physical punishment of children. McGee (2000) found violent men less involved in childcare, less affectionate to their children and more likely to use physical punishment, and Kerker et al (2000) reported that

mothers experiencing domestic violence were significantly more likely to report hitting their children hard enough to leave a mark, compared with those not experiencing violence. Of concern, where both parents use physical punishment, children in two-parent families could experience significantly more physical punishment than those in single parent families.

From a legal and constitutional perspective Lyon (2007) discusses the absurdity behind the decision of the government to enact section 58 of the Children Act 2004 which legally allows parents to physically discipline children, while in the same year they also passed the Domestic Violence Crime and Victims Act to protect women from domestic violence. Perhaps even more remarkable is how women figure significantly among those who support parental right to continue to use physical punishment. However, it must be remembered that questions used to assess public views on smacking are often couched in terms of removal of personal rights and few individuals vote to have their rights curtailed, making it difficult to accurately ascertain public opinion.

Feminism also informs the cultural theory of child abuse, and maintains that violence by men against women and children in the family reaffirms the male position of power in society. This patriarchal view stems from a belief that men are of a higher order, which allows them greater power and control over women, who are lower in the social hierarchy (Browne and Hamilton-Giachritsis 2007). Feminists maintain that society condones these attitudes, and warns that ignoring family violence, particularly abuse towards women, may well perpetuate the cycle of family violence.

The influence of sociological factors on child physical abuse

Social and economic factors play a crucial role in child abuse, and are closely related to degrees of poverty, in that the more extreme poverty families are subjected to, the greater the likelihood of child abuse occurring (Corby 2005). Generally, studies find stronger correlations between poverty and physical abuse than sexual or emotional abuse, and when considering there are approximately 3.8 million children currently living in poverty in the UK, this is of concern (Dyson 2008). Choices are constrained for people on a low income, which in turn reduces opportunities for social contact. This can result in social isolation and poor social contacts for families who live on the 'bread line', increasing a family's vulnerability to child abuse (Browne and Hamilton-Giachritsis 2007).

Although it is known that the most severe injuries to children occur in the poorest families, the research base to support a single cause-and-effect relationship in the absence of other factors is sparse. Studies have found a positive correlation between factors such as poverty, unemployment, poor housing, low educational levels, lower social class and the abuse of children (Bentovim 2007). However, other authors suggest the relationship between socio-economic status and child maltreatment is inconclusive (Browne and Hamilton-Giachritsis 2007). Ultimately, poverty environments do tend to be chaotic, more highly stressed and lack resources; however, an assumption cannot be made that all children from lower socio-economic groups will be abused (Dyson 2008). Other social factors associated with an increased vulnerability to child maltreatment include social isolation, out of home placements, step-parents and spiritual possession.

Social isolation

Social isolation and lack of a supportive network have been recognized as risk factors and the nuclear isolated family identified as being at greater risk of abusing their children (Corby 2005). The 'quality' of social support is probably more important than the quantity, as a protective factor for parents. Social isolation may be more common in single female parents, who tend to be at greater risk of abusing their children, with over 40% of single parents represented in British studies of abused children (Browne and Saqi 1988).

Out of home placements

A retrospective survey by Hobbs et al (1999) of children in care requiring paediatric report for suspected, probable or confirmed physical or sexual abuse, provided details on a series of disturbing findings. Of 103 fostered children, 51 were diagnosed as suspected, 66 as probable or confirmed and 40 as having experienced physical and sexual abuse. Boys experienced greater levels of physical abuse whereas girls experienced greater levels of sexual abuse. One 2-year-old child died after being shaken by a foster parent. The authors' records indicated that children in foster care were 7–8 times more likely to be assessed by a paediatrician for abuse than a child in the general population.

Step-parents

Physical abuse of children is more common by step-parents, particularly fatal abuse, compared with that of natural parents. Egan-Sage and Carpenter (1999) cites step-fathers as being responsible for abuse of the child in 14% of referrals to social services, and 16% of those entered on the child protection register. The reason for this may relate to an inability of the step-parent to form an attachment relationship with the step-child.

Spiritual possession

Physical child abuse is associated with carers' belief in spirit possession of a child. Belief in spirit possession is defined as 'the belief that an evil force has entered a child and is controlling him or her' (Department of Health 2007: 5). A child may also be perceived as a witch and this is defined as 'the belief that a child is able to use an evil force to harm others' (Welsh Assembly Government 2007: 5). Alternative terminology and labels include black magic, kindoki, ndoki, the evil eye, djinns, voodoo, obeah and child sorcerers. The number of confirmed cases of this type of abuse is small; however, it is likely that a significantly larger number of cases remain undetected. Where it is present the impact on the child is considerable and the child faces risks which could result in significant harm. The most common forms of physical abuse include beating, burning, cutting, stabbing, semi-strangulating, tying up the child, or rubbing chilli peppers or other substances on the child's genitals or eyes. The abuse normally takes place in the child's home but it also occurs in places of worship where 'exorcisms' are conducted (Welsh Assembly Government 2007). The physical experience of abuse may be severe. However, such children also suffer psychologically, especially if ostracized by their family or community.

The influence of structural characteristics and environmental stress on child physical abuse

The United Nations Children's Fund (UNICEF; 2003) reminds how the transition to parenthood is an overwhelming experience for the majority of parents, who suddenly find themselves faced with the responsibility for the well-being of a small, often demanding and dependent infant. Adjusting to a new social role, while feeling exhausted, and add to that the stress from any financial and/or relationship difficulties, compounds feelings of inadequacy and can contribute to anxiety and depression. For the majority of parents, such feelings are transitory, aided by a social environment that is warm, supportive and which helps to instil confidence and raise self-esteem. Others, however, already familiar with a life characterized by emotional and environmental poverty, now face a mountain of new pressures 'ill-equipped, ill-prepared and unsupported' (UNICEF 2003: 11).

The result can be catastrophic, when feelings of intense frustration and stress can result in aggressive and violent outbursts, directed at partners and children. In the majority of cases the perpetrator of violent acts is the man, and in the worst cases, deaths of women or children are the tragic consequences of uninhibited aggressive outbursts. Two children die from homicide each week in the United Kingdom, mostly at the hands of their biological parents (Krug et al 2002). For children, the possibility of death by maltreatment is approximately three times greater for those less than 1 year old than for those aged 1 to 4, who in turn experience double the risk of those aged 5 to 14 (UNICEF 2003). The stress of caring for infants together with their fragility undoubtedly accounts for the raised mortality in this age range, providing a strong rationale to target support for parenting in the formative years of a child's life.

The frustration–aggression hypothesis (Frude 1991) may partially explain the large number of perpetrators from lower social groups who direct their aggression at innocent victims such as children. Frude (1991: 196) outlines the possible association between social class and child abuse as what he terms a 'distal causal factor'. This is described in the following manner: an individual's attitude, perceptions and behavioural patterns will be formed as a result of the situational stresses placed upon them. For example, being raised in a poor household, exposed to aggressive behaviour that is considered acceptable, surrounded by relatives and friends who share the same value systems and lack of exposure to the media or education which challenges these views, may well affect the child's perceptions of child rearing as an adult. As Frude points out, this person may be authoritarian and their childhood experience may

increase the risk of them abusing their children. Others dispute this explanation and comment on a 'subculture of violence' which maintains there is greater acceptance of violence and aggression in the lower classes, which leads to violence being considered a 'way of life' (Barnett et al 1997). However, little empirical evidence supports either the frustration–aggression hypothesis or the subculture of violence (see Chapter 11 for further information).

As can be seen, there are numerous macrotheoretical perspectives presented that attempt to explain reasons why children are physically abused. Causes are multifactorial and incorporate a complexity of interactions between the individual, family, community and society, and in most instances causation cannot be isolated to one determinant. However, as well as these macrotheories, microtheoretical explanations also exist which require consideration.

A microtheoretical perspective on child physical abuse

The majority of theories pertaining to child physical abuse have historically focused on the perpetrator as the causal agent. Microtheoretical perspectives follow this thinking and identify factors related to the individual, blaming them for the consequences of their actions. They fail to take cognizance of external variables that can influence, for example, parental disciplinary patterns and subsequent physical injuries (Watkins and Cousins 2005). Microtheory incorporates parental biological and lifestyle factors, biological differences in the child and the socialization experience of parents.

Parental biological factors: the psychopathic model

This approach to determining the cause of child physical abuse explains it in terms of psychological malfunction or psychiatric illness in the abusing parent, and it ignores socio-economic factors, or other possible causes of stress in the family, as contributing factors. It concentrates on psychopathology, that is abnormal behaviour or a mental disorder as the cause of child abuse. This follows a 'disease model' where the abusing parent is considered to have certain personality or character traits which predispose them to violent behaviour (Browne and

Saqi 1988). This predisposition may be genetic or acquired through personal socialization, such as experience of being abused or neglected as a child, continually observing violence, or through experience of being involved in aggressive interactions (Bentovim 2007).

Bird (1999) is positive regarding the ability of mothers with mental health problems to care adequately for their children. However, she acknowledges there are those who will be unable to cope, and at the extreme those who are capable of killing their children. In contrast with this view, others believe parents with chronic mental health problems may well affect their children's health. Parents who delude become a concern, as some may include the child in their delusions, or expect the child to behave in a way that is compatible with their thoughts. This can lead to confusion and fear with 'children becoming involved in a mad world where reality and unreality become confused and uncertain' (Parker 1999: 26). Psychological abuse in these instances may be unwittingly administered by a parent with a mental health disorder, resulting in possible psychological disturbances for the child. However, it should be emphasized that socio-economic disadvantage such as poverty, unemployment, poor housing, marital discord, etc. are often associated with mental health problems. As discussed, these issues also contribute to child abuse, and thus must be considered in the context of parents with mental health disorders.

The development of a 'secure' attachment between mother and child is extremely important, as it is predictive of the mother's behaviour with the child. Research indicates that in instances where a secure attachment is not formed, the child is more at risk of abuse from the mother (Ghate et al 2003). An inability to form a secure attachment has been linked to the mother's own experience of childhood, where a secure attachment between herself and her mother (or another carer) has failed to develop. This can result in 'transgenerational child abuse' that frequently occurs between mother and child across generations (Belsky and Stratton 2002).

Parental lifestyle factors: drug and alcohol dependency

The Advisory Council on the Misuse of Drugs (ACMD; 2003) reported that there are between 250 000 and 350 000 children of problem drug users in the UK, which equates to approximately 1 child for every problem drug user. The Council notes how problem drug use in parents has the potential to causes serious harm to children at every age from conception to adulthood. For younger, vulnerable children this can manifest as inadequate access to basic health services, even when ill, accidental smothering when unconscious due to drug intoxication, abandonment when parents go off to seek drugs or money, insufficient food, shelter and clothing and a greater tendency by parents to adopt authoritarian or neglecting parenting styles. The ACMD (2003) notes how the heavier the drug use, the poorer the parenting skills are likely to be.

A study by Wasserman and Leventhal (1993) set out to identify whether women who were cocaine dependent were more likely to physically abuse their children. A cocaine-dependent group was matched with a control group and the results demonstrated that by 2 years of age, 23% of children in the cocaine-dependent group sustained physical abuse compared with 4% in the control group. There was no documented evidence of neglect in the control group, while 11% suffered neglect in the cocaine-dependent group. Heavy drug use is linked with poverty, social isolation, traumatic histories, young age at the birth of the first child and minimal education. Thus, Hampton et al (2002) conclude that drug use may both reflect and exacerbate many other adversities, all of which impact upon parenting ability and capacity.

Biological differences in the child

Biological factors are thought to increase the potential for child abuse. Browne and Saqi (1988) discuss low birthweight and the premature infant as possible risk factors, in relation to the increased difficulties associated with feeding and handling small infants. The ill or disabled child is likely to make greater demands on parents, who may not be able to cope with the level of care required. The National Working Group on Child Protection and Disability (2003) reports that children with physical or mental disabilities form a large proportion of children abused and that children born 'different' for whatever reason may be more susceptible to parental abuse.

Biologically, children are probably born different, and according to the early work of Thomas and Chess (1977) they quickly exhibit different temperaments. The authors outline three distinct categories of temperament: the first category includes children who cope with changes easily, are placid by nature, adaptable and contented. These children quickly establish good routines in relation to eating and sleeping and are termed the 'easy' child. The second category relates to children who are more 'difficult', react less positively to changes, and are slow to establish eating and sleeping routines. They are more irritable than the easy child and cry more often. Once these children have adapted to something new then they become positive, although the process of adaptation may have been difficult for both the parents and the child. The third category is that of the 'slow to warm up' child. These children often have a passive resistance or ambivalence to change, showing neither a negative nor a positive reaction. Research indicates that children who fall into the 'difficult' category are criticized and experience more physical punishment than those who fall into the other two categories (Ghate et al 2003). However, not all difficult children are subjected to criticism and punishment by their parents; some skilled parents manage any demanding situations in a positive manner.

Socialization of parents

Social learning theorists suggest we learn through observing and then 'model' the behaviour of others, particularly those we hold in high esteem (Bandura 1973). Children who observe or experience violent behaviour in the home may learn this and model it throughout childhood and later adult life. The theory postulates that children exposed to parental violence as a method of resolving conflict learn this mechanism for dealing with difficult situations. Unfortunately it is unlikely that children who observe or experience violence are provided with opportunities to learn non-violent assertive behaviour as an alternative (see Chapters 10 and 11 for further information).

It is important that professionals appreciate how parents start from different places, encountering life experiences and circumstances that help or hinder them in their parenting role (Moran et al 2004). Sutton and Murray (2004) explain that where parenting beliefs are harsh and punitive, targeting interventions at improving parents' understanding and knowledge of child development and child care is beneficial. Similarly, Harker and Kendall (2003) conclude how a crucial step in preventing child

abuse is for professionals to support parents in their parenting role, suggesting that 'support should be early, be developed in partnership with parents, be intense, be targeted at those most needy and be home-based using appropriately qualified staff' (p. vii, Executive Summary). Practitioners wishing to promote safe parenting practices may find the following framework useful in the planning of therapeutic interventions.

A framework for the prevention of child physical abuse

An analysis of the many theories formulated to explain child abuse leaves little doubt that it occurs as a result of a complex interaction of individual, social and environmental influences that require an integrated approach to prevention. Browne (1988) discusses the association between social factors and relationships to child abuse. This author proposes that violent behaviour is influenced by:

1. Situational stressors – this may include difficult family relationships, unwanted or problem children, low self-esteem.
2. Structural stressors – this would incorporate poverty, poor housing, financial problems, unemployment, social isolation and health problems.

Browne (1988) expands on the effects of structural and situational stressors and suggests that the 'chances of structural and situational stressors resulting in family violence depend on the interactive relationships within the family' (p. 22). Good secure relationships may well act as a 'buffer' even in circumstances where the structural and situational stressors would appear to be raised. These protective relationships may well lead to a reduction in stress, and result in coping, caring behaviour. When the opposite occurs and insecure relationships are present within the family, then the effects of structural and situational stressors may be heightened, resulting in an attack of violence against a family member. The effect of the 'buffering' process is then further reduced, resulting in what Patterson (1976) describes as a 'coercive spiral of violence' (Browne 1988: 22). The family may become overloaded, as each aggressive and violent attack further aggravates the situation, leading to an increase in situational stressors.

Table 12.1 Situational and structural stressors of theoretical perspectives

Macrotheories	Microtheories
Society's view of child abuse	Individual differences in parent and child (to include physical, social and psychological)
Cultural norms and values	Parent–child interaction
The legal and political framework	Relationships between parents and significant others
Socio-economic factors	Psychopathic states
Structural characteristics of the family	Socialization experience (to include acquired models of parenting and methods of conflict resolution)
Quality of social support	↓
↓	**Structural stressors**
Situational stressors	

Adapted from the work of Browne and Saqi (1988), Cooper (1993) and Barnett et al (1997).

Table 12.1 summarizes the theoretical perspectives explored earlier in the chapter and categorizes them into situational and structural stressors.

Obviously any strategy aimed at the prevention of child physical abuse would need to incorporate the above stressors. One such model is that proposed by Cooper (1993), which specifically relates to child abuse. This ecological model, originally based on the work of Bronfenbrenner (1979), seeks to encompass the macro- and microtheories mentioned previously and tries to address these within a framework based on human ecology that values the importance of social contexts as influences on human development. Cooper's model consists of the following interrelated dimensions:

- the microsystem
- the mesosystem
- the exosytem
- the macrosystem.

The microsystem includes relationships, and the close 'day-to-day' experiences of an individual. In some instances this may only include the relationship between the child and parents; however, in other situations, relationships with others, such as grandparents or siblings, may be extremely influential. There may be someone else who is not part of the nuclear or extended family who would be included in the microsystem if they have a significant relationship with the child. The mesosystem refers to close relationships the child may have with those outside the home, for example nursery school or school. The child's experiences in these settings may link closely to the microsystem. The exosystem is seen to incorporate 'others' involved with the family who are influential, but whom the family may have little control over; however, they influence family functioning, for example social worker, health visitor, police, etc. The macrosystem includes the broader cultural, social and political perspectives regarding child abuse. It is inclusive of historical perspectives on child rearing, family norms and values, and legislation regarding child abuse, as society's view of abuse will influence all other systems (Cooper 1993).

This model attempts to incorporate the wider influences on child abuse, and prevents cause being attributed to one particular theory. It also highlights that child abuse is not static, but a dynamic changing situation, influenced by the interaction between the different systems. It should influence practitioners to move away from a narrow knowledge base and to look beyond the individual to the situational dynamics that influence child abuse. Table 12.2 links the theories reviewed to the ecological model discussed, outlining preventative strategies.

Table 12.2 Child abuse preventative strategies and ecological models

Ecological model	Preventative strategy
Macrosystem	i. Engage in political action to change legislation that bans 'smacking' and physical punishment of children ii. Work with the United Nations Convention on the Rights of the Child to protect children from all forms of physical punishment iii. Tackle domestic violence through developing a national strategy iv. Coordinate multiagency working in relation to protecting women and children from domestic abuse v. Work to change society's view of children and punitive discipline vi. Reduce the coverage of violence in the media as an accepted form of dealing with conflict situations vii. Tackle poverty through working at a national, local and community level to change policy and establish programmes to assist with financial hardship, e.g. food cooperatives
Mesosystem	i. Work collaboratively and in partnership with communities to identify health and social needs and establish community development programmes ii. Identify families in need of social support and establish community-based networks to help combat social isolation iii. Communicate effectively with nursery, school, general practitioner, paediatrician, etc.
Exosystem	i. Develop a multiagency team approach to working with families and children ii. Engage constructively with voluntary groups and services in the community iii. Perform accurate needs assessment and clarity in definition and reporting between agencies iv. Promote excellence in communication between agencies involved with the child and family v. Work in partnership with parents vi. Develop quality assurance mechanisms and measure the process and outcome of professional practice vii. Engage in multiagency collaborative policy development and research to further the evidence base on the prevention of child abuse
Microsystem	i. Identify mothers in the antenatal period who would benefit from parenting programmes ii. Identify those children who may be vulnerable to abuse because of prematurity, physical or mental health problems or disability and provide these families with multiagency support iii. Work in partnership with mothers to build self-esteem and confidence in child rearing iv. Establish home visiting programmes that concentrate on developing a relationship with the mother, reviewing their own child-rearing histories, and promoting sensitive, responsive and engaged caregiving to the child (Olds et al 1997) v. Establish parenting programmes in the community and on a one-to-one basis that seek to build the mother's self-efficacy (a belief in one's own ability to make life changes and succeed), promote the attributes of attachment between mother and child and provide education on appropriate modes of discipline vi. Diagnose postnatal depression quickly and treat as appropriate vii. Provide extra support to mothers and families with disabilities, physical or mental illness, or drug and alcohol misuse

Conclusion

The theories reviewed assist our understanding of how child abuse can occur. However, they are by no means inclusive, and do not account for all cases. The vicious unprovoked attack on a child, the deliberate affliction of burns and the sexual abuse of children are more difficult to explain, and certain types of abuse could well be attributed to psychopathic tendencies. However, some instances of physical abuse directed towards children may occur as a result of an accumulation of extrinsic and intrinsic factors.

It would appear that society's acceptance of violence may well lay the foundations for child abuse. Although as mentioned at the beginning of this chapter it is unlikely that cultural factors in isolation of other determinants would result in abuse of children, society's attitudes towards physical discipline most certainly contribute to child physical abuse and are an issue that must be addressed in the United Kingdom.

In the face of adversity, families living in poverty will be subjected to greater situational stress. While the literature suggests no direct cause and effect, the distal causal relationship cannot be ignored, presenting opportunities for prevention. The solutions to inadequate housing, low educational levels and poverty lie in a more equitable distribution of income, a redistribution of power and resources and an involvement in political activities by nurses. One should not ignore the social context in which child physical abuse occurs, and the dangerous circumstances in which people live and, against all odds, try to successfully rear their children. While we know the distribution of abuse to children is higher in lower socio-economic groups, it is important to pay due regard to the bias which may exist in the patterns of abuse seen among the lower social strata.

SUMMARY

- Child physical abuse is difficult to define within the realms of what might be considered 'normal discipline' of children.
- The predisposing factors are multifactorial and include the broader environmental issues and individual factors within the child and parent (or carer).
- Prevention needs to focus on an ecological framework that seeks to address the macro-, meso-, exo- and microsystems that exist within society today.

DISCUSSION POINTS

1. Consider factors that may predispose families to physically abuse their children.
2. What could be the contribution of policy makers and politicians to the prevention of child physical abuse and how could you work proactively to bring about this political change?
3. As a community nurse how could you work in a preventative manner with families, to help prevent physical abuse of children?

References

Advisory Council on the Misuse of Drugs 2003 Hidden harm – responding to the needs of children of problem drug users. HMSO, London

Bandura A 1973 Aggression: a social learning analysis. Prentice Hall, Upper Saddle River, NJ

Barnett OW, Miller-Perrin CL, Perrin RD 1997 Family violence across the lifespan. Sage Publications, California

Belsky J, Stratton P 2002 Ecological analysis of the etiology of child maltreatment. In: Browne KD, Hanks H, Stratton P, Hamilton C (eds) 2002 Early prediction and prevention of child abuse: a handbook. John Wiley & Sons, Chichester

Bentovim A 2007 Working with abusing families. In: Wilson K, James A (eds) The child protection handbook, 3rd edn. Baillière Tindall, Edinburgh

Bird A 1999 Families coping with mental health problems: the role and perspective of the general adult psychiatrist. In: Weir A, Douglas A (eds) Child protection and adult mental health. Butterworth Heinemann, Oxford

Bronfenbrenner U 1979 The experimental ecology of human development. Harvard University Press, Cambridge, MA

Browne K 1988 The nature of child abuse and neglect: an overview. In: Browne K, Davies C, Stratton P (eds) Early prediction and prevention of child abuse. John Wiley & Sons, Chichester

Browne K, Hamilton-Giachritsis C 2007 Child abuse: defining, understanding and intervening. In: Wilson K, James A (eds) The child protection handbook, 3rd edn. Baillière Tindall, Edinburgh

Browne K, Saqi S 1988 Approaches to screening for child abuse and neglect. In: Browne K, Davies C, Stratton P (eds) Early prediction and prevention of child abuse. John Wiley & Sons, Chichester

Cawson P, Wattam C, Brooker S, Kelly G 2000 Child maltreatment in the United Kingdom: a study of the prevalence of child abuse and neglect. NSPCC, London

Cooper D 1993 Child abuse revisited: children, society and social work. OUP, Buckingham

Corby B 2005 Child abuse: towards a knowledge base, 3rd edn. Open University Press, Maidenhead

Cousins J, Watkins D 2005 Macrotheories: child physical punishment, injury and abuse. Community Practitioner 78(8): 276–279

Creighton SJ 2007 Patterns and outcomes. In: Wilson K, James A (eds) The child protection handbook, 3rd edn. Baillière Tindall, Edinburgh

Department for Children, Schools and Families 2007 Referrals, assessments, and children and young people who are the subject of a Child Protection Plan or are on Child Protection Registers, England – year ending 31 March 2007. Online: http://www.dfes.gov.uk/rsgateway/DB/SFR/s000742/index.shtml

Department for Education and Skills 2006 Working together to safeguard children: a guide to inter-agency working to safeguard and promote the welfare of children. HMSO, London

Department of Health 2007 Safeguarding children from abuse linked to a belief in spirit possession. HMSO, London

Dyson C 2008 Poverty and child maltreatment. National Society for the Prevention of Cruelty to Children. Online: http://www.nspcc.org.uk/Inform/research/Briefings/povertyPDF_wdf56896.pdf

Egan-Sage E, Carpenter J 1999 Family characteristics in cases of alleged abuse and neglect. Child Abuse Review 8(5): 301–313

Frude N 1991 Understanding family problems. Wiley, Chichester

Gershoff ET 2002 Corporal punishment by parents and associated child behaviours and experiences: a meta-analytic and theoretical review. Psychological Bulletin 128(4): 539–579

Ghate D, Hazel N, Creighton S, Finch S, Field J 2003 The national study of parents, children and discipline in Britain. Economic and Social Research Council, London

Hampton RL, Senatore V, Gullotta TPE 2002 Substance abuse, family violence and child welfare: bridging perspectives: Vol. 10: Issues in children's and families' lives. Sage, Thousand Oaks, CA

Hanks H, Stratton P 2007 Common forms and consequences of child abuse. In: Wilson K, James A (eds) The child protection handbook, 3rd edn. Baillière Tindall, Edinburgh

Harker L, Kendall L 2003 An equal start: improving support during pregnancy and the first 12 months. Institute for Public Policy Review, London

Hester M, Pearson C, Harwin N (with Hilary Abrahams) 2007 Making an impact: children and domestic violence, 2nd edn. Jessica Kingsley, London

Hobbs C 2003 Physical abuse. In: Bannon MJ, Carter YH (eds) 2003 Protecting children from abuse and neglect in primary care. OUP, Oxford

Hobbs FA, Hobbs CJ, Wynne JM 1999 Abuse of children in foster and residential care. Child Abuse and Neglect 23(12): 1239–1252

Kanoy K, Ulku-Steiner B, Cox M, Burchinal M 2003 Marital relationship and individual psychologic characteristics that predict physical punishment of children. Journal of Family Psychology 17(1): 20–28

Kempe C, Silverman F, Steele B, Dregemueller W, Silver H 1962 The battered child syndrome. Journal of the American Medical Association 181: 17–24

Kerker BD, Horwitz SM, Leventhal JM, Leaf PJ 2000 Identification of violence in the home: pediatric and parental reports. Archives of Pediatric Adolescent Medicine 154(5): 457–462

Krug EG, Dahlberg LL, Mercy JA, Zwi AB, Lozano R (eds) 2002 World report on violence and health. World Health Organization, Geneva

Korbin JE 2007 Issues of culture. In: Wilson K, James A (eds) The child protection handbook, 3rd edn. Baillière Tindall, Edinburgh

Lyon CM 2007 Child protection in the international and domestic civil legal context. In: Wilson K, James A (eds) The child protection handbook, 3rd edn. Baillière Tindall, Edinburgh

McGee C 2000 Childhood experiences of domestic violence. Jessica Kingsley, London

Moran P, Ghate D, van der Merwe A 2004 What works in parenting support? A review of the international evidence (Research Report No 574). HMSO, London

Mullender A 2004 Tackling domestic violence: providing support for children who have witnessed domestic violence. Home Office Practice and Development Report 33, Home Office, London

National Working Group on Child Protection and Disability 2003 It doesn't happen to disabled children. NSPCC, London

NCH Action for Children 1994 The hidden victims: children and domestic violence. NCH, London

NSPCC 2008 Physical abuse. Online: http://www.nspcc.org.uk/helpandadvice/whatchildabuse/physicalabuse/physicalabuse_wda33606.html

Olds D, Eckenrode J, Henderson C, Kitzman H 1997 Long-term effects of home visitation on maternal life course and child abuse and neglect. Journal of the American Medical Association 278(8): 637–643

Parker E 1999 Professional challenges and dilemmas. In: Weir A, Douglas A (eds) Child protection and adult mental health. Butterworth Heinemann, Oxford

Parton N 1985 The politics of child abuse. Macmillan Press, Houndsmills

Patterson GR 1976 The aggressive child: victim and architect of a coercive system. In: Hamerlynck LA, Mash EJ, Handy LC (eds) Behaviour modification and families. Brunner/Mazel, New York

Phillips M 2007 Issues of ethnicity. In: Wilson K, James A (eds) The child protection handbook, 3rd edn. Baillière Tindall, Edinburgh

Royal College of Paediatrics and Child Health 2006 Safeguarding children and young people: roles and competences for health care staff. Online: http://www.rcm.org.uk/info/docs/safeguarding_children.pdf

Royal College of Psychiatrists 2004 Mental health and growing up: domestic violence – its effects on children, Factsheet 17. Online: http://www.rcpsych.ac.uk/pdf/Sheet17.pdf

Smith M, Bee P, Heverin A, Nobes G 1995 Parental control within

the family: the nature and extent
of parental violence to children.
In: Messages From Research.
Department of Health, London

Sutton C, Murray L 2004 Birth to two
years: risk and protective factors. In:
Sutton C, Utting D, Farrington D
(eds) 2004 Support from the start:
working with young children and
their families to reduce the risks
of crime and anti-social behaviour.
Department for Education and
Skills, London

Thomas A, Chess S 1977 Temperament
and development. Brunner/Mazel,
New York

United Nations Children's Fund 2003
A league table of child maltreatment
deaths in rich nations: Innocenti
Report Card No. 5. UNICEF,
Florence

Wasserman DR, Leventhal JM 1993
Maltreatment of children born
to cocaine dependent mothers.
American Journal of the Disabled
Child 147(12): 1324–1328

Watkins D, Cousins J 2005 Child
physical punishment, injury and
abuse (part two). Community
Practitioner 78(9): 318–321

Welsh Assembly Government 2007
Safeguarding children from abuse
linked to a belief in spirit possession:
draft guidance for consultation.
HMSO, Cardiff

Recommended reading

Corby B 2005 Child abuse: towards
a knowledge base, 3rd edn. Open
University Press, Maidenhead
*This is the third edition of a
bestselling text. This edition covers
aspects of abuse including
institutional abuse, preventative
approaches to protect children
from abuse and contemporary
research evidence on the effect on
children from abuse. A valuable text*
*for all practitioners working with
children.*

Howe D 2005 Child abuse and neglect:
attachment, development and
intervention. Palgrave Macmillan,
London
*For those students wishing to gain a
greater appreciation of associations
between attachment theory and child
abuse, this text will introduce key
theories and concepts and will enable*
*students to gain a broader
appreciation of this subject.*

Wilson K, James A (eds) 2007 The
child protection handbook, 3rd edn.
Baillière Tindall, Edinburgh
*An excellent source of information.
Students will find this work both
comprehensive and informative,
covering research, policy and
practice.*

Section **Four**

Shifting the boundaries of public health and community practice

This section explores the boundaries of practice in specialist community public health nursing as outlined by the Nursing and Midwifery Council (NMC) in 2004 and the areas included in the Community Specialist Practice Framework outlined by the United Kingdom Central Council for Nursing, Midwifery and Health Visiting (UKCC; now the NMC) in 1996. There is an addition to this section, over and above that presented in the second edition of the book. The area of occupational health nursing has been included as it is now considered part of the specialist community public health nursing framework provided by the NMC.

The first chapter provides an overview of the changing role of the practice nurse, following its interesting evolution, through to present-day practice. This is followed by a chapter that focuses on district nursing and how it can rise to the challenge of providing nursing care to patients with complex health needs.

The next three chapters discuss the three strands of specialist community public health nurse practice, namely that of health visiting, school nursing

and occupational health nursing. The chapter on health visiting outlines the role and discusses the tensions between empowerment and risk management that practitioners face when working to promote health, while protecting the health of vulnerable groups in society. The school nursing chapter discusses the constraints on the development of the profession, the diversity of the role and the potential for school nurses to contribute to the public health agenda. The chapter on occupational health nursing introduces the broad remit of this role and debates how the NMC has fitted this discipline into a public health nursing framework.

Following on from this, the chapter on community mental health nursing discusses policy development and how it has shaped current practice. The next chapter on community learning disability nursing describes the needs of clients with a learning disability, the move to community care and the role of the community learning disability nurse in empowering clients. Finally the chapter on community children's nursing outlines various models of service provision across the United Kingdom and discusses the concept of family nursing. This section is by no means inclusive of all issues influencing public health and community nursing practice. It is meant to provide a 'springboard' for discussion and debate and to promote an understanding of the dimensions of nursing currently practised in community, primary care and workplace environments.

References

Nursing and Midwifery Council 2004 Standards of proficiency for specialist community public health nurses: protecting the public through professional standards. The Stationery Office, London

UKCC 1996 Council's standards for education and practice following PREP: transitional arrangements – Specialist Practitioner Title/ Specialist Qualification. UKCC, London

Practice nursing

Judith Carrier

KEY ISSUES

- Historical development
- Education
- Policy and practice across the four nations
- Future developments

Introduction

When Linda Carey last updated this chapter in 2003, she wrote that 'practice nursing has reached an important pinnacle in its development; no longer struggling to identify a clear role for itself, it has emerged as a discipline in its own right, acknowledged as making a significant contribution to the provision of care' (p. 211). For many years practice nurses strove to develop their own voice and identity, the role being viewed for a long time as one that was pursued only by part-timers and a role that was inferior to the more fashionable nursing roles in other areas of the NHS, particularly the acute sector. Indeed Martin (2007) cites Baker (1988) who once made the comment that practice nursing was 'not a step forward in a progressive career'! In part this was due to the origins of practice nursing, the role originally evolving from GPs' wives, who were nurses, assisting them in their everyday practice and also from the 'treatment room' services provided by district nursing teams. In the community sector, roles such as district nursing and health visiting (now designated specialist practitioners in community public health nursing) were seen as having more defined career pathways and were thus a more fashionable calling. This view has now

changed; the Department of Health (1990) GP contract provided the first impetus for nurses interested in a primary care career to move away from other nursing roles into general practice. Because of both practice nurses themselves who have lobbied to ensure they are a recognized discipline, and the influence of subsequent governmental healthcare policy, the role has continued to expand. Practice nursing is now seen as a popular career choice, not only for those well established in their nursing career, but also for those newly qualified nurses just starting out in their profession. A valid career pathway is rapidly developing, enabling those who enter the profession to have specific goals towards which they can aim, planning their personal and educational development needs towards a definite purpose. Without doubt it is a role that is shifting the boundaries of community practice.

Historical development

General practice nursing has evolved rapidly over the past 16 years, with numbers across the UK increasing from 3500 in 1990 to 24 959 in 2003 (Royal College of General Practitioners (RCGP) 2004). The United Kingdom Central Council for Nursing, Midwifery and Health Visiting's (now the Nursing and Midwifery Council, NMC) acknowledgement of general practice nursing as a community specialism in 1994 gave recognition to the role, ensuring qualified practice nurses had equality with other community nurses, such as district nurses, specialist community public health nurses and community mental health nurses, as specialist practitioners. Individual practice nurses themselves, however, have much to be proud of, having adapted and shaped their role to meet the needs of care provision in primary care and consequently having developed their role from one of delegated work to that of provider of specialist healthcare (Carey 2003). The role has continued to evolve and, with the current focus on the moving of services from secondary to primary care, is now viewed as increasingly important, practice nurses often taking on the 'gatekeeping' role, triaging patients requesting same-day care (Cullen 2005) in addition to their more traditional roles. The practice nurse role is varied and diverse but remains one that is continually growing, from originally concentrating on delegated general treatment room duties (e.g. wound management, venepuncture, injections and ear care) to the current picture of nurse-run clinics in areas such as public health and long-term conditions management. In addition, there is a recently increasing emphasis on providing first contact care in the form of triage, advanced assessment, management of minor illnesses and injuries, and since the advent of independent nurse prescribing yet another new role is opening up, that of medicines management.

The new General Medical Services (nGMS) contract (Department of Health 2003) created a further expansion of the role, with practice nurses increasingly taking on the responsibility of meeting the demands of the Quality and Outcomes Framework (see Chapter 2 for further information on developments in primary care). This has created new challenges for practice nursing along with further opportunities. An emphasis on skill mix has been seen as an integral feature of NHS reform and is seen as being particularly relevant in the context of the primary healthcare team. An RCGP information sheet on practice nurses, published in 2004, suggested that an estimated 10% of workload could be transferred from GPs to nurses by 2007/2008 with a consequent increase in the ratio of practice nurses to GPs from 60 per 100 to 70 per 100. More recent figures have indicated that practice nurses cover an estimated 28% of total patient contacts in practice, compared to 60% covered by GPs (Technical Steering Committee 2006/2007) and work an average of 22.8 hours a week in comparison to the 38.2 hours per week worked by GPs. An emerging picture of skill mix among practice nurses themselves is now being seen, with many practices now employing a team of nurses from healthcare assistants to

Table 13.1   Nursing skill mix in primary care

Nurse practitioner/specialist practitioner General practice nursing Band 7/8 (G/H grade)	Degree/masters level education specific to general practice nursing/primary care
Specialist practitioner: general practice Nursing/practice nurse Band 6 (E/F grade)	Diploma level education specific to general practice nursing/primary care
Practice nurse Band 5 (D grade)	Registered nurse, no qualifications specific to general practice nursing
Healthcare assistants Band 3	NVQ or other qualification specific to working in primary care
Healthcare assistants Band 2	No qualifications specific to working in primary care

specialist practice nurses and nurse practitioners (Table 13.1).

Cross (2006) noted that the Wanless Review suggests that up to 70% of the work currently undertaken by GPs might be moved to general practice nurses with the expectation that nurses working in these extended roles will:

- enhance the quality of services provided by doctors
- safely substitute for doctors in a wide array of services, thus reducing demand for doctors
- reduce the direct costs of service. (Cross 2006: 420)

Carey (2003: 213) commented that 'delegation and relinquishment of traditional roles is crucial to the provision of primary care'. However, she argued that while taking on these delegated duties, it is important that practice nurses furthermore continue to establish their own knowledge base and define their own role, determining how they can contribute to care delivery in primary care, rather than the role becoming one that is simply based on delegation of GPs' work.

This chapter will provide a four-nation perspective, first discussing educational preparation for the role, then providing an overview of the NHS policies that have both shaped and had an impact on practice nurse development. Case studies are included to demonstrate good practice and to encourage reflection. The reader will be updated regarding the latest NHS reforms that have influenced practice nursing in recent years, referring to Carey's 2003 chapter. There will be an update on the current position in which practice nurses find themselves and finally there will be a discussion as to how the role may look in the future.

Education

General

Preparation for the role of general practice nurse is wide-ranging, with practice nurses possessing a variety of educational qualifications varying from attendance on study days and foundation programmes to diploma qualifications specific to practice nursing (for example, asthma, diabetes and coronary heart disease), to degree level specialist practitioner preparation. Unlike other community specialisms, there is no mandatory training requirement to adopt the title of 'general practice nurse', other than initial registration with the NMC as a registered nurse. The same applies to those practice nurses adopting the title 'nurse practitioner'; some have been prepared at diploma, degree and masters level but others have received only in-house training, adopting the title without having a specific qualification in order to undertake the role. The NMC specialist practitioner programme made transitional arrangements for experienced practice nurses to acquire a recordable qualification when its policy for community nurse education came into operation in 1996; since this time the route to specialist practitioner qualification has been at degree level provided by higher education institutions (HEIs). However, in light of the NMC's current review of the specialist practice qualification (SPQ), many HEIs are revisiting their current programmes and will need to ensure that future programmes meet the needs of nurses both working in and new to general practice.

The RCN (2004a) guidance on good employment practice notes that the nGMS contract provides for resources to support role development and higher quality services and enables practice nurses to expand their interest in general practice in a variety of ways including:

- becoming more involved in the business side of the practice
- taking a strategic role within primary care
- becoming partners within the practice. (RCN 2004a: 8)

In addition to this, the RCN (2004a) guidance notes that the nGMS contract opens up other new opportunities to practice nursing such as becoming sub- or specialist providers of services such as sexual health, minor surgery and vaccinations and immunizations (see Case study 13.1). However, in order for practice nurses to develop apposite skills, education providers need to offer a suitable curriculum.

England

Many HEIs in England have discontinued, or are reviewing, their SPQ programmes and are instead developing new curricula that embrace the wider range of clinical competencies required to meet the needs of today's practice nurses, recognizing the evolution of practice nursing into a more integrated primary care role (Ruscoe 2006).

Although small, a study undertaken by Crossman (2006) to investigate the impact of the nGMS contract on the role and educational needs of practice nurses working in one primary care trust (PCT) in England is worth noting, as this appears to be an area in which little research has been undertaken. The results indicated that the practice nurse participants reported a definite change in their role since the advent of the contract, but felt that there was a lack of support available for them to explore new roles. Regarding the training topics they requested, to support the role developments they identified, training in minor illness and injuries was given maximum priority, with chronic disease topics also being high on the agenda. Surprisingly, there was less demand for training in mental health, particularly as the Mental Health Foundation (2006) note that one in four people experience some kind of mental health problem in the course of a year and nearly a third of all patients seen by GPs have common mental health problems such as depression and anxiety. Mental health and depression have been included in the 2006 Quality and Outcomes Framework in the nGMS contract and will increasingly become part of the practice nurse role. Initiatives to improve practice nurses' knowledge in this area are already being developed with a distance learning course on mental health and well-being

Case study 13.1

Jill, a practice nurse with 15 years' experience, first took on the role as a part-time post when her children were small as the hours suited her family life and a local practice was recruiting nurses to provide extra health promotion services following the 1990 GP contract. Over the years Jill has undertaken numerous courses, initially occasional study days but as the children grew older and she had more time to spend on her career she undertook diploma level courses related to her role as a practice nurse.

One area in which she became particularly interested was that of sexual health; working in a socially deprived area with a large adolescent population, this was something where she felt the need wasn't being met. With the support of the practice that part funded her, she commenced and successfully completed a master's degree in sexual health issues.

With the experience she gained on the course she was able to set up a sexual health service for the patients within her practice, providing not only advice but also screening services. This enabled prompt treatment for patients and reduced the pressure on the genitourinary medicine clinic at the nearest district hospital, which was 20 miles away. With the advent of the nGMS contract in 2004 the five local practices in Jill's area decided to opt out of providing this more specialized sexual health care, feeling that they had enough to do meeting the requirements of the Quality and Outcomes Framework.

The local primary care trust, as part of their sexual health strategy, invited local providers to tender for the service. Jill, seeing an opportunity, put forward a business plan to provide specialized sexual health services to the local population. Jill's offer was accepted and she now runs a very successful sexual health service covering the population of all five practices.

Discussion points

1. What specialist skills, knowledge or interest do you have that could be used to develop local enhanced services?

2. What knowledge do you have of the population needs in your area; have you undertaken a recent practice profile?

---

specifically aimed at practice nurses now available (Scanlan 2007).

A significant development in practice nurse education (Cross 2006) has been the commissioning by The Working in Partnership Programme (WIPP) in 2006 of the development of an online, interactive toolkit to highlight good practice in general practice nursing. This comprises a number of tools to provide practical guidance about improving clinical practice. Campbell (2007: 2) highlights the six key areas that are addressed within the toolkit:

- *The development of the general practice nurse role*: this embraces national polices, career structures, role definitions, maximizing staff potential, bank staff and skill mix.
- *Employment of general practice nurses*: this includes advertising, recruitment and retention, contracts, terms and conditions of employment, appraisals and facilitating the adoption of Agenda for Change.
- *Competence of general practice nurses*: this provides examples of competence at varying levels linked to the Knowledge and Skills Framework and defines and measures competency.
- *Career, education and professional development of general practice nurses*: this advises on

formal and informal ways of learning, identification of development needs, learning opportunities, clinical supervision and career pathways.

- *Integration of general practice nurses into the wider community nursing workforce*: this discusses integrated teams, various models to promote integration, liaison with the voluntary and independent care providers.
- *Quality improvement and evaluation*: this draws attention to the importance of team and individual appraisal, clinical governance and patient satisfaction.

Since its launch in October 2006 the WIPP website notes that there have been over 200 000 downloads and that it is increasingly being recognized as one of the most influential developments in general practice nursing (WIPP 2007). The WIPP programme of work was formally completed in June 2008; resources remain live and are available on new host sites.

Scotland

The Framework for Nursing in General Practice (Scottish Executive 2004) indicated that practice nurses wanted education which:

- was consistent and comprehensive
- reached a nationally agreed standard
- was flexible and work based
- was supported through mentorship and clinical experience. (http://www.scotland.gov.uk/Publications/2004/09/19966/43287)

The educational standards for the initial preparation of general practice nurses were drawn up and published by the NHS Education for Scotland (NES) in 2006. To implement the initial preparation of general practice nurses, NES facilitated a 1-year pilot in 2006–2007 to support initial preparation for practice nurses in defined areas across Scotland.

A national learning and network coordinator, located within NES and supported by the Scottish Executive, has been appointed (Bell 2007). The aim of this initiative is to provide national coordination of education and practice development initiatives related to practice nursing and to develop collaborative links with stakeholders. Bell (2007) notes that information about general practice nurses in Scotland thus far has been limited and professional support and access to practice nurse groups has been inconsistent for Scottish practice nurses. This new role aims to find out what nurses in Scotland believe they need and allow future education and networking to be targeted towards meeting these needs.

Wales

The Welsh Assembly Government (WAG) continues to fund degree education leading to the NMC general practice nurse specialist practitioner qualification, undertaken in Welsh HEIs, for both existing and new practice nurses, through the National Leadership and Innovation Agency for Healthcare (NLIAH) (see Case study 13.2). A review of primary care and community nursing in Wales commissioned by WAG (Williams 2004), however, recommended:

> … a move away from a competency based framework of educating nurses to an education that prepares nurses to deal with uncertainty, manage complexity and respond to changing service needs in such a way that avoids the need to radically re-write nursing curricula in response to the inevitable evolution and change of the service … (p. 10)

A similar message came out of a review of district and practice nursing undertaken by Caerphilly Teaching Local Health Board (TLHB; 2007), who recommended that education at both pre- and post-registration needs to change to produce autonomous practitioners who are fit for purpose. They also noted that the role of practice nursing would continue to develop in the future as fewer GPs are recruited and the role of advanced practice nurse will become the standard for all practice nurses to achieve. HEIs are currently reviewing their programmes to ensure they meet the needs of the developing role of the practice nurse. A Community Nursing Strategy for Wales, including recommendations on future education for all community nurses, is due for publication in 2009.

Case study 13.2

Amy had worked in intensive care since her initial registration as a nurse. During her pre-registration community placement she had spent time with a practice nurse and felt that this was a career she wished to pursue. She applied unsuccessfully for some posts, as they all wanted prior experience, difficult to obtain before actually being in post.

Amy met a colleague who had completed a degree leading to the NMC specialist qualification of practice nurse at a local university. The degree was funded by WAG for nurses working in Wales and, being 50% theory, 50% practice, enabled Amy to gain the practical experience she needed to obtain a position as practice nurse. Amy successfully applied for the programme, covered all the theory required for her new career at the university, including that relating to the management of

long-term conditions. Under the supervision of her practice tutor, an experienced practice nurse, she was able to relate theory to practice and gain the valuable practical experience she needed.

At the end of the course she applied for and successfully obtained a position as a practice nurse and is enjoying her new career while appreciating that she still has much to learn.

Discussion points

1. What skills and knowledge do you think you need to become a practice nurse?
2. What education is available locally to help you achieve the skills and knowledge required to work as a practice nurse?

Northern Ireland

Northern Ireland produced a position paper (Department of Health, Social Services and Public Safety (DHSSPS) Nursing and Midwifery Advisory Group 2003), *Strategic Direction in Community Nursing in Northern Ireland*, in which a recommendation was made that there should be a review of education for nurses who work in the community and primary care, suggesting that new combinations of skills are needed and a 1-year community nursing qualification for life may be less useful than a build-up of skills in response to the clinical and social setting. The final report on the review, *Regional Redesign of Community Nursing Project* (DHSSPS 2006), made a number of recommendations for education, and this can be accessed at http://www.dhsspsni.gov.uk/print/regional_redesign_of_community_nursing_project-4.pdf.

Policy and practice

General

Carey (2003) in her chapter discussed the influence of central government funding on UK healthcare provision and how 'the specific nature of care delivery and the roles of the practitioner are shaped by politicians and dependent on the prevailing political ideology'. She also noted how for many practitioners the political agenda is far removed from the day-to-day issues surrounding care delivery, but emphasized that the development of the role of the practice nurse has been shaped, more than any other, not by 'the needs of the population, or through the impact of nursing as a profession, but as a response to the healthcare political agenda'. This section will refer to Carey's original chapter detailing the government policies that shaped the practice nurse role and then bring the reader up-to-date with the health policies across the four nations that continue to influence practice nurse development.

The 1990 GP contract (Department of Health 1990) laid the foundations for practice nursing by moving primary care services away from a curative, illness-led service to that of a preventative health-promotion-led service. GPs were encouraged to promote health, as well as treating illness, through a system of financial reimbursement for providing services such as well person health checks and chronic disease management clinics. In order to provide these services GPs employed more practice nurses. Although some practice nurses had been employed directly by GPs in the late 1960s/early 1970s it was the 1990 contract that provided nurses with the opportunity to develop a new role 'unconstrained by traditional NHS nursing management hierarchy' (Carey 2003). Parallel to the introduction of the contract, GPs were given the opportunity to take control of their own budgets under GP fund-holding (abolished by central government in 1997), which gave them further flexibility in employing staff to meet the needs of their particular practice population.

Atkin et al (1993) carried out some seminal work in a national census of practice nurses, identifying their role as ranging from chronic disease management and health promotion to more practical tasks such as venepuncture and wound care. Considerable diversity was noted in roles and responsibilities, educational preparation and grading. In 2001 Eve and Gerrish, reporting on the results of two studies of practice nursing in Sheffield, noted that practice nurse roles and responsibilities had undergone spectacular development with nurse triage, nurse practitioner roles and clinical governance becoming an established part of the scenery. They added a cautionary note, however, that the variety of work seemed to be more dependent on historical precedent than in direct response to the needs of the population. Practice nurse activity continued to fall into four broad areas: chronic disease management, health promotion, treatment room activities and domiciliary visiting. Reassuringly, Eve and Gerrish noted that nearly three-quarters of practice nurses had undergone a validated practice nursing course and study days attended had gone up to an average of 8.5 days a year, a considerable improvement from Atkin et al's (1993) survey, which reported that only 36% of nurses had attended more than five study days in the previous year.

The nGMS contract (Department of Health 2003), implemented in 2004, gave practice nurses the chance to further extend their roles. The contract, for the first time, was practice based rather than an individual doctor contract, opening up the possibility of nurse-led services and allowing nurses (and other disciplines) to enter into partnerships with GPs, rather than be employed by them (see Case study 13.3) (see Chapter 2 for further information on the nGMS contract). The RCN (2004b) has provided guidance on this role and

Case study 13.3

Philippa worked as a practice nurse in a South Wales practice for a number of years. During this time the nursing team expanded and she became senior nurse leading a team of three qualified nurses and two healthcare assistants. She achieved her practice nurse specialist qualification at diploma level during the NMC interim arrangements before degree level study became mandatory. She then obtained her degree in respiratory health.

Her responsibilities included supervising the training of the healthcare assistants. During this time she noticed the lack of accredited training available for them to carry out their role. She was appointed as the nurse member of the local health board and began to explore possibilities for developing suitable training programmes with a local further education provider. With the support of the board she was able to secure a contract to ensure that all future healthcare assistants employed in the area would be able to undergo a programme, relevant to the needs of primary care, leading to the qualification of NVQ Level 2.

Following on from this the GP partners in the practice had the opportunity to tender for a local practice where the GP had recently retired. Knowing the skills that Philippa would bring to the role, they asked her to become a partner in the new practice, taking a lead on clinical issues and taking responsibility not only for the nursing team but also for the salaried GPs they were employing to work in the new practice.

Discussion points

1. What are the benefits and risks of becoming a practice partner?

2. What other non-clinical issues would you be involved in, and how would you prepare yourself for this new role?

practice nurses considering partnership are strongly advised to refer to it. The guidance notes, however, that current nurse partners have reported a number of personal and professional benefits including:

- a sense of ownership of the practice and stronger teamwork between nurse partner and GPs
- having an equal say in decision-making
- finances that can be enhanced through profit sharing, but with this also lies possible financial risk. (http://www2.rcn.org.uk/pcph/resources/a-z_of_resources/general_medical_services_contract)

With the nGMS contract came the Quality and Outcomes Framework (QOF), which provided practices with financial reimbursements (rewards for quality) for meeting targets in a number of designated areas: clinical, organizational, additional services, patient experience and holistic care. The clinical areas included were expanded in the 2006 revision of the contract (NHS confederation/BMA 2006) and can be found in Table 13.2. Much of the work involved in meeting the targets fell to practice nurses, but the contract also had an impact on recruitment, with many practices employing more practice nurses in order to meet their quality goals. NB: QOF is subject to regular updates, and was revised in 2008/2009, at which time the clinical areas remained the same. Readers should access the most recent version.

Table 13.2 Quality and Outcomes Framework

Quality indicator	Clinical domain
CHD (coronary heart disease)	Mental health
Heart failure	Asthma
Strokes and TIAs (transient ischaemic attacks)	Dementia
Hypertension	Depression
Diabetes mellitus	CKD (chronic kidney disease)
COPD (chronic obstructive pulmonary disease)	Atrial fibrillation
Epilepsy	Obesity
Hypothyroidism	Learning disabilities
Cancer	Smoking indicators
Palliative care	

Practice nurses had already demonstrated their ability in chronic disease management (now referred to as long-term conditions), specifically in conditions such as asthma, diabetes, hypertension and coronary heart disease. The importance of strategic and systematic care of patients with these conditions, including regular recall and review, which began with the 1990 GP contract, was further emphasized with the publication of national service frameworks (NSFs), the first of which to be introduced was the NSF for coronary heart disease (Department of Health 2000b). The rise of the clinical governance agenda (Department of Health 1998) put an increasing emphasis not only on the provision of evidence-based care, but also on procedures such as audit in order to monitor the quality of the care provided to patients and the quality of the organizational set-up providing this care. In the primary care setting practice nurses took much of the responsibility for providing this quality, developing their skills and knowledge accordingly. The QOF requirements brought with it new challenges for practice nurses to become involved with conditions that had not always been a routine part of their day-to-day practice. For individual practice nurses to become knowledgeable in such a variety of subjects is difficult; many practices expanded their nursing teams, encouraging individual nurses to concentrate on particular fields and take on a more specialist role. Carey (2003) stresses the importance, however, of practice nurses developing their own distinct knowledge base, as the reality of nurses continuing to be employed and using the title 'practice nurse' without this knowledge base raises doubts concerning the power base through which they practise. She continues to say that the influence of individual GPs in shaping the boundaries of their practice has prevented them developing their skills to their full potential. With primary care trusts (PCTs), local health boards (LHBs), community health partnerships (CHPs) and local commissioning groups (LCGs) employing and supporting practice nurses it is hoped that in the future support will be given to further develop practice nursing into a coherent discipline.

England

Practice nurses had already taken on delegated duties following the Department of Health (1990) GP contract. A number of innovative nurse-led schemes began to develop following the Primary Care Act (Department of Health/NHS Executive 1997), which allowed a departure from the national General Medical Services contract. Personal medical services practices developed, providing general practice services via contracts with health authorities, this responsibility later being devolved to primary care organizations (PCOs), which eventually merged with social services departments to form PCTs. Practice nurses were for the first time able to employ salaried GPs, contracting to deliver services to either specific population groups, for example the homeless, or in areas of GP shortage. As it was a local arrangement it enabled new services to be developed around the specific needs of populations, thus allowing practice nurses who took on this new role to become highly

specialized and develop their skills away from the traditional influence of general practitioners.

The NHS Plan (Department of Health 2000a) set out to reconfigure healthcare delivery. In primary care this meant modernizing GP practices, improving IT systems and delegating the traditional roles undertaken within general practice to other disciplines. Traditionally practice nurses had been employed by GPs rather than by a community or hospital trust. With the advent of PCOs and then PCTs practice nurses also became employed by them in a variety of roles, some to work in PCT-managed practices or teams, but also in new practice nurse roles within the PCT, such as educational and organizational support roles. Support for practice nurses from individual PCTs, as from GPs, however, continues to vary.

The Department of Health (2002) document *Liberating the Talents* emphasized the need for nurses to break down boundaries, working to provide seamless care for patients, and described three core functions for community nurses, all of which are services that practice nurses provide:

* public health
* first contact work
* management of long-term conditions. (p. 8)

The *NHS Improvement Plan* (Department of Health 2004) continued to emphasize the central role of primary care in the new NHS. The importance of meeting the needs of patients with long-term conditions was accentuated, along with stressing the importance of prevention of illness and keeping people healthy. Although roles such as community matrons have evolved using case management techniques to care for patients with complex needs relating to long-term conditions, regular monitoring for the majority of patients with long-term conditions and support to assist them with developing self-management skills will continue to be delivered by practice nurses.

Practice-based commissioning as set out in the White Paper *Our Health, Our Care, Our Say. A New Direction for Community Services* (Department of Health 2006) also offered new opportunities for practice nurses, both as alternative providers of services based on local need and as part of practice-based commissioning groups. The Queen's Nursing Institute (2006) has provided a briefing paper for nurses in primary care about practice-based commissioning which should be accessed by those requiring further information on this topic.

Scotland

The Scottish Executive (2000) set out a plan to provide an NHS focused on health improvement and meeting the particular health needs of local communities and excluded groups, with unified NHS boards developing local health plans. Community health partnerships were established in 2004 to provide a more consistent and enhanced role in service planning and delivery.

A Framework for Nursing in General Practice was published in 2004 by the Scottish Executive, which provided a resource for practice nurses and practices to aid the development of nursing roles in individual general practices. Eleven standards in total, covering six areas, form the structure of the framework:

- fair and consistent treatment
- induction and initial preparation for role
- developing the nursing team
- learning and development
- communication and teamwork
- accountability for professional practice. (http://www.scotland.gov.uk/Publications/2004/09/19966/43287)

The framework is intended to be a resource for practice, with community health partnerships (CHPs) having a crucial role in providing local leadership and support, promoting good practice and supporting practices that wish to use it as a developmental tool. The review of community nursing in Scotland (Scottish Executive 2006) suggested a new role, the community health nurse (CHN), who will work closely with practice nurses to assess nursing needs and plan care for patients on a practice list, including planning public health activities, and caring for those who are ill or have a long-term condition.

Wales

In Wales, following the White Paper *Putting Patients First* (Welsh Assembly Government 1998), local health groups (LHGs) were established to provide a more local focus to healthcare provision, identifying need, determining priorities and commissioning services accordingly. For practice nurses this was a noteworthy development as each LHG board was to appoint two nurse members, one of whom was expected to be a practice nurse. Although the boards were heavily weighted towards GP representation, for the first time practice nurses had the chance to have their say on local healthcare service delivery.

Improving Health in Wales (Welsh Assembly Government 2001) set out a 10-year plan for health services in Wales, which involved abolishing the health authorities and devolving further responsibilities to LHGs, which would evolve into local health boards (LHBs). Primary care would be strengthened with investments in infrastructure and the workforce, with a further increase in collaborative working between providers of health and social care. Each LHB would have one nurse board member, who could be working in any of the community nursing disciplines. However, many practice nurses retained their board membership. LHBs also began to employ nurses in various roles, including practice nurse facilitators. As in the PCTs in England, support for practice nurses from LHBs across Wales varied widely. In some areas practice nurses were directly employed by LHBs in either managed practices, or as supernumerary nurses to provide support to practices to assist them in meeting their quality targets and to provide cover for educational leave. Some LHBs identified budgets to support practice nurses in gaining necessary educational qualifications while others provided no financial support, leaving this to individual practices. Support for practice nurses currently varies in Wales and is an area that needs to be addressed in order for practice nursing to continue developing as a coherent discipline.

The review of primary care and community nursing in Wales recommended that:

- nurse-led, first contact primary care would be coordinated and, effectively, led by highly skilled generalist nurse practitioners/practice nurses
- careful consideration should be given to the designation given to the lead, coordinating, generalist role in first contact care (options include 'practice nurse', 'nurse practitioner'). (Williams 2004: 11)

Designed for Life (Welsh Assembly Government 2005) further emphasized that patients should have access to an appropriate member of the primary care team within 24 hours, which has had further impact on the role of the practice nurse in delivering first contact care. If practice nurses are to continue to develop their role and deliver effective services, as set out in the current health agenda, then appropriate support systems need to be put in place.

Addendum

Since writing this chapter the Minister of Health for Wales unveiled plans to simplify the NHS structure in Wales. Following a 12-week consultation in early 2008 the emerging view was to create single local health organizations that would be responsible for delivering all healthcare services within a geographical area, rather than the trust and local health board system currently operating. In November 2008, the Health Minister confirmed that the new NHS local bodies in Wales would be established as local health boards (LHBs). A simplified structure was proposed for the NHS in Wales which involves the dissolution of 21 LHBs (all except Powys LHB), and seven NHS trusts in Wales. A second consultation paper, 'Delivering the new NHS for Wales', provides details of the proposed model, membership and functions of the seven LHBs, which will be operational by autumn 2009.

Readers are advised to refer to the Health of Wales website at http://www.wales.nhs.uk/ for up-to-date information regarding the changes.

Northern Ireland

Unlike England and Scotland, no specific frameworks have been developed in Northern Ireland for practice nursing. However, within the government health policy documents setting the way forward for primary care there is much that will impact on the role. The Department of Health, Social Services and Public Safety (DHSSPS 2005) published a primary health and social care strategic framework: *Caring for People Beyond Tomorrow*. This framework was developed as an integral component of the regional strategy *A Healthier Future* (DHSSPS 2004) and stressed a greater emphasis on health promotion, enhanced social well-being and disease prevention. In order to help people make lifestyle changes to reduce future levels of chronic illness, and support them in managing their own condition, it was noted that multidisciplinary primary care teams with greater specialization in areas such as diabetes, respiratory illness and heart disease needed to be in place. Although practice nurses are not specifically mentioned, a number of goals were set out, many of which are relevant to practice nurses. These included:

- 24-hour access to primary care services
- development of multidisciplinary assessment and treatment services in primary care

- improved management of chronic conditions in the community
- development and implementation of a strategy to enhance the skills base in the primary care workforce (http://www.dhsspsni.gov.uk/primarycare05.pdf).

The position paper: *Strategic Direction in Community Nursing in Northern Ireland* (DHSSPS Nursing and Midwifery Advisory Group 2003) set out a strategy for nursing that considered the delivery of nursing services in both community and primary care. The paper proposed that an adapted strategy similar to that presented in *Liberating the Talents* (Department of Health 2002) would be useful. The modified model included:

- first contact care
- continuing care
- public health.

The paper suggested that nurses be given the freedom and support to work with GPs and to take on more advanced and specialized roles in first contact care, chronic disease management and preventative services. The final report, *Regional Redesign of Community Nursing Project* (DHSSPS 2006), can be accessed at http://www.dhsspsni.gov.uk/print/regional_redesign_of_community_nursing_project-4.pdf.

Conclusion

Practice nursing has continued to grow and develop; indeed the practice nurse association is one of the largest of the RCN forums. The RCN has produced a general practice nursing tree to demonstrate the diversity of the role. Both as individuals and as a group, practice nurses have fought long and hard for the role to be recognized. Many new challenges await them with the movement of healthcare services from secondary to primary care and they need to continue to meet these challenges head on. HEIs also need to be prepared to provide practice nurses with the appropriate education for them to continue to expand the services they provide. The future will see practice nurses taking an increased role in providing services such as sexual health, advanced assessment, triage, minor illness and injuries as well as becoming further involved with providing care to those with learning disabilities and mental health problems. Practice nurses have already demonstrated their ability in managing long-term conditions and providing health promotion services and are equally able to rise to the new challenges they are presented with. England and Scotland have led the way in developing frameworks for both practice nurses and their employers and to highlight good practice. The RCN (2007) is continuing to lobby the government to include practice nurses in Agenda for Change. Primary care trusts, local health boards, community health partnerships and local commissioning groups need to provide support and direction for practice nurses to ensure that they can continue to provide valid healthcare services based on the needs of the population in conjunction with other community practitioners.

SUMMARY

- The role of the general practice nurse (GPN) has undergone rapid expansion and continues to evolve, with GPNs rapidly moving towards the 'gatekeeper role' in primary care.
- Educational preparation for the role has been diverse; higher education institutes (HEIs) should continue to provide adequate educational programmes to enable GPNs to fulfil their role.

- Practice nurses need to continue to expand their knowledge base and define their own role.
- Supporting frameworks for GPNs and their employers vary in the four nations of the UK, with England and Scotland currently leading the way forward.

DISCUSSION POINTS

1. Do you feel that you have been adequately prepared for the role of GPN?
2. Should there be a minimum educational requirement for the GPN role, and if so at what level?
3. What policies and frameworks need to be put in place by primary care trusts, local

health boards, community health partnerships and local commissioning groups to support GPNs?
4. Has the nGMS contract helped or hindered the development of the GPN role?

References

Atkin K, Lunt N, Parker G, Hirst M 1993 Nurses count: a national census of practice nurses. Social Policy Research Unit, University of York, York

Baker J 1988 What now? Post basic opportunities for nurses. Macmillan, Basingstoke

Bell F 2007 Improving education and peer support. Practice Nursing 18(3): 114–115

Caerphilly Teaching Local Health Board 2007 District and practice nursing review evaluation report. Caerphilly Teaching Local Health Board

Campbell 2007 Background to creating the general practice nursing toolkit and commissioner's guide to general practice nursing. New@WIPP (Working in Partnership Programme) Issue 7. Online: http://www.wipp. nhs.uk/uploads/pam_campbell_

background_to_toolkit.doc (accessed 7 August 2007)

Carey L 2003 Practice nursing. In: Watkins D, Edwards J, Gastrell P (eds) Community health nursing: frameworks for practice, 2nd edn. Baillière Tindall, Edinburgh

Cross 2006 Supporting an evolving nurse role. Practice Nursing 7(9): 420–422

Crossman S 2006 Practice nurses' needs for education since the advent of the new GMS. Practice Nursing 17(2): 87–91

Cullen J 2005 Gatekeeping part 3: results and practice recommendations. Practice Nursing 16(12): 611–617

Department of Health 1990 General Medical Services Council – new GP contract. HMSO, London

Department of Health/NHS Executive 1997 Personal medical services under the NHS (Primary Care) Act 1997. HMSO, London

Department of Health 1998 A first class service: quality in the new NHS. HMSO, London

Department of Health 2000a The NHS plan – a plan for investment, a plan for reform. HMSO, London

Department of Health 2000b National Service Framework for coronary heart disease. HMSO, London

Department of Health 2002 Liberating the talents. HMSO, London

Department of Health 2003 Delivering investment in general practice: implementing the new GMS contract. HMSO, London

Department of Health 2004 NHS improvement plan 2004: putting people at the heart of public services. HMSO, London

Department of Health 2006 Our health, our care, our say. A new direction for community services. HMSO, London

Department of Health, Social Services and Public Safety Nursing and Midwifery Advisory Group 2003 Strategic direction in community nursing in Northern Ireland – a position paper. Online: http://www.dhsspsni.gov.uk/nursing_strategic_direction.pdf (accessed 14 Aug 2007)

Department of Health, Social Services and Public Safety 2004 A healthier future. Online: http://www.dhsspsni.gov.uk/healthyfuture-main.pdf (accessed 14 Aug 2007)

Department of Health, Social Services and Public Safety 2005 Caring for people beyond tomorrow. Online: http://www.dhsspsni.gov.uk/primarycare05.pdf (accessed 14 Aug 2007)

Department of Health, Social Services and Public Safety 2006 Regional redesign of community nursing project. Nursing And Midwifery Group. Online: http://www.dhsspsni.gov.uk/print/regional_redesign_of_community_nursing_project-4.pdf (accessed 14 Aug 2007)

Eve R, Gerrish K 2001 Roles, responsibilities and innovative capacity: the case of practice nurses. JCN online 15(9). Online: http://www.jcn.co.uk/journal.asp?MonthNum=09&YearNum=2001&Type=backissue&ArticleID=384 (accessed 7 Aug 2007)

Martin J 2007 The next generation. New@WIPP (Working in Partnership Programme) (Issue 7). Online: http://www.wipp.nhs.uk/uploads/jeanett_martin_article.doc (accessed 7 Aug 2007)

Mental Health Foundation 2006 Statistics on mental health. Online: http://www.mentalhealth.org.uk/information/mental-health-overview/statistics/# (accessed 8 Aug 2007)

NHS confederation/BMA 2006 New GMS contract 2006/2007. Online: http://www.dh.gov.uk/PolicyAndGuidance/OrganisationPolicy/PrimaryCare/PrimaryCareContracting/GMS/fs/en (accessed 7 Aug 2007)

NHS Education for Scotland 2006 Initial preparation for practice nurses: educational standards. Online: http://www.nes.scot.nhs.uk/nursing/practice_nursing/ (accessed 8 Aug 2007)

Queen's Nursing Institute 2006 Briefing no. 4. Practice based commissioning. Online: http://www.qni.org.uk/pdfs/Briefing%20%20Practice%20Based%20Commissioning.pdf (accessed 7 Aug 2007)

RCGP 2004 RCGP information sheet no.19. Practice nurses. Online: http://www.rcgp.org.uk/pdf/ISS_INFO_19_AUG%2004.pdf (accessed 7 Aug 2007)

RCN 2004a Nurses employed by GPs: RCN guidance on good employment practice. Online: http://www.rcn.org.uk/publications/pdf/nurses_employed_by_gps.pdf (accessed 14 Aug 2007)

RCN 2004b RCN zones, primary care public health. General Medical Services contract. Online: http://www2.rcn.org.uk/pcph/resources/az_of_resources/general_medical_services_contract (accessed 7 Aug 2007)

RCN 2007 Agenda for change: practice nursing. Online: http://www.rcn.org.uk/agendaforchange/independentsector/practicenurses.php (accessed 14 Aug 2007)

Ruscoe D 2006 Education, education, education! Practice Nurse Feb 24, p. 6

Scanlan M 2007 Mental health training for practice nurses. Practice Nursing 18(5): 224–227

Scottish Executive 2000 Our national health: a plan for action, a plan for change. Scottish Executive, Edinburgh

Scottish Executive 2004 Framework for nursing in general practice. Online: http://www.scotland.gov.uk/Publications/2004/09/19966/43287 (accessed 14 Aug 2007)

Scottish Executive 2006 Improving health by providing visible, accessible, consistent care. Scottish Executive, Edinburgh

Technical Steering Committee 2006/2007 2006/2007 UK general practice workload survey. Online: http://www.ic.nhs.uk/webfiles/publications/gp/GP%20Workload%20Report.pdf (accessed 8 Jan 2009)

Welsh Assembly Government 1998 Quality care and clinical excellence – putting patients first. Welsh Assembly Government, Cardiff

Welsh Assembly Government 2001 Improving health in Wales: a plan for the NHS with its partners. Welsh Assembly Government, Cardiff

Welsh Assembly Government 2005 Designed for life: creating world class health and social care for Wales in the 21st century. Welsh Assembly Government, Cardiff

Williams A 2004 Review of primary care and community nursing in Wales: summary and recommendations. Welsh Assembly Government, Cardiff

Working in Partnership Programme (WIPP) 2007 General practice nursing – getting it right for patients and public health. Online: http://www.wipp.nhs.uk/22.php (accessed 7 Aug 2007)

Recommended reading

Carey L (ed.) 2000 Practice nursing. Baillière Tindall, Edinburgh
A comprehensive textbook developed to reflect the community specialist practitioner role for practice nurses.

Edwards M (ed.) 2008 The informed practice nurse, 2nd edn. John Wiley & Sons, Chichester

The Informed Practice Nurse offers both new and experienced practice nurses the opportunity to reflect on their current practice.

Hampson G 2006 Practice nurse handbook, 5th edn. Blackwell Publishing, Oxford

The Practice Nurse Handbook is an essential guide to all aspects of clinical practice, health promotion and practice management, for nurses in general practice.

District nursing

Carol Alstrom and Pat McCamley

KEY ISSUES

- The evolving role of the district nurse
- First assessment
- Influences on practice
- Changing demands
- Interdisciplinary working

Introduction

The role of the district nurse is evolving to care for patients with complex nursing needs in the community setting, and in striving to achieve this, it is essential for district nurses to work as proactive members of the primary healthcare team. This chapter provides an insight into the history and the evolving role of the district nurse, outlines some of the challenges faced by district nurses and discusses managing a team in the changing context of modern healthcare.

The evolving role of the district nurse

The role of the district nurse is constantly changing and a look back in recent history provides an insight into how fast those changes have occurred. District nursing has evolved from its origins that can be traced back to the mid 19th century. Before formal training and registration were developed for nurses working in the community, standards were variable (Baly et al 1987). During the early 19th century the old Poor Law committees often employed nurses to care for the sick in their own home. Even following the Poor Law amendment in 1834 and the advent of the workhouse this practice continued. During the mid 19th century some charities provided a more well-to-do class of women with some training in nursing to provide care. However, this arrangement was not successful as there was no systematic approach to training and care provision.

The work of William Rathbone in establishing the first nurse training school in Liverpool in the 19th century specifically to train nurses for the 'districts' of the city did much to promote recognition of the role and to improve the quality of care. This followed his personal experiences of employing a nurse to care for his terminally ill wife, within the home. His work and the support of senior nurses of the time, including Florence Nightingale, established the foundation of the service that can be seen today. The first trained nurses were educated at Liverpool Infirmary and they began working in the homes of Liverpool in 1863 (Baly et al 1987). In 1887 the Queen Victoria Jubilee Institute for Nurses was established and district nursing associations were offered the opportunity to affiliate to this organization providing they could meet the high standards required for the training of nurses. Out of this organization came a new breed of district nurses known as Queen's Nurses. These nurses were often superintendents of services and some districts could not afford to employ them. By 1902 the Institute had established examinations and created a community nurse who dealt with a whole range of health and social needs.

In 1919 state registration as a nurse become mandatory and was a prerequisite to undertaking training as a district nurse with the Institute. The Queen's Nursing Institute (QNI), as it became known, continued to be the training organization until 1968. Various changes continued to affect the training of district nurses until in 1981 new mandatory training was introduced before a nurse could use the title 'district nurse' (Baly et al 1987). Since that time the training of district nurses has moved into universities and in 1994 the introduction of the community specialist practitioner qualification meant academic recognition at degree level. This move was seen as a positive step and welcomed by the profession.

Traditionally the key role of the district nurse is as the expert in the care of the sick at home. This remains predominantly true. However, the remit has extended to incorporate health promotion and a focus on independence, supporting individuals to reach their personal optimum potential within their health status, and avoiding dependence on both nursing and other services where possible. This concept supports a clear ethic, to respect and maintain the dignity and the individuality of patients and manage care collaboratively in a holistic and proactive way.

Education and training in preparation for district nursing remains a topic for debate, highlighted at QNI conferences; views and opinions are wide and varied, with some feeling that there is not a need to train district nurses as specialists, while others feel strongly that specialist training is essential. One suggestion has been made that pre-registration nurses should be trained in the community, with hospital care being the specialist element, particularly with the move towards care closer to home (Butterworth 2007). In November 2007 the Nursing and Midwifery Council (NMC) and Department of Health commenced consultation on potential changes to pre- and post-registration education, including a shift to community nursing being a first post option for staff (Department of Health 2007a, NMC 2007).

The core elements of the district nursing role are to hold the continuing responsibility for the assessment and provision of care to a group of patients within a chosen locality. This involves planning, implementation and evaluation of the care provided, ensuring at all times that an evidence base underpins practice (Audit Commission 1999). District nurses also require management and leadership skills to promote effective teamwork within a multidiscipli-

nary setting, across the boundaries of health and social care, facilitating the identification of complementary approaches to meet individual need.

The remit of the district nurse has changed significantly in recent years and will continue to evolve in response to changes in the provision of health and social care, such as shorter hospital stays, technological developments and increased life expectancy with its associated morbidity (Audit Commission 1999). The Commission also informs on how the district nursing services nationally undertake more than 36 million contacts each year and have approximately 2.75 million patients on their caseload, the majority of these patients being elderly people. A report by the QNI in 2006 reviewed the changes in district nursing over the last 5 years and presented a view on the changes required in next 5 years to enable the service to deliver high-quality care in the future (QNI 2006). The key messages included:

At national level:
- Establish and publish a consensus about the values, purpose, boundaries and functions of the district nurse role.
- Clarify its relationship to other community nursing roles and establish its place in the wider primary care team.
- Locate it in the wider family of nursing.
- Agree the most appropriate form and level of educational preparation.
- Develop a national vision for district and community nursing and a strategy to deliver that vision to ensure that district nursing is fit for the future.

At local level:
- Help community nurses engage with local commissioning and planning groups.
- Provide the strong local leadership that makes a noticeable difference.
- Address the technology issues: phones that work and access to computers.
- Consult staff genuinely about the best forms of team working.
- Work with community nurses to explain to the public and other staff how different roles fit together in the local model of community nursing (QNI 2006).

The reinstatement of Queen's Nurses was a direct response to the loss of identity expressed by nurses in the meetings conducted to inform this report. In May 2007 the first group of new Queen's

Nurses were announced; these nurses came from a wide range of community nursing disciplines, including two from district nursing (QNI 2007).

Leadership has become a key focus since the launch of *The NHS Plan* in 2000. Recognizing the need for leadership skills, district nurses have found themselves alongside other nursing team and ward leaders on courses such as Leading Empowered Organizations (LEO) and the Royal College of Nursing Leadership Programme. However, it would appear that in many NHS trusts in England only senior nurses are attending these programmes. This may make the introduction of new skills difficult as colleagues and others may not have a shared understanding of the leadership concepts presented. However, a few NHS trusts have been innovative, bringing LEO programmes into the whole organization, and have employed a training facilitator to cascade the information. The focus of leadership is now on empowering nurses and ultimately patients to facilitate high-quality care in a partnership relationship. This is ideally undertaken utilizing a transformational leadership style (Davidhizar 1993), in which leaders seek to understand the problems and issues affecting both nurses and patients and then support them through changes and developing new ways of working. The concept of leadership has been enhanced further by other national initiatives including the Leadership at the Point of Care programme, aimed at nurses working directly with patients and focusing on relationship based accountability, enabling nurses to take appropriate responsibility for patient experience (NHS Leadership Centre 2004).

First assessment: a review of district nursing

In 1999 a key document was published which continues to have a direct impact on district nurses: *First assessment: a review of district nursing services in England and Wales* (Audit Commission 1999). This provided an insight into the pressures on the district nursing service and highlighted that there is often a discrepancy between resources, skills and demand for service provision. The report made a series of recommendations for district nursing providers including the need to set clear service objectives, set referral criteria, establish systematic methods of caseload review, improve the management of patient demands and ensure the appropriate targeting of resources.

This report presented a challenge to district nurses, service managers and trusts to review ways in which district nursing services are organized, managed and delivered. The report also spelt out key messages about integrated working, self-managed teams and the way services are developed and provided. The Audit Commission (1999) also highlighted the following variations that exist in district nursing services across the country:

- some areas provide 24-hour cover
- some only provide daytime and evening services
- variation in the numbers of patients per whole time equivalent district nurse
- inconsistency in the roles undertaken by the district nurse and members of the nursing team
- variations in the provision of continence and leg ulcer care in clinic settings.

It looked critically at service provision, and following publication of the report, every district nursing service in England and Wales was evaluated against the report; how improvements in the services could be made for the benefit of patients was also investigated. One of the key issues identified was the need to ensure that the patients being cared for by the district nurse were the right patients. The scope of district nursing practice, if not clearly defined, can lead to inappropriate referrals, and ultimately inefficient and ineffective management of resources (Seccombe 1999). By developing locally agreed, clearly stated service definitions, referral criteria and documentation, district nurses can ensure that they are delivering appropriate and high-quality care.

Caseload review

An area of weakness identified by the Audit Commission was the need for caseload review in order to improve the management of patient demands and the allocation of resources. The review process allows the opportunity for:

- comparing the numbers of patients on an active caseload
- profiling the gender, age, frequency of visits and dependency of patients
- estimating the overall workload
- comparing the caseload at practice level.

By providing district nurses with information about their caseload, service leaders can support district nurses in:

- encouraging patient discharge or transfer to other more appropriate services
- regularly monitoring change in casemix to ensure effective use of resources
- identifying the type of care patients are receiving
- developing core competencies for assessment and delivery of packages of care.

Few areas have undertaken this type of work and there is little published research in this field, yet the understanding of the types of care packages required can assist service leaders to identify training needs to meet patient care requirements. On a day-to-day basis caseload analysis can support nurses in prioritizing visits, justify need for temporary staff and support appropriate care for the patient in the right setting.

Work in one district nursing service resulted in the development of a casework management tool that is able to provide information about the increased demands on district nursing services. Its emphasis is on defining the complexity of patient care and the equal distribution of the workload within a district nursing team. It also aims to identify areas of inequality between the resourced nursing time and the actual time required to undertake care, and indicators of when a team has reached its patient capacity (Frame and O'Donnell 1996). However, this project did not state the types of nursing care being provided or if other services were involved and it did not identify a core caseload.

Another dependency tool has been developed to identify the needs of patients and indicate the care that they were receiving (Freeman et al 1999). This has been used as an audit tool for the management of certain conditions. One of the key aspects of this tool is that it can be used to identify district nursing teams which are under pressure, and therefore identify the appropriate distribution of staff. It provides an ongoing profile of the demands on the service and allows informed discussion about the development of services. This tool needs to be evaluated, as no evidence of comparison or transfer to another area is demonstrated. Indeed, the effectiveness and validity of these tools need to be explored, as they may not meet the needs of every district nursing service.

The Audit Commission report and subsequent service reviews have provided district nursing serv-ices with an effective plan for the future and with achievable goals to enable the provision of a service that can demonstrate high quality while offering effective and equitable care.

Influences on practice

Influences on practice for the district nurse come from a wide variety of sources including the Department of Health, Audit Commission, Queen's Nursing Institute and most importantly the patients themselves. *Liberating the talents. Helping primary care trusts and nurses to deliver the NHS Plan* (Department of Health 2002) was driven by the Chief Nursing Officer's 10 key roles for nurses and the new General Medical Services (GMS) contract and details how the roles of nurses and midwives are changing. It is aimed at discovering how the talents of nurses and midwives working in primary care settings can be used to best advantage in improving the health and healthcare of the population.

Whatever the title, employer or setting there are three core functions to be provided by nurses, midwives and health visitors:

- first contact/acute assessment, diagnosis, care, treatment and referral
- continuing care, rehabilitation, chronic disease management and delivering national service frameworks (NSFs)
- public health/health protection and promotion programmes that improve health and reduce inequalities.

These three core functions overlap and should form the basis for planning services across primary and community care utilizing the following framework:

- planning services in a new way
- developing clinical roles
- securing better care.

One major impact for the future is the implementation of the NHS Care Records Service. This will connect more than 30 000 GPs and all acute, community and mental health NHS organizations in a single, secure national system and provide all 50 million NHS patients with an individual electronic NHS care record detailing key treatments and care within either the health service or social care. The

NHS Care Records Service will ensure that the right information is available to the right people at the right time (Department of Health 2003). For nurses working in primary care, access to accurate and timely information is key to delivering patient-centred care. The introduction of this national system has not been without its challenges but once in place will provide a vital communication tool for district nurses and other healthcare professionals.

Safeguarding adults has become an issue that has affected and changed practice across many aspects of health and social care work. In 2000, the government published a national framework, 'No Secrets', so that local councils with social services responsibilities, local NHS bodies, local police forces and other partners could develop local multiagency codes of practice to help prevent and tackle abuse. Codes of practice were to be in place by October 2001 (Department of Health and Home Office 2000).

Having previously raised awareness of domestic abuse, the Community and District Nursing Association (CDNA) recognized that elderly people were often forgotten by other members of society and were particularly vulnerable to abuse. Feeling that something needed to be done on this issue the CDNA focused its efforts on elder abuse. The report *Responding to Elder Abuse* helped raise awareness and provided guidance to practitioners recognizing and dealing with elder abuse (CDNA 2003). This was a major step forward in the protection of those who suffer from abuse and many of the recommendations from the report are being implemented across the country. Following the publication of this document the CDNA provided evidence to a House of Commons Select Committee investigation into elder abuse.

The CDNA is continuing to further develop its role, working to highlight the issues of abuse to any member of society and looking to its members to work actively to prevent abuse of their patients. Government recognition and support for safeguarding adults has grown; this is reflected in standards of care through national frameworks, human rights legislation and the regulation of care providers. The Safeguarding Vulnerable Groups Act 2006 sees the introduction, in the early part of 2009, of a new vetting and barring scheme for those who work with children and vulnerable adults covering both health and social care services. A review of 'No Secrets' commenced during 2008.

Box 14.1

Vignette: safeguarding adults

A district nurse visits a residential home to undertake an urgent review of a client who has fallen. She realizes that in the last 3 weeks she has seen six different clients in this particular home who have all experienced a fall. While the injuries the clients have sustained have been minor, she is concerned that clients in the home are at risk. Following a discussion with the home's registered manager she is still not confident that mechanisms are in place to ensure the safety of clients within the home and that appropriate falls risk assessments are in place. She discusses the case with her line manager and decides to refer the home to the adult services duty team within the local authority for a review under the safeguarding adults procedure. The district nurse attends the strategy meeting, outlining her concerns, and a joint visit is undertaken between health and social care to review care provision in the residential home. A plan is put in place to support the registered manager and her team to ensure the safety of clients is maintained. The district nurse participates in providing that ongoing support.

1. Consider different populations of patients who may be considered at greater risk for vulnerability.
2. What circumstances are commonly present in cases involving the protection of vulnerable adults?
3. What national and local policies exist to guide your practice and inform you of your professional responsibilities when caring for vulnerable adults?

The changing context of healthcare finds district nurses in leading positions within primary care. Through the White Paper *The New NHS. Modern, Dependable* (Department of Health 1997) the government provided the opportunity for nurses working in the front line of the primary healthcare team to become clinical strategists. The creation of primary care trusts (PCTs) opened the way for the direct involvement of nurses on the executive board of these organizations. As a result of these changes, community nurses now find themselves working as employees of primary care organizations that are focused on the commissioning services. In 2005 further changes to the NHS structure were announced as part of commissioning a patient-led NHS (Department of Health 2005), which reduced the numbers of strategic health authorities and the number of PCTs in England, with in some areas large numbers of PCTs coming together to form county-wide organizations. As part of this process the role of the Professional Executive Committee (PEC) was also reviewed with the following guiding principles laid down by the Department of Health:

- PECs need to be patient-focused and promote the health and well-being of communities, as well as addressing health inequalities.
- PECs need to be drivers of strong clinical leadership and enablers of clinical empowerment.
- PECs need to be decision-making and firmly part of the governance and accountability framework of the PCT.
- PECs will be expected to reflect a range of clinical professionals and the wealth of experience this brings.
- PCTs will have the freedom to determine how PECs operate according to local circumstances (Department of Health 2007b).

Some NHS managers may have interpreted these principles as removing the opportunity to have nurses in the PEC, but in the autumn of 2007, when the changes to the legislative framework that support PCTs were enacted, it became clear that there was still an expectation that nurses would continue to be a vital part of PECs.

District nurses have become key workers and coordinators of care for those patients who have complex health and social care needs being cared for in the community. Their assessment of the ability and capacity of staff to accommodate care and their organizational skills will often be the key to deciding whether it is possible for a patient to remain in their own home setting. The new national framework for NHS continuing healthcare and NHS funded nursing care was implemented in October 2007. The changes mean that more people are likely to meet the criteria and many more of these patients will be living in the community in their own homes. The expectation is that the process will now be completed in 2 weeks including assessment, decision, funding and care package provided; this will have a huge impact on the capacity of staff to undertake this work and will mean more involvement for district nurses (Department of Health 2007c).

District nursing waited patiently for the introduction of nurse prescribing, which was first mentioned in the Cumberlege Report over 20 years ago (Department of Health and Social Security 1986). In 1999 a 2-year roll-out of nurse prescribing education began to allow nurses holding a district nursing or health visiting qualification to undertake this new role. The products available for district nurses were fairly limited but allowed them to prescribe frequently used items such as wound dressings, catheter products, stoma care products and compression hosiery. The ability to prescribe has helped to improve patient care by saving time, promoting continuity of care and enabling a more responsive service (Berry and Hurst 1999). With changes over time to the legislation, nurses and other non-medical prescribers, after appropriate training, are now able to prescribe from the *British National Formulary* within their sphere of practice, as both independent prescribers and as supplementary prescribers working to a management plan agreed between the medical practitioner, patient and supplementary prescriber. This fundamental change in clinical practice must be seen as a key method of improving the patient experience of district nursing services, and reinforces the need for strong interprofessional working to ensure all healthcare professionals understand the role of the independent non-medical prescriber.

Another dimension impacting on how nurses provide care is the analysis and review of patient views and satisfaction with services provided. District nurses need to explore how they can gather views on the services to inform practice and to develop new ways of working. Satisfaction surveys help to provide an insight into patients' understanding of how services are delivered. One survey has found that: patients are unaware of how to access the service until they are referred; have a perception that nurses are too busy; that they spend too much time on nursing administration; and that visits can be interrupted by mobile phones (Cusick 1998). Another survey indicated that patients wanted a nurse they could trust and who would visit them in their own home; they also wanted to be able to establish a good relationship with that nurse. It went on to highlight that the majority of patients wanted to know what time the nurse would visit, to enable them to be ready and so that they could plan other events in their day (Bartholomew et al 1999). Further concerns relate to a lack of understanding of the role of the district nurse on the part of patients, some of whom have an expectation that care will be provided in the home, even if it is more appropriately provided in another setting. The district nurse can use the development of service definitions, referral criteria and patient information leaflets to help educate patients and other healthcare professionals accordingly. District nurses need to take advantage of patient and public involvement activity, ensuring that they understand the views of patients and the public, to enable them to influence services in a proactive and informed way.

Changing demands

District nurses are no strangers to change, the current role being very different to its origins (Baly et al 1987). However, the current demands on the service are constantly changing due to influences in society, political and medical developments and patient expectations. Government White Papers are providing the drivers and influencing the transition of care in to the community; the Department of Health held a listening exercise, which took place between September and November 2005. This consultation asked the public, patients and service users and staff for their views on how to improve the services provided in the community by the NHS and social care. This resulted in the White Paper *Our Health, Our Care, Our Say* (Department of Health 2006) highlighting a new strategic vision and direction for health and social care services in local communities. People wanted their local services to:

- understand how they live and support them to lead healthier lives
- help them to live independently if they have ongoing health or social care needs
- be easy to get to and convenient to use
- be nearer to where they live, or easily available in the areas they work.

The proposals in the White Paper aim to:

- change the way these services are provided in communities and make them as flexible as possible
- provide a more personal service that is tailored to the specific health or social care needs of individuals
- give patients and service users more control over the treatment they receive
- work with health and social care professionals and services to get the most appropriate treatment or care for their needs.

The increasing number of older people in the population is now well recognized (Department of Health 2001a), and the publication of the National Service Framework for Older People (Department of Health 2001a) reflects the recognition that this group have specific needs which need to be addressed across all areas of health and social care. Older people experience more social and healthcare needs (Department of Health 2001a) and as a consequence there has been an increased demand for district nursing services. The range of skills required for the management of chronic ill health and the older person has become more diverse as many more people are cared for at home and in other community settings.

A multidisciplinary approach to the care of the older person and the introduction of the single assessment process (Department of Health 2001a) may in some areas require the district nurse to develop better understanding of care management skills and financial assessment. This may be compromising for some nurses and lead them to question the fundamental principles of the provision of health service free at the point of delivery. However, the single assessment process should ultimately ensure that the patient receives a more effective service which avoids duplication.

Since 1990 there has been no significant growth in the number of district nurses (Ross and Corbett 2005) and a total of 17% of nurses in England work in a primary care setting. The ageing profile of the district nursing workforce is an issue that continues to be raised (QNI 2006), particularly since there has been a drop in the numbers of places being commissioned for district nurse training. This comes at a time when the elderly population is increasing and there is a declining proportion of the population aged under 16.

With the government placing high priority on waiting list initiatives, there is a great deal of pressure on acute services to achieve a higher level of patient throughput. This has led to early discharge of patients from hospital and a wider use of day surgery which has also placed an increasing demand on district nursing services. With the drive to reduce waiting lists, the focus is now on patients completing their journey from referral to treatment within 18 weeks; this has resulted in an increase in the pressure on district nursing services to accept patients home with more complex care requirements than in the past. The need for hospital-at-home care, intravenous therapy in the home and other traditionally hospital-based services will continue to grow.

The change in demand for services is accompanied by the requirement for district nurses to possess and use a broad range of skills in order to meet needs and manage a wide range of chronic illnesses. They also care for patients who may require more technical and specialized nursing than previously. Physical assessment and history taking, and clinical decision-making have now become a fundamental component of district nursing education. The public also has a higher level of expectation and understanding of healthcare provision and this is no less true of the district nursing service. *The Patients' Charter* (Department of Health 1995) supported patients having a clear say in care provision and invited their involvement in the evaluation of care received. A more informed public demands a service that they perceive will meet their needs and offer a partnership approach to care.

As the provision of healthcare changes, so too must the roles of those delivering care change. One of the most significant changes is that of the healthcare support worker. The scope of roles undertaken by this group of staff ranges from a generic role to undertaking tasks that have traditionally been the province of the registered nurse, including wound care and continence assessments. This role has been developed in all healthcare settings, working with therapists, in GP practices and with district nurses. Education programmes such as the Foundation Degree have been developed to support this role and to give career structure and recognition with a qualification. This enables a support worker or assistant practitioner to be banded up to and including Band 4. In response to issues regarding accountability and delegation, the NMC has published guidance relating to this issue (NMC 2007).

Interdisciplinary working

In recent years health and social services have been encouraged to work together to meet the needs of local populations and to provide effective patient-centred care. The concept of collaborative working to meet patient needs is not new to primary care. The Harding Committee (Standing Medical Advisory Committee 1981) provided a definition of a primary healthcare team and stressed the need to understand the varying roles and responsibilities of healthcare staff in the community setting. District nurses have a long tradition of working together with other healthcare professionals to determine care provision, often in informal ways due to variations of employment and management (Young 1997). However, government policy has advocated community staff move beyond the informal approach and towards a more structured strategy in an endeavour to ensure a cohesive approach to care.

This would incorporate a wide range of staff from health and social care sectors. *The New NHS. Modern, Dependable* (Department of Health 1997) identified that integrated teams were the way forward, citing the need for healthcare professionals not only to work more closely but also to work across boundaries between health and social care. *Making a Difference* (Department of Health 1999a) stated that interdisciplinary working was important for all professionals but that nurses would have the skills to support the process. Much work had already been undertaken to develop closer working practices in localities with the creation of self-managed and integrated nursing teams (Gerrish 1999). The Audit Commission (1999) acknowledged that district nurses have played a significant part in the development of these teams, defining clarity and understanding of nurses' roles and working in more coordinated and complementary ways to meet the needs of the patients.

The success of self-managed and integrated teams seems dependent on a willingness to work together and establish a shared vision that is owned by all members, ensuring a cohesive approach towards the service to be provided. An understanding of roles is vital and communication at all levels is seen as an essential component (Audit Commission 1999). Rowe (1998) recognized that these teams needed to have the power to make change, but argues that to function effectively it is vital that district nurses have the skills of team coordination as well as clinical skills. Many services now devolve aspects such as budgetary management and collective decision-making to teams. This move away from traditional ways of working can enable district nurses at all levels to influence future developments (Gerrish 1999) and make a difference to the local provision of care. The concept of team working which crosses boundaries may, however, be challenging for nurses as boundaries become blurred and traditional roles are questioned. The district nurse's role has needed to be responsive to change and evolve and transform progressively, but it is not a generic role and the nature of district nursing could be challenged if the professional boundaries are not clear (see Chapter 21 for further information on partnership working in health and social care).

Leadership may also be an area for concern. District nurses traditionally undertake post-registration qualifications and many expect to engage in a team leader role. Studies relating to self-managed and integrated teams have differing views when considering the need for a team leader (Owen 1998). With the need for collaborative working, the role of coordinator is often adopted to ensure the team democratically makes decisions. This may challenge the traditional hierarchical approach within district nursing. The development of integration and future team working in primary care goes beyond nursing, with many integrated teams already involving care managers.

Challenges for the future

The NHS is currently going through a period of transition and the government's agenda would indicate that this is set to continue. District nurses need to be proactive, accept the challenges they are presented with and find new and innovative ways of incorporating these to ensure that they remain fit for practice. Extended nurse prescribing (Department of Health 1999b), *The Essence of Care – Patient Focused Benchmarking* (Department of Health 2001b), the national service frameworks (Department of Health 2001a), *Our Health, Our Care, Our Say* (Department of Health 2006), *Vision and Values* (QNI 2006), *The Future of Pre-registration Nursing Education* (NMC 2007) and *Towards a Framework for Post Registration Nursing Careers* (Department of Health 2007a) will all change the way that district nursing provides care for patients. District nurses have to be ready to accept the challenges to traditional ways of working and demonstrate that they are both partners and leaders in the provision of primary care nursing.

Conclusion

District nursing is constantly evolving and must be prepared to meet the challenges it faces. Influences from national and local initiatives are impacting on working practices and the skills required to meet patient need. District nurses must ensure that the team is able to embrace the challenges faced. Working in new ways in a community setting will offer exciting opportunities for district nurses as they work more collaboratively with health and social care practitioners. This may also lead to a review of current working methods and to the abandonment of some of the traditional aspects of their role. The Audit Commission report, *First Assessment* (1999), provided a framework for district nursing to build on and the more recent *Vision and Values* (QNI 2006) provides a vehicle for dialogue to move district nursing forward for the 21st century. The ever-changing context of healthcare provision will mean district nurses have to ensure that they are key players in future decision-making and they should ensure that their voice is heard.

SUMMARY

- This chapter has explored the evolving role of the district nurse, the changes in healthcare policy and how this impacts on district nursing. It considers how good leadership skills can enable district nurses to undertake key roles.
- The need for caseload review is explored to support the ability of district nursing to demonstrate high-quality service provision.
- The need for collaborative multiagency working is also explored with particular reference to safeguarding adults.

DISCUSSION POINTS

1. How realistic is the concept of caseload management/analysis? How can it support district nurses in practice?
2. How realistic is the aim to provide district nursing services that are equitable country-wide?
3. How do district nurses maintain their profile as key providers of care for patients in the community?
4. It has been suggested that district nurses do not use their prescribing powers to the full; how can nurses change this perception?
5. Have NHS leaders and the profession grasped the challenges of *Vision and Values* to make district nursing fit for the future?

References

Audit Commission 1999 First assessment: a review of district nursing services in England and Wales. Audit Commission, London

Baly ME, Robottom B, Clark JM 1987 District nursing. Heinemann Nursing, Oxford

Bartholomew J, Britten N, Shaw A 1999 What they really, really want. Nursing Times 95(12): 30–31

Berry L, Hurst R 1999 Nurse prescribing: the reality. In: Humphries JL, Green J (eds) Nurse prescribing. Macmillan, Basingstoke: 90–106

Butterworth T 2007 QNI website, QNI 120th Anniversary Conference. Online: http://www.qni.org.uk/eforum.htm

Community and District Nursing Association 2003 Responding to elder abuse. Community and District Nursing Association, London

Cusick K 1998 User views of the district nursing service. British Journal of Community Nursing 3(2): 74–81

Davidhizar R 1993 Leading with charisma. Journal of Advanced Nursing 18: 675–679

Department of Health 1995 The patients' charter. HMSO, London

Department of Health 1997 The new NHS. Modern, dependable. Department of Health, London

Department of Health 1999a Making a difference. Department of Health, London

Department of Health 1999b Review of prescribing supply and administration of medicines. Department of Health, London

Department of Health 2001a National service framework for older people. Department of Health, London

Department of Health 2001b The essence of care – patient focused benchmarking for health care

practitioners. Department of Health, London

Department of Health 2002 Liberating the talents. Helping primary care trusts and nurses to deliver the NHS Plan. Department of Health, London

Department of Health 2003 Press release – national programme for IT announces further contracts to run NHS care records service. Online: http://www.dh.gov.uk/en/Publicationsandstatistics/Pressreleases/DH_4064974

Department of Health 2005 Commissioning a patient-led NHS. Department of Health, London

Department of Health 2006 Our health, our care, our say: a new direction for community services. Department of Health, London

Department of Health 2007a Towards a framework for post-registration nursing careers. Department of Health, London

Department of Health 2007b Primary Care Trust Professional Executive Committees. Fit for the future. Department of Health, London

Department of Health 2007c The national framework for NHS continuing healthcare and NHS funded nursing care. Department of Health, London

Department of Health and Home Office 2000 No Secrets: guidance on developing and implementing multi-agency policies and procedures to protect vulnerable adults from abuse. Department of Health, London

Department of Health and Social Security 1986 Neighbourhood nursing: a focus for care, report of the Community Nursing Review (The Cumberlege Report). HMSO, London

Frame G, O'Donnell P 1996 Community nursing. Weight-lifters. Health Service Journal 19: 30–31

Freeman S, Shelley G, Gay M, Ingram B 1999 Measuring services: a district nursing tool. Nursing Standard 13(47): 39–41

Gerrish K 1999 Teamwork in primary care: an evaluation of the contribution of integrated nursing teams. Health and Social Care in the Community 7(5): 367–375

NHS Leadership Centre 2004 Leadership at the point of care. Participant guide. Department of Health, London

Nursing and Midwifery Council 2007 The future of pre-registration nursing education. NMC, London

Owen A 1998 Self managed teams, the West Berkshire approach. Health Visitor 71(1): 23–24

Queen's Nursing Institute 2006 Vision and values. A call for action on community nursing. Queen's Nursing Institute, London

Queen's Nursing Institute 2007 Online: http://www.qni.org.uk/pdfs/nQNnamesconference15.5.07.pdf

Ross F, Corbett K 2005 Primary care nursing: education for changing roles and boundaries. Education for Primary Care 16: 246–255

Rowe A 1998 Self-management in primary care. Nursing Times 94(29): 60–62

Safeguarding Vulnerable Groups Act 2006. Online: http://www.opsi.gov.uk/ACTS/acts2006/ukpga_20060047_en_1

Seccombe I 1999 Listening exercise. Nursing Times 95(25): 56–58

Standing Medical Advisory Committee 1981 The primary health care team: report of a joint working group (Harding Report). Department of Health, London

Young L 1997 Improved primary healthcare through integrated nursing. Primary Health Care 7(6): 8–10

Recommended reading

Audit Commission 1999 First assessment: a review of district nursing services in England and Wales. Audit Commission, London
This document provides a strategy for the future of district nursing services and practical tips on how to implement the changes required.

Covey SR 1992 The 7 habits of highly effective people. Simon & Schuster, London
This book is a tool kit for life and leadership, but also provides the principles of adapting to change, and the understanding and power to take advantage of the chances that change can generate.

Department of Health 2001 National service framework for older people. Department of Health, London
This document provides a framework for the future provision of health and social care for the older person, promoting working across boundaries to ensure needs are most effectively met.

Queen's Nursing Institute, 2006 Vision and values. A call for action on community nursing. Queen's Nursing Institute, London
This report looks at the experience of district and community nurses to better understand their role in contemporary healthcare and provides a starting point for debate about how district nurses can be prepared, supported and developed in the future.

Specialist community public health nurse: health visiting

Dianne Watkins and Lorraine Joomun

KEY ISSUES

- History and development of health visiting
- Current specialist community public health nursing professional practice and the principles of health visiting
- Family health visiting
- The specialist community public health nurse: health visitors' role in safeguarding children
- Emerging opportunities for specialist community public health nurse: health visitors in public health

Introduction

The 21st century provides opportunities for specialist community public health nursing, health visiting, to reaffirm its public health role and make an active and visible contribution to meeting the public health agenda in the United Kingdom. Health visiting has always been firmly rooted in promoting the health of the public with a particular emphasis on maternal and child health (Council for the Education and Training of Health Visitors (CETHV) 1977). However, a more interprofessional approach to public health is now required to address the gross inequalities in health between social groups in society and to work in a proactive manner. This ideology is clearly directed by government policy in the present-day National Health Service (NHS) (Department of Health 1999a, 1999b, 2001, 2003a, 2003b, 2004a, 2004b, 2007, Home Office 1998, 1999, SNMAC 1995, Welsh Assembly Government 2005a, 2005b, Welsh Office 1998a, 1998b, 1999) and in the past history of the development of health visiting (CETHV 1977, Ministry of Health 1948).

Health visiting encompasses an individualistic and a structuralist approach to its work that seeks to empower individuals and communities to achieve their full potential for the achievement of health, through actions directed at biological, socio-economic, lifestyle and environmental determinants of health. The focus of practice is the promotion of health and well-being, protection and prevention (Nursing and Midwifery Council (NMC) 2004). The contribution of health visiting to the public health agenda has been reaffirmed by the House of Commons Health Committee (2001) and is further supported by the Royal College of General Practitioners (RCGP; 2001). They are considered 'major contributors to improving health and to the broader social inclusion agenda' (United Kingdom Central Council for Nursing, Midwifery and Health Visiting (UKCC) 2001: 2) and a key resource on public health issues in the community (House of Commons Health Committee 2001).

This chapter will provide a brief overview of the history of the profession and discuss the origin of the current specialist community public health nurse, the health visitor's role in public health, maternal and child health, and the protection of children under the age of 5 years in the United Kingdom. It will briefly explore the concept of public health, with an emphasis on health visitors' work in relation to primary, secondary and tertiary prevention. The chapter will conclude with identifying the emerging opportunities for health visitors to expand their public health role, discussed in the context of current health and social policies. It is important to note that although health visitors are renamed specialist community public health nurses, at this present time they are still annotated on the register as health visitors. Therefore to avoid confusion they will be referred to as health visitors throughout this chapter.

Historical perspective

The origins of health visiting practice began in 1862 with the formation of the Manchester and Salford Ladies Sanitary Reform Association. Respectable women were appointed to 'teach hygiene and social welfare, give social support and teach mental and moral health' (Robinson 1982). The notion of household hygiene was one echoed by Florence Nightingale; even in those early days of nursing she recognized the link between child mortality and cleanliness:

The same laws of health or of nursing, for they are in reality the same, obtain among the well as among the sick. The causes of the enormous child mortality are perfectly well known, they are chiefly want of cleanliness, want of ventilation, careless dieting and clothing, want of whitewashing; in one word defective household hygiene. (Florence Nightingale 1858 cited in CETHV 1977: 12)

Although Florence Nightingale felt this was a call to the nursing profession, she was able to make the division between nursing the sick and nursing the well. She acknowledged the importance of a 'non-judgemental' home visiting service, which would prevent the service becoming unpopular or seen as interference in the lives of families (CETHV 1977: 12). In 1892 the first health visiting training programme was established. However, it was not formally recognized as such until 1919 when the Ministry of Health and the Board of Education jointly validated a 2-year course of study.

During these early years of health visiting, the emphasis was on promoting public health, through teaching and helping the poor, with activities more related to social work, and improving sanitary conditions, than it was to nursing. However, the importance of maternal and child health grew, influenced by the many recruits to the Boer War who were unfit for military service. This led to a realization that investing in the health of children was important for the economy and productivity of the country, and consequently the infant welfare movement emerged. Clinics were established to teach mothers how to care for their babies, and in 1925 the Ministry of Health recommended that all health visitors possess a midwifery qualification. This was influential in promoting the health visitors' role in working primarily with mothers and children, and health visiting became a universal home visiting service extended to middle class families.

The health visitor's work continued to retain a child and maternal health perspective. However, it also focused on the field of social medicine and the numbers of health visitors were increased in an effort to reduce child mortality and morbidity. There was a fall in maternal and child mortality between 1901 and 1971, which can be attributed in part to improved maternal nutrition, legal abortion, extending the period of breastfeeding, and improved living conditions. Although medical advances, such as immunization and antibiotics, made some contribution to improving the health of the nation, this was considered small in comparison with the impact of efforts to improve environmental and social conditions (Ashton and Seymour 1988). As the health of mothers and children improved, so the need for health visitors appeared to decline. However, Beveridge (Ministry of Health 1948) reinstated the role which reinforced the maternal and child health component, and also widened the scope of the health visitor's work. The NHS Act (Ministry of Health 1948) defined health visitors as:

Women employed by local authority for visiting persons in their homes for the purpose of giving advice as to the care of young children, persons suffering from illness, and expectant and nursing mothers, and as to the measures necessary to prevent the spread of infection. (Wilkie 1979)

Although the focus was primarily mothers and young children, the scope of health visiting practice expanded during the early years of the NHS in an attempt to meet the above description of the role. This led to some difficulties in health visitors clearly defining their work and disparities were evident throughout the UK. Some health visitors were 'triple duty' nurses engaged in health visiting, district nursing and midwifery duties, others were working directly in the school health service and some were working with the elderly or diabetics (CETHV 1977).

As a result of the inequities in service delivery and poor recruitment to health visiting training, an investigation was commissioned. The Jameson Report (Ministry of Health 1956) was published as a result of this investigation, which advocated a number of changes for the profession. It stated that health visitors must retain their focus with families where there were young children. However, they should become family visitors with a primary function of social advice and health education.

Present-day specialist community public health nursing: health visiting practice

In 1962 the Health Visiting and Social Work Act set up the Council for the Training of Health Visitors (later known as the Council for the Education and Training of Health Visitors (CETHV)). They offer the following definition for health visiting:

the professional practice of health visiting consists of planned activities aimed at the promotion of health and prevention of ill health. It therefore contributes substantially to individual and social well-being, by focussing attention at various times on either an individual, a social group or a community. (CETHV 1977: 8)

This definition is one that is still used today and it outlines the complex nature of health visiting, in that the focus for promoting health is not just the individual, i.e. the child, mother or family, but also social groups and communities. Health visitors assess the health needs of community populations, groups and individuals and establish appropriate programmes of prevention which contribute to social well-being, as well as physical and emotional health (NMC 2002, 2004, Quality Assurance Agency for Higher Education (QAA) 2001, UKCC 2001). Health visiting differs from other dimensions of nursing because of its emphasis on working with communities to address issues of health and social inequalities and social exclusion (see Chapter 23 for further information). This dimension of their work clearly fits into the remit of public health, although it is different from other professionals who practise within this field. Health visitors usually hold a caseload made up of individual clients who are either registered with a general practitioner to whom the health visitor is attached, or make up a defined community, allocated to them on a geographical basis. This allows for personal individual contact, as well as opportunities to work on public health issues with specific groups and communities, such as Sure Start and Flying Start.

In 2004 the NMC made changes to the current register, with the formation of three registers, one each for nursing, midwifery and specialist community public health nursing. All health visitors were migrated to this register. The formation and naming of this register had implications for health visiting, in light of the name change and protection of the public. Standards of proficiency for specialist community public health nursing were developed by the NMC in 2004. These standards also incorporated school nursing and occupational health nursing. All three disciplines were registered on the third register under the title 'Specialist Community Public Health Nurse'. Each discipline would be annotated on the register according to the route that was undertaken within an educational programme. New educational programmes were designed to meet this new structure.

The public health role of the health visitor

Public health has been defined as 'the science and art of preventing disease, prolonging life and promoting health through organized efforts and informed choices of society, organizations, public and private, communities and individuals' (Wanless 2004: 27). The science and art of preventing disease in health visiting practice has been described by Twinn (1991), who discusses how health visitors combine a scientific approach with the art of health visiting. The scientific basis to their work encapsulates epidemiology, and the evidence base for practice is extracted from research. This is combined with the art of professional judgement based on intuition, the complexities of families and communities, past experiences and the unique situations health visitors find themselves in. There is an art in synthesizing this information, reflecting on and in action and understanding and helping clients to achieve health. Health visiting as previously mentioned is also concerned with 'planned activities aimed at the promotion of health and prevention of ill health' (CETHV 1977), which has a positive effect on the health of individuals and society.

The public health role of the health visitor is reaffirmed by the NMC in its standards of proficiency for specialist community public health nursing when 'health visiting' was renamed 'SCPHN' (NMC 2004). This is further supported by the QAA, who developed 'benchmarking standards for health visiting education and practice' that clearly articulate the public health dimension of their work (QAA 2001). The latter document uses the following health visiting principles developed in 1977 (CETHV 1977) to underpin professional practice, which provide a sound basis for public health and are now firmly rooted in research. The NMC adopted these principles and adapted them to support their standards for practice (CETHV 1977: 9, Cowley and Appleton 2000, Cowley and Frost 2006, Twinn and Cowley 1992):

1. The search for health needs.
2. The stimulation of an awareness of health needs.
3. The influence on policies affecting health.
4. The facilitation of health-enhancing activities.

The search for health needs

One of the unique functions of health visiting is searching for health needs, some of which may be self-declared by individuals or communities, while others may be unrecognized and require skill by the health visitor to identify. This search, or proactive investigation, is essential before an assessment of health needs and planning to meet these can take place. It is working at this stage of 'pre-need' when trying to prevent needs arising in relation to social and health issues (Standing Nursing and Midwifery Advisory Committee (SNMAC) 1995) that makes health visiting practice different to any other health professional working within primary or community

care and also adds to the complexities of measuring the effectiveness of their practice (Campbell et al 1995, McHugh and Luker 2002). The universal nature of the health visiting service places health visitors in an excellent position to identify the wider needs (Cowley and Frost 2006) which may otherwise have remained suppressed or concealed. Some examples of this work include detecting and working effectively with women suffering postnatal depression (MacInnes 2000), working with children and families 'in need' and identification of child neglect or abuse (Appleton and Clemerson 1999), identifying and working with parents on child-feeding issues, nutrition, behavioural or sleep problems, all of which affect child and family health (Acheson 1998, Olds et al 1997, Seeley et al 1996).

Health visitors are also concerned with the broader issues that influence health, for example poverty, housing, unemployment and infrastructures supporting communities, such as public transport. A more recent finding is the effect that 'place' has on health improvement (Popay et al 2003). The search for health needs involves looking at these external factors that affect health, which individuals ultimately may have little control over, and working at a political level to try to positively influence these issues (see Chapter 7 for further information).

The work of health visitors in searching for health needs in communities primarily revolves around creating a profile of the local community that takes cognizance of epidemiological data, local information, community and individual needs (see Chapter 6 for further information on health needs assessment). This information is used to inform the Health Improvement Programme (HImP) for that area and ultimately to influence resource allocation (United Kingdom Standing Conference for Health Visiting Education (UKSC) 2001). Sharing of information

 Activity box 15.1

Sharon is a single parent with two children under 3 years. She lives in rented accommodation on a deprived housing estate. Sharon has recently moved to the area. There is a lack of provision and a shop that sells a small variety of groceries is available. The area is particularly run down, with graffiti over the walls and burnt out cars in the streets.

Q. What knowledge and skills do you have that could identify the immediate needs of this family?

 Activity box 15.2

Sharon is socially isolated, lacking friends or family in the vicinity; she only goes out to the local shop when necessary, and she is fearful of some of the local youths that hang around. The children are kept inside and they never socialize with other children. Sharon is finding it difficult to cope, especially as the older child is displaying behaviour problems.

Q. What knowledge do you have of the local community and what services are on offer for families?

especially in safeguarding children is an important part of this process and the common assessment frameworks (CAF) have been identified in searching for these health needs.

The stimulation of an awareness of health needs

The stimulation of an awareness of health needs refers to helping people become aware of what may be possible to achieve in an effort to improve their personal health, or the health of the community (CETHV 1977, Twinn and Cowley 1992, UKSC 2001). This can also include working with disadvantaged groups in society who may have limited access to health information and resources (QAA 2001, UKSC 2001). Cowley and Frost (2006) suggest that stimulating an awareness of health needs should be extended to three different levels:

- to clients, individuals and communities
- to those who take responsibility for the commissioning of health services (health authorities, primary care trusts, local health boards)
- to politicians and policy makers.

In working with all of the above groups, the health visitor may stimulate an awareness of health needs through the provision of knowledge, recognizing that the way in which this is delivered is dependent upon the situation. When working with individuals and communities it is essential to take cognizance of social, educational and cultural backgrounds and people's personal experiences, and consider how they affect individual perceptions of health. Empowering individuals and communities to gain control over factors that influence their health underpins the application of this health visiting principle in practice and demonstrates the approach used by health visitors when engaging in 'health promotion' as seen in its broadest sense. This is encapsulated in the definition given by the World Health Organization (1986), which states that 'health promotion is about enabling people to increase control over and so improve their health'. The QAA (2001: 7) emphasizes this point when it describes health visiting as using a 'partnership approach to practice, through which clients are empowered to address issues influencing their health'. This is an essential element of promoting health and preventing ill health and places health visitors in a central position to deliver a public health agenda, based on identified health needs.

Activity box 15.3

Sharon's accommodation consists of a flat on the third floor; she has no garden for the children to play in, and there are no park facilities in the neighbourhood.

Q. What specialist skills and knowledge do you have to influence the local authority in developing safe play areas for children?

It is worth exploring 'empowerment' in more detail in an effort to describe the way in which health visitors undertake practice. Empowerment is a two-way process between professional and client, where the client's needs take priority, and goals are negotiated (Naidoo and Wills 2000). The principles revolve around fostering informed choice, supporting change rather than coercing clients, the provision of knowledge and allowing people to make up their own mind (Tones and Tilford 1994: 11). Persuasion, instruction or propaganda do not form part of the process; however, clarifying values, building self-esteem, and developing supportive environments and services to achieve well-being are essential ingredients of this approach (Cowley and Frost 2006). It is important to consider that some families lead complex and deprived lives; these often hard to reach families have hidden needs which can be identified by the health visitor.

When working with politicians and policy makers to stimulate an awareness of health needs it is essential to ensure that links, whether overt or covert, are made with the political agenda. To inform this process health visitors need to ensure that health profiles are compiled based on epidemiological data and client experiences, and clearly identify the issues for the community, such as housing or safe play areas for children. Action taken to improve communities must be undertaken in partnership with other agencies, as no one agency can be effective alone.

The influence on policies affecting health

Cowley and Frost (2006: 32) suggest that this principle can be implemented through three interwoven mechanisms:

- information/health intelligence
- innovation and change within the NHS/health sector
- acting as a resource.

Activity box 15.4

Sharon and the children would benefit from groups and activities that would enable her to meet people and socialize her and the children into the community.

Q.   What knowledge and skills do you have that could be used to develop interventions to address the needs for this family?

Health visitors influence policies on a national and local level and this is pivotal to promoting health and preventing ill health (QAA 2001, UKSC 2001). They are ideally placed in the heart of the community to identify health and social needs, by identifying problems early, and to develop policies to prevent these problems (Wanless 2004). Information about emerging health needs in the community should be disseminated to health commissioners; health visitors collate such information, and therefore it would make sense for health visitors to become actively involved in primary care trusts or local health boards to influence healthcare planning based on accurate needs assessments, ensuring that strategies include issues for prevention (SNMAC 1995). This would incorporate taking part in strategy development that may impact on the health of the community. Examples relate to influencing health improvement plans, health action zones (HAZs) or contributing to services in relation to healthy living centres. Working at an international and a national level with organizations such as the Community Practitioner and Health Visitor Association and the Royal College of Nursing is an effective way to influence policy development and the future profession of health visiting.

The facilitation of health-enhancing activities

Facilitating health-enhancing activities is a major part of health visiting professional practice and includes the broad remit of public health inclusive of environmental changes, personal preventative activities and therapeutic endeavours (Cowley and Frost 2006). This may take place through encouraging and enabling individuals to take responsibility for their own health, through facilitating health-enhancing activities which could be community or family based, or by influencing policy formation which positively affects health. Campaigning to establish

services in deprived or disadvantaged areas such as nursery school provision, or activities for teenagers are examples of facilitating health-enhancing activities. Monitoring health needs and acting as an agent who mediates between agencies on behalf of families and individuals and promotes health-enhancing activities is another element of health visiting.

Sure Start, and more recently Flying Start, is the cornerstone of the government's drive to tackle child poverty and social exclusion (Home Office 1998, Welsh Office 1999, Welsh Assembly Government 2005b), and provides excellent examples of health-enhancing activities by health visitors (Bidmead 1999, Daniel 1999). There is substantial evidence to support early interventions with children and much of the work in the United States by Olds et al (1986, 1997) and Kitzman et al (1997) demonstrated the benefits of home visiting in the pre- and postnatal period. The results of these studies indicate programmes can reduce child abuse and neglect, improve parenting skills and the quality of child interactions, reduce subsequent pregnancies and, in the long term, reduce criminal behaviour of mothers and children (Olds et al 1998). This evidence base has been used as the basis for Sure Start programmes, which are multiagency and set about to improve the health, intellectual and social development of children; pilot sites have been set up in England to implement parenting programmes using the Olds methods (Home Office 1998, 1999).

The principles of health visiting can be traced through professional practice as demonstrated in the above discussion. However, it is worth clearly articulating their role in family visiting and child protection. This vital work continues to dominate health visiting practice, and although in some areas different models of health visiting are being implemented, the universal service of home visiting continues in one form or another. The term progressive universalism was defined by the Department of Health (2007: 25) as 'those with the greatest risks and needs receive more intensive support', which idealizes the more targeted approach. The NHS Executive (1996) recommended that all families should receive a visit from a health visitor following the birth of a baby and that future visits after this time should be needs led and left to the discretion of the health visitor. This has resulted in NHS trusts setting their own frameworks and standards for health visiting practice (McHugh and Luker 2002). However, experience and research confirm that the focus of their work remains with children under 5 years and their families (Appleby and Sayer 2001, Department of Health 2007, House of Commons Health Committee 2001, NMC 2004).

Family health visiting

The nature of home visiting health visitors undertake can be categorized into primary, secondary and tertiary prevention, although Downie et al (1996) warn against the difficulties in defining any health promotion work in this way. They comment on the disease focus, the lack of standard definitions for these three areas thus categorizing prevention in the absence of meaning, and the continued debate over what constitutes primary and secondary prevention. Hall and Elliman (2003) attempt to attach definitions to the three areas and describe primary prevention as reducing the incidence of a given disease or condition. Examples of the health visitor's work in primary prevention would be the promotion of immunization programmes to reduce the incidence of communicable diseases; promotion, education and advice regarding breastfeeding to promote child immunity and protect from infection and atopic conditions (Latham 1999, Lawrence 2000); education related to the prevention of childhood injuries and home accidents and parenting programmes aimed at enhancing parents' confidence and self-esteem (Department of Health 1998, Home Office 1998, Kitzman et al 1997). The latter improves children's health and educational attainment and reduces juvenile delinquency and mental health problems in later life, which demonstrate excellent examples of primary prevention (Olds et al 1998).

Secondary prevention is aimed at reducing the prevalence of diseases or conditions, that is reducing the impact, shortening the duration, and early detection of abnormalities resulting in prompt intervention (Hall and Elliman 2003). Health visitors engage in secondary prevention by early referral to speech therapy for speech problems in children; working with parents in relation to child sleep difficulties (Kerr et al 1997); detection and prompt management and treatment of postnatal depression thus avoiding the potential adverse consequences on child health and development (MacInnes 2000, Seeley et al 1996); identification of child feeding problems and children who fail to thrive; early detection and management of child development and behaviour problems (Sutton 1995) and prompt referral to other professionals.

Tertiary prevention is identified as reducing the impact of disease or disabilities, and assisting people to live within the confines of a disease or condition (Hall and Elliman 2003). Health visitors have a limited role in tertiary prevention, compared to other nurses who work in the community, particularly the district nurse whose role includes working with terminally ill patients and those with chronic diseases. The majority of the health visitors' work in tertiary prevention relates to working with families where there is a child with special needs.

As previously mentioned, the division between primary and secondary prevention remains blurred and is open to criticism no matter how one defines these elements of prevention. Perhaps a useful way to clarify their meaning is to consider primary prevention as activities undertaken with a particular group or population in which there is no identified risk. Once risk has been identified then activities fall into secondary prevention. An example of this is screening for cardiovascular risk factors such as smoking, obesity and raised blood pressure. Identification is primary; however, once any one of these risks has been identified and is treated or monitored, then it becomes secondary prevention, e.g. monitoring and treatment of hypertension, smoking cessation programmes. Tertiary prevention would relate to working with clients post-myocardial infarction in relation to cardiac rehabilitation. Heartline, an initiative by health visitors in Lincolnshire, has adopted an approach to prevention of coronary heart disease that encompasses primary, secondary and tertiary prevention. It includes working with families with a new baby, work with schools on lifestyle issues and post-coronary care (Ching and Pledge 1996).

Domiciliary health visiting has been scrutinized over recent years, in relation to its effectiveness and cost efficiency, and a systematic review was completed by Elkin et al (2000) and Bull et al (2004). When considering the results of this review, it is important to note that many of the studies included were American and so may be atypical of health visiting in the United Kingdom. Robinson (1999) reviewed the draft report of the systematic review and commented on the paucity of British research in relation to health visiting, particularly the lack of randomized controlled trials. The results must therefore be viewed with trepidation. Home visiting effectiveness was demonstrated in (Robinson 1999: 16):

- improved parenting skills and quality of home environment
- amelioration of child behaviour problems
- improved child intellectual and motor development, especially in low-birthweight children and failure to thrive
- increased immunization uptake
- reduced use of medical services
- reduced unintentional injury and the prevalence of home hazards
- improved detection and management of postnatal depression
- enhanced quality of social support to mothers
- improved breastfeeding rates
- initiatives limiting family size.

Both reviews were inconclusive in demonstrating effectiveness in reducing child abuse and neglect. However, surveillance bias was a particular problem in determining the effectiveness of home visiting in this area. Home visiting of the older person was proven as effective in relation to reducing carers' coping stress, enhancing carers' quality of life and reducing mortality and hospital admissions in elderly people. Cost-effectiveness was based on six studies from the USA, five of which produced favourable results, with the costs of home visiting offset by savings in reduced inpatient and outpatient care and/or reduced welfare provision (Robinson 1999).

The specialist community public health nurse's role in safeguarding children

Whilst health visiting was developing as a profession, in the background there was concern over protecting children's interests. The National Society for the Prevention of Cruelty to Children (NSPCC) campaigned for legislation to protect children who were the victims of ill treatment by parents or caretakers (Dingwall 1982).

Parental 'duty' and the 'right' to punish children prevails through the history of child rearing, and has been influential in shaping the construction of childhood and child abuse, and consequently the health visitor's work in working with families to safeguard children. Advice to parents in the postwar period referred to not picking up youngsters for fear of spoiling them, and the parent's duty to 'discipline'

the child is referred to in present-day literature. The fine line between leniency and discipline is difficult to determine for some, with others basing their child-rearing practice on transgenerational family cultures, which may date back to the middle years of the 20th century. Some parents believe they have a right to discipline their child in whatever way they wish (Mayall and Foster 1989). However, there has been a move away from parents 'owning their children, to do with as they wish', towards state protection of children as an investment for the country. It was felt that parents held their children in trust, and should they betray that trust, then the state had the right to intervene and monitor the parents to ensure they carried out their duties.

The maternal and child welfare service that developed in response to the above philosophy was seen as best delivered by the health visiting service. It was seemingly non-stigmatizing and the health visitor was considered a 'friend' rather than an inspector (Newman 1980). Dingwall (1982) comments on the suitability of the health visiting service delivering a surveillance service into the 'very heart of every family home in the country', because of 'its compromise between enforcement and libertarian values' (Dingwall 1982: 340). Although health visitors had no legal right of entry into families, they rarely made this fact known, they were accepted by communities, and the principles they adhered to revolved around respect, waiting for an invitation to enter, and not acting as an inspector (Dingwall 1982). These values remain inherent today in the professional practice of health visiting.

The health visitor's role in safeguarding children has now become a major one, and in recent years particular emphasis has been placed on the profession promoting and protecting the health of children under the age of 5 years. This includes the prevention, detection and management of child abuse and neglect (Department for Education and Skills 2003, Department of Health 1999a, 2003b, Welsh Office 1998a, 1998b). Deaths of children caused by child abuse or neglect have heightened public awareness of the problem and there is acceptance that health visitors intervene in the private life of families, on behalf of the state (Dingwall and Robinson 1993).

The main agencies and professionals who work together in the prevention and identification of child abuse include: National Health Service trusts (particularly health visitors and school nurses), social services, the police and the NSPCC. Health visitors and school nurses do not have legal right of access to households, while all other professionals mentioned have statutory powers to investigate cases of actual or suspected child abuse (Department of Health 1989, Home Office, Department of Health, Department of Education and Science 1991).

The Health Visitors Association (HVA; 1994) describes the work of the health visitor in the prevention of child abuse as one of observation, assessment, recording and referring. They note that it is 'not the responsibility of the health visitor to diagnose, nor to investigate child abuse' and categorize the role into (HVA 1994: 17):

1. the prevention of abuse and neglect
2. the identification and assessment of children causing concern
3. the referral for investigation of children who are at risk of or subject to abuse or neglect.

A variety of interventions are undertaken by health visitors that aim to prevent the abuse and neglect of children, and these may take place through the universal home visiting service, or community-based work. Mayall and Foster (1989: 64) define intervention as: 'any unsolicited action taken by health visitors to concern themselves with the way parents bring up their children'. It is recognized that home-based interventions by health visitors may stretch across a continuum, depending on the needs of the family. It may extend from 'compulsory supervision of households to ensure children are not being ill treated (initiated by a Court Order), to monitoring health, to promoting development of the child's full potential' (Mayall and Foster 1989: 66). The surveillance role of health visitors would also fit into this continuum; although comparable with monitoring it appears to have more of a custodial meaning. This is illustrated by the *Collins English Dictionary* (1993) definition which refers to surveillance as 'close observation of a person in custody or under suspicion', while monitoring is to 'observe or record the condition or performance of a person or thing'.

Many authors comment on the important surveillance role of health visitors (Dingwall 1982, Hall and Elliman 2003, HVA 1994), which some authors interpret as a 'policing role' (Dingwall 1982), and others as secondary prevention (Hall and Elliman 2003). The HVA (1994) remark on the health visitor's prime responsibility revolving around child health surveillance, based on the monitoring of child health, identifying families who may be vulnerable

to abuse and agreeing a programme of intervention which assists parents in providing 'more adequate care for their child' (HVA 1994: 19). Health promotion theorists may dispute whether surveillance, interpreted as 'policing' and 'compulsory supervision of households', performed by health visitors is comparable with the main principle of health promotion, namely empowerment.

Relating this to the prevention of child abuse and neglect raises some interesting dilemmas for health visitors. It may be necessary to have a hidden agenda and to work towards this when trying to oversee the welfare of children, although health visitors may wish to empower mothers. This raises the question of whether prevention using an empowerment approach and protection, using the definition for surveillance, can take place in tandem.

Taylor and Tilley (1989) discuss the difficulty health visitors encounter between establishing a trusting confidential relationship with families, and their policing role. They suggest the problem may be resolved by accepting that the child has priority over the carer, whose needs must take precedence over all other factors. This view is supported by De La Cuesta (1994), who remarks that the family is the secondary concern and the child the primary client. She states the health visitor's relationship or friendship with the mother may continue in a confidential manner, until the primary client is threatened, and it then becomes a policing role on behalf of the state.

Work by Appleton and Clemerson (1999) suggests that 'children in need' may stretch across a continuum, with low need at one end and high at the other. Low need would indicate the family are functioning well and require limited intervention by the health visitor. The focus may be on health promotion activities using an empowerment approach. Children on the child protection register would constitute the highest point on the continuum and would require professional intervention based on protection of the child. Here health visitors may be required to work in a different way with families, which involves adopting a far more directive approach. A truly empowerment approach to protection work is difficult when a child's life may be at stake.

Although there is diversity, and sometimes confusion, in approaches used by health visitors, safeguarding children forms a major element of their role. They act as an advocate for the child, and sometimes this conflicts with parental views.

UK policy and the challenges for specialist community public health nursing: health visiting

The *Independent Inquiry into Equalities in Health Report* (Acheson 1998) coupled with the 'New Labour' government has placed public health at the top of the NHS agenda. The evidence base to support prevention is strengthened by the research conducted over the last decade into the impact of poverty on maternal and child health and the implications of poor nutrition, housing, unemployment and poverty on health outcomes for all ages in the population (Acheson 1998). More recent policies commissioned by the government into the population's health (Wanless 2004) have advocated more interagency working and better involvement with communities.

Health visitors have been identified as a professional group who have close contact with the well population and are in a position to assess need and initiate appropriate programmes of prevention. The House of Commons Health Committee (2001) previously indicated that health visitors have a key role in advising community healthcare professionals and acting as a public health resource. Assessing health needs and taking an active part in commissioning health services that are responsive to local need should also comprise a major part of their work (Department of Health 2001).

The RCGP was asked how it saw the future role of the health visitor and outlined five future roles (RCGP 2001):

- protection of the vulnerable in society (not only children)
- health needs assessment and commissioning
- action to reduce inequalities
- health promotion
- primary and secondary prevention.

It proposes that training for health visitors should encompass a wider public health role, which allows them to develop the knowledge and skills to lead in the above five elements. This is supported by the government in *Saving Lives: Our Healthier Nation* (Department of Health 1999a), *Making a Difference* (Department of Health 1999b) and the *NHS Plan* (Department of Health 2001), all of which recommend a public health role for health visitors

that moves away from an individualistic approach to practice and concentrates on reducing health inequalities in a wider arena.

Although there are moves in some parts of the UK to shift the focus of health visiting from working primarily with the under-5s and their families into community- and population-based practice, barriers in terms of time and resources remain in some areas. Clark et al (2000) conducted a review of health visiting and school nursing in Wales and found that health visiting was 'under-developed, under-managed and under-resourced' (p. 36). Health visitors are faced with competing demands associated with managing caseloads and undertaking community-based interventions, as well as providing a service to vulnerable groups in society, e.g. travellers. Clark et al (2000: 37) recommend that health visiting should be reorganized to support the following three roles:

- a generalist health visiting service to families with children
- a generalist health visiting service to particular groups identified by the assessment of local needs (e.g. older people, travellers, asylum seekers)
- a public health and community development role.

In 2007 a review of health visiting was undertaken in England (Department of Health 2007), which formed part of a wider review of the nursing workforce, *Modernising Nursing Careers* (Department of Health 2006); two primary roles were identified by this review:

1. leading and delivering the child health promotion programme using a family-focused public health approach
2. delivering intensive programmes for the most vulnerable children and families (p. 23).

The review also identified that health visitors would fit into a specific role, either a wider public health role or concentrate on primary care services for children and families. Unlike the NMC (2004) who supported a cradle to grave philosophy, they advocated that health visitors should be entirely child focused, work in teams and focus more on public health from an individual and population perspective. Health visitors are beginning to work geographically and not linked to a specified GP practice. Corporate caseloads are becoming more common and teams are emerging with health visitors taking the lead.

The House of Commons Health Committee (2001) has also raised questions as to whether all health visitors can continue to work with individuals, families, groups, communities and populations. They also question whether health visitors can continue to include in their role, acting on the determinants of health, empowerment, protection of children, and working at a political level as well as influencing policy. Some decisions need to be made as to how health visitors are used effectively to meet the public health agenda. Opportunities to expand their work in public health relate to the access they have to the population through being placed in primary care, and the interdisciplinary nature of the work they undertake, which puts them in frequent contact with other professionals and agencies who serve the community.

Conclusion

This chapter set out to examine the history of health visiting and link current practice with social and health policies. It has outlined the health visitor's work with reference to the existing evidence base, recognizing that health visiting is difficult to measure in some instances because of the nature and diversity of practice, searching out and meeting needs at a pre-need level.

It would be true to say that the future looks bright for health visiting under 'New Labour' where the government's focus is on reducing inequalities and promoting health. Although the rhetoric found in recent government policies supports the health visitor's role in making a contribution to the nation's health, the conflict in paradigms between individual practice and community and population work needs to be addressed. Health visitors are unable to meet the competing demands associated with managing a caseload, child protection work and public health until extra resources are injected to support the profession. The Department of Health, in its review *Facing the Future* (2007), suggests that the time has come to develop different models of health visiting to meet all demands. Health visitors would be employed either to visit families and provide one-to-one advice and support, or to work with communities using a community development approach. All models would encompass a social and medical model of health, working towards promoting health in a number of different ways, all of which work towards meeting the public health agenda in the United Kingdom.

SUMMARY

- Health visiting has its roots in public health and continues to address the public health agenda in the United Kingdom.
- Health visitors' work is primarily focused on primary and secondary prevention with limited tertiary practice.
- Safeguarding children continues to be a major part of the role of the health visitor, although the focus of activity may need to change from prevention to protection, when the health of a child is at risk.
- The political agenda supports health visitors refocusing some of their individualistic practice to working with communities and populations.
- The time has come to re-evaluate health visiting and encourage employers to clearly articulate the service they require in line with the health needs of local populations.

DISCUSSION POINTS

1. Compile a profile of your local community using both a social and medical model of health. Identify issues you feel could influence the health of the people residing there and discuss how health visiting could contribute to enhancing the health of the community.

2. Discuss the dichotomy between 'empowerment' and 'policing' families and consider how you may deal with the dilemmas this brings when working with children and families at risk of child abuse or neglect.

3. Government policy places 'public health' at the top of its agenda. Consider how you would prioritize issues for prevention.

References

Acheson D 1998 Independent inquiry into inequalities in health report. The Stationery Office, London

Appleby F, Sayer L 2001 Public health nursing – health visiting. In: Sines D, Appleby F, Raymond E Community health nursing. Blackwell Science, Oxford

Appleton J, Clemerson J 1999 Family based interventions with children in need. Community Practitioner 72(5): 134–136

Ashton J, Seymour H 1988 The new public health. Open University Press, Milton Keynes

Bidmead C 1999 Bidding for success; making a Sure Start application. Community Practitioner 72(6): 166–167

Bull J, McCormick G, Swann C, Mulvihill C 2004 Ante- and post-natal home-visiting programmes: a review of reviews. Evidence briefing. Health Development Agency, London

Campbell F, Cowley S, Buttigeg M 1995 Weights and measures: outcomes and evaluation in health visiting. Health Visitors' Association, London

Ching A, Pledge F 1996 A lifelong approach to coronary heart disease prevention. Health Visitor 69(7): 278–279

Clark J, Buttigeg M, Bodycombe-James M, et al 2000 A review of health visiting and school nursing in Wales. University of Swansea School of Health Care Science, Swansea

Council for the Education and Training of Health Visitors (CETHV) 1977 An investigation into the principles of health visiting. CETHV, London

Cowley S, Appleton J (eds) 2000 The search for health needs. Macmillan, Basingstoke

Cowley S, Frost M 2006 The principles of health visiting: opening the door to public health practice in the 21st century. CPHVA, London

Daniel K 1999 Working in partnership. Community Practitioner 72(5): 117–118

De La Cuesta C 1994 Relationships in health visiting: enabling and mediating. International Journal of Nursing Studies 31(5): 451–459

Department for Education and Skills 2003 Every child matters. HMSO, London

Department of Health 1989 The Children Act 1989 – an introductory guide for the NHS. HMSO, London

Department of Health 1998 Our healthier nation: a contract for health. HMSO, London

Department of Health 1999a Saving lives: our healthier nation. HMSO, London

Department of Health 1999b Making a difference: strengthening the nursing, midwifery and health visiting contribution to health and health care. HMSO, London

Department of Health 2001 Investment and reform for NHS staff – taking forward the NHS plan. HMSO, London

Department of Health 2003a Liberating the public health talents of community practitioners and health visitors. HMSO, London

Department of Health 2003b Every child matters. HMSO, London

Department of Health 2004a National service framework for children, young people and maternity services. HMSO, London

Department of Health 2004b Choosing health: making healthier choices easier. HMSO, London

Department of Health 2006 Modernising nursing careers – setting the direction. DH, London

Department of Health 2007 Facing the future: a review of the role of health visitors. HMSO, London

Dingwall R 1982 Community nursing and civil liberty. Journal of Advanced Nursing 7: 337–346

Dingwall R, Robinson K 1993 Policing the family? Health visiting and the public surveillance of private behaviour. In: Beattie A, Gott M, Jones L, Sidall M (eds) Health and wellbeing: a reader. The Open University Press, Basingstoke

Downie R, Fyfe C, Tannahill A 1996 Health promotion models and values, 2nd edn. Oxford Medical Press, Oxford

Elkin R, Kendrick D, Hewitt M, Robinson J, Tolley K, Blair M 2000 The effectiveness of domiciliary health visiting: a systematic review of internal studies and a selective review of British literature. Health Technology Assessment 4(13)

Hall D, Elliman D (eds) 2003 Health for all children, 4th edn. Oxford University Press, Oxford

Health Visitors Association 1994 The health visitor's role in child protection. HVA, London

Home Office 1998 Supporting families: a consultation document. The Stationery Office, London

Home Office 1999 Supporting families: summary of responses to the consultation document. The Stationery Office, London

Home Office, Department of Health, Department of Education and Science 1991 Working together under the Children Act 1989. HMSO, London

House of Commons Health Committee 2001 Inquiry into public health. House of Commons, London

Kerr S, Jowett S, Smith L 1997 Education to help prevent sleep problems in children. Health Visitor 70(6): 224–225

Kitzman H, Olds D, Henderson C, et al 1997 Effect of prenatal and infancy home visitation by nurses on pregnancy outcomes, childhood injuries, and repeated childbearing. Journal of the American Medical Association 278(8): 644–652

Latham M 1999 Breast feeding reduces mortality. British Medical Journal 318: 1303–1304

Lawrence R 2000 Breastfeeding: benefits, risks and alternatives. Obstetrics and Gynaecology 12: 519–524

McHugh G, Luker K 2002 Users' perceptions of the health visiting service. Community Practitioner 75(2): 57–61

MacInnes A 2000 Findings of a community based group for women with PND. Community Practitioner 73(9): 754–756

Mayall B, Foster M 1989 Child health care. Heinemann Nursing, Oxford

Ministry of Health 1948 National Health Service Act. Ministry of Health, London

Ministry of Health 1956 An inquiry into health visiting. HMSO, London

Naidoo J, Wills J 2000 Health promotion foundations for practice, 2nd edn. Baillière Tindall, Edinburgh

Newman B 1980 The Betty Newman health care systems model. In: Riehl J, Ray C (eds) Conceptual models for nursing practice. Appleton Century Crofts, New York

NHS Executive 1996 Child health in the community: a guide to good practice. Department of Health, London

Nursing and Midwifery Council 2002 Requirements for pre-registration health visitor programmes. Nursing and Midwifery Council, London

Nursing and Midwifery Council 2004 Standards of proficiency for specialist community public health nurses. NMC, London

Olds D, Henderson C, Chamberlin R, Tatenbaum R 1986 Preventing child abuse and neglect: a randomised trial of nurse home visitation. Paediatrics 78(1): 65–78

Olds D, Eckenrode D, Henderson C, et al 1997 Long-term effects of home visitation on maternal life course and child abuse and neglect. Journal of the American Medical Association 278(8): 637–643

Olds D, Henderson C, Cole R, et al 1998 Long-term effects of nurse home visitation on children's criminal and antisocial behaviour. Journal of the American Medical Association 280(14): 1238–1244

Popay J, Thomas C, Williams G, Bennett S, Gatrell A, Bostock L 2003 A proper place to live: health inequalities, agency and the normative dimensions of space. Social Science and Medicine 57: 55–69

Quality Assurance Agency for Higher Education (QAA) 2001 Benchmark statement: healthcare programmes; health visiting. QAA, Gloucester

Robinson J 1982 An art and a science. Nursing Mirror 3rd November: 24–27

Robinson J 1999 Domiciliary health visiting: a systematic review. Community Practitioner 72(2): 15–18

Royal College of General Practitioners 2001 The future roles of health visitors: a position statement. RCGP, London

Seeley S, Murray L, Cooper P 1996 The outcome for mothers and babies of health visitor intervention. Health Visitor 69(4): 135–138

Standing Nursing and Midwifery Advisory Committee (SNMAC) 1995 Making it happen. Public health – the contribution, role and development of nurses, midwives and health visitors. Department of Health, HMSO, London

Sutton C 1995 Educating parents to cope with difficult children. Health Visitor 68(7): 284–285

Taylor S, Tilley N 1989 Health visitors and child protection: contradictions and ethical dilemmas. Health Visitor 62(9): 273–275

Tones K, Tilford S 1994 Health education: effectiveness, efficiency, equity, 2nd edn. Chapman and Hall, London

Twinn S 1991 Conflicting paradigms of health visiting: a continuing debate for professional practice. Journal of Advanced Nursing 16: 966–973

Twinn S, Cowley S 1992 The principles of health visiting: a re-examination.

Health Visitor Association and UK Standing Conference on Health Visiting Education, London

United Kingdom Central Council for Nursing, Midwifery and Health Visiting (UKCC) 2001 Developing standards and competencies for health visiting. UKCC Prime Research and Development Ltd, London

United Kingdom Standing Conference for Health Visiting Education (UKSC) 2001 Position statement: health visiting in the 21st century. UKSC, London

Wanless D 2004 Securing good health for the whole population. HMSO, London

Welsh Assembly Government 2005a National service framework for children, young people and maternity services in Wales. WAG, Cardiff

Welsh Assembly Government 2005b Flying start. WAG, Cardiff

Welsh Office 1998a Better health, better Wales. Welsh Office, Cardiff

Welsh Office 1998b Strategic framework: better health, better Wales. Welsh Office, Cardiff

Welsh Office 1999 Sure Start: a programme to increase opportunity for very young children and their families in Wales. Welsh Office Circular 21/99. Welsh Office, Cardiff

Wilkie E 1979 The history of the Council for the Education and Training of Health Visitors. George Allen and Unwin, London

World Health Organization (WHO) 1986 Ottawa Charter for Health Promotion. WHO, Geneva

Recommended reading

Acheson D 1998 Independent inquiry into inequalities in health report. The Stationery Office, London
This report provides an excellent insight into the inequalities in health that exist in the United Kingdom and outlines opportunities for preventative work.

Cowley S, Appleton J (eds) 2000 The search for health needs. Macmillan, Basingstoke
This book is based on sound research into health visiting practice and provides evidence to outline the work

health visitors undertake in searching out health needs.

Cowley S, Frost M 2006 The principles of health visiting: opening the door to public health practice in the 21st century. CPHVA, London

Specialist community public health nurse: school nursing

Ros Godson

KEY ISSUES

- School nursing: a historical perspective
- Development of different models of school nursing in the four countries of the UK
- Examining the role and challenges associated with school nursing
- Promoting the value of school nursing

Introduction

The school nurse role has changed considerably over the years and the stereotypical image of the school nurse checking for head lice is fast disappearing. Contemporary school nursing has received significant attention arising from the realization of the potential for school nurses to make significant contributions to the public health agenda, especially to the health of school-aged children. The word 'school nurse' in this chapter is a generic term, which can apply to any nurse who works in the field of public health with school-aged children, whether or not they are at school. This chapter will inform on the historical background of school nursing and provide an insight into school nursing services in the four countries of the UK. The school nursing role is explored and the chapter concludes by examining a range of opportunities and challenges facing the professional.

Historical perspectives

The Education Act of 1907 gave local education authorities the duty to provide for the medical inspection of children at admission to public ele-
mentary school and on other such occasions as the board directed (Harris 1995). This was a medical model of care, based upon screening, which showed up many clinical problems. But these were the days before the National Health Service (NHS), and so effective treatment was not available to all families, although school nurses were expected to do home visits and 'follow up' children, especially in regard to hygiene issues. Furthermore, schooling was not compulsory or accessible to every child until after the 1944 Education Act (Department of Education 1944), which also placed a duty on local authorities to contribute towards the mental and physical development of children. The doctor-led school health service was transferred to district health authorities under the NHS in 1974 and from this time became more universal. It was still a screening service but by now it encompassed vision and hearing tests, height and weight recording as well as immunization. Further Education Acts in 1981 (Department of Education 1981) and 1993 (Department of Education 1993) placed a statutory requirement on local education authorities to notify health services when a child needed special services in order to access education. This multiagency working has continued and expanded. Gradually the school nurse service has moved from being a task-orientated service that adopted a medical model approach to service delivery, to a public health social model approach, using health education and promotion alongside clinical interventions to improve the health of the school-aged child. School nursing is not, and has never been, the same service across the UK, and now with the four countries developing their own health services, the situation remains diverse.

School nursing: a four nation perspective

In England, school nurses are largely employed by primary care trusts (PCTs), although some are employed by secondary care trusts (hospitals) and others are employed or seconded into the local authority or a social enterprise. It is seen as a public health role, centring on health education and promotion. Independent schools, particularly secondary schools and boarding schools, usually employ their own school nurse to do first aid and caring for children who become sick at school, as well as day-to-day health administration, and sometimes health promotion work. Occasionally, the 'school nurse' is not a registered nurse, but individuals call themselves by this name as the title is not protected by statute.

The policy drivers behind school nursing in England are *Every Child Matters* (Department for Education and Skills (DfES) 2003); the *National Service Framework* (NSF) *for Children, Young People and Maternity Services* (Department of Health (DH) 2004a); *Choosing Health* (DH 2004b) and the *Healthy Living Blueprint for Schools* (DfES 2004). The Children Act (2004) provides the legal underpinning for the Every Child Matters: Change for Children (DfES 2003) programme in England and Wales. It places a legal duty on local authorities to cooperate with statutory bodies (e.g. police, probation, Connexions, NHS) to develop a single children's plan, based on the five outcomes: be healthy; stay safe; enjoy and achieve; make a positive contribution; achieve economic well-being. This is the basis for children's trusts. *The Children's Plan* (Department for Children, Schools and Families 2007) has brought these and other guidance into one document.

Currently many PCTs are undertaking service redesign in order to align school nurses more closely with health visitors and other primary care staff in children's trust formats. Children's trusts are multiagency working agreements to deliver the outcomes of *Every Child Matters* (DfES 2003). They can be 'virtual' arrangements or properly constituted trusts; each area can decide how to do this.

The NSF (DH 2004a) is a model of assessment and early intervention to improve health outcomes, which extols the role of school nurses as they play an essential role in promoting the health of school-aged children, and providing confidential healthcare advice and support. School nurses are part of a team in schools who can support the attainment of national targets such as those on child and adolescent mental health services, teenage pregnancy, child obesity and school attendance (DfES, DH 2006b). It flags up the certificated training for Personal, Social and Health Education (PSHE) which is available to all community nurses so that they can help deliver PSHE in schools (National PSHE CPD Programme 2008). The NSF (DH 2004a) states the Chief Nursing Officer's (CNO) recommendation of a minimum of one full-time, whole-year, qualified school nurse in every secondary school and its cluster primary schools, to lead the delivery of effective public health programmes and states that additional funding has been made available to PCTs to employ additional school nurses where needed.

The *Healthy Living Blueprint for Schools* (DfES 2004) includes school nurses among other health promotion staff and reiterates the CNO's recommendation to increase numbers. *Choosing Health* (DH 2004b) heralded an enhanced role for school nurses as leaders to support the health environment of schools, and again mentioned new funding which had been given to PCTs so that they could employ extra staff. School nurses would have roles in early detection and prevention and referral of problems, and health promotion regarding sexual health, obesity and mental and emotional well-being. The tool for this would be children's health guides; an extension of the Personal Child Held Record (known as the 'red book'), which the parent would fill in with the child, who would increasingly take responsibility for his/her own health, in conjunction with advice and support from the school nurse. The CNO would lead work to modernize and promote school nursing and develop a national programme for best practice.

The deputy CNO did indeed undertake a review of school nursing with stakeholder involvement which resulted in *Looking for a School Nurse* (DfES, DH 2006b). This non-statutory guidance was intended for head teachers and school governors to explain the skills and services which school nurses can bring to schools and the potentially improved health and well-being outcomes for pupils. However, as schools do not directly employ school nurses, and do not usually put aside any funding to do so, it was limited in use. At the same time the *School Nurse Practice Development Resource Pack* (DfES, DH 2006a) was republished. This gives lots of practical advice to school nurses to improve and define their practice in order to 'sell' their service to schools.

There are significant public health problems in Scottish children and young people: risk-taking behaviours such as smoking, drinking alcohol to excess and drug taking; teenage sexual health and pregnancy; poor dental health; obesity; lack of exercise, etc. (Scottish Executive 2007). The policy background for children's health services in Scotland is *Getting it Right for Every Child* (Scottish Executive 2006a). This sets out a programme of reform placing a duty on statutory agencies to enhance cooperation and information sharing and develop integrated service plans, putting the needs of children at the centre. *Delivering a Healthy Future* (Scottish Executive 2007), the action framework, states that services must be designed to protect and promote health as well as treating disease, targeted to the health challenges of the 21st century, and equitable across the country.

All schools in Scotland should be Health Promoting schools (Barnekow et al 2004). This overarching programme covers physical and emotional health and well-being in a whole school dimension. However, these initiatives have shown up the problem of a lack of children's health workforce across primary and secondary care, especially Child and Adolescent Mental Health Services (CAMHS). Scotland is now trialling a community health nurse role (Scottish Executive 2006b) which will be a combined health visitor/school nurse/district nurse public health job. This will need new university training courses to be developed, alongside existing training courses, and will need extra funding from health boards. It is difficult to see how one nurse could fulfil and maintain the competencies to the required standard across such a wide spectrum of work. Some community health partnerships have decided to keep the different public health nurse disciplines separate as before, so there is a patchwork of services across the country.

A review of school nursing in Wales (Allen et al 2004), based on representative sample data, showed an ageing, underdeveloped, under-resourced service, with disparity of practice and lack of policy direction. This was followed by a re-examination of the review of health visiting and school nursing undertaken by the National Assembly for Wales in 2000 (Irvine and Kenkre 2004). The recommendations included:

- The assembly should adopt the targets and strategies set out by the World Health Organization (WHO; 1998) in Health 21 as a framework for action.

- The school health service should be a year round service for all children and young people.
- The name 'school nurse' should be changed to 'school health nurse' to reflect the specialist public health role.
- Every school should have a designated school health nurse, but no nurse should have to serve more than five schools, depending on the health needs and location, and presuming average sized schools.
- An urgent need to map training requirements.

The Welsh government has committed to provide a minimum of one 'family nurse' per secondary school by the end of the assembly term (Welsh Assembly Government 2007) and has consulted with stakeholders regarding the scope of this role, which is an enhanced school health nurse reaching out to families and the community.

The Department of Health, Social Services and Public Safety (DHSSPS) in Northern Ireland commissioned a report on community health nursing (DHSSPS 2003) to review the current practice and possible future direction of the services. School nurses were found to have low status and low staffing levels (only 93), but no specific plans were identified for them.

All four countries are reviewing their school nurses, with the aim of involving them more in public health work streams. However, these plans have become tied up with the CNO's Modernising Nursing Careers (DHSSPS et al 2006) programme, which suggests generic roles rather than specific ones, with skills and competencies as the benchmark for employment, and not a specific school nurse qualification. This is a joint project with each country leading on a specific theme, and will result in new training routes and possibly better career progression.

Meanwhile, NHS workforce census figures show that there are only just over 1000 whole-time equivalent qualified school nurses for over 3000 secondary schools in England. Even taking into account other registered nurses working in school health teams, the total numbers remain disappointing at around 2000 whole-time equivalent nurses. These numbers include those registered nurses who only work in special schools, so the numbers available for mainstream schools are under 2000. The result is that school nurses are increasingly frustrated because they are unable to perform their public health functions owing to over-large caseloads, while all the

Case study 16.1

Laura had worked as a children's nurse in a hospital for several years, during which time she had her own three children, and became interested in working in the community. She applied to become a school staff nurse, and thoroughly enjoyed the work. Her caseload consisted of a mixed comprehensive secondary school of 1200 pupils aged 11–16, and four primary schools of 240 children each, on three days a week, term time only. The schools were delighted by the proactive way in which she approached the role, and were only too happy to have her expertise on all health matters. She set up regular 'drop-in' sessions for students at the secondary school, liaised with staff at the attached autistic unit, worked with teachers to deliver puberty talks in the primary schools, promoted the healthy schools agenda in all schools and became heavily involved with child protection concerns. However, she became increasingly frustrated by the fact that her caseload was too large for her to be effective in a public health sense, and she realized that there were limits to her knowledge. She had a previous degree in politics and could see that the best way forward for her to remedy the situation was to get her specialist community public health nurse qualification, go into management and advocate for more staff.

Discussion points

1. What transferable skills could you bring to the position of community staff nurse in a school nursing team? What attributes are needed to work within a mixed inner city comprehensive secondary school?

2. Think about an area of work where you have been frustrated because you felt unable to do your best for your patients. Is 'going into management' the only way forward, or can you think of other strategies which could improve the working environment?

time schools and PCTs find new streams of work which they should do (Ball and Pike 2005) (see Chapter 23 for further information on barriers and facilitators to nurse practice in public health). In many areas their involvement in health promotion activities has ceased as resources have been diverted to the National Child Measurement Programme and new immunization schedules. This has dire consequences, as England is forging ahead with commissioning of primary care services, and school health teams will be expected to produce results in line with Every Child Matters outcomes (DfES 2003) and government and local public service agreement targets. Contracts are being framed within the current under-resourced climate and it is difficult to see how the 'step change' in public health outcomes for school-aged children can be achieved.

The school nurse role

The first prerequisite to becoming a school nurse is to be a registered nurse who likes working with children, especially adolescents. Preferably the nurse would have an additional qualification in areas such as child development, family planning or health education. Registered nurses can apply to join a school nurse service as a community staff nurse, and once experience in this role has been gained, practitioners may go on to do the postgraduate qualification in Specialist Community Public Health Nursing, which is a 1-year, full-time programme at university.

These courses are sponsored by the strategic health authorities in the different countries. Ongoing training to become fully competent would include PSHE certificate, sex and relationships education, mental health and well-being of young people, nurse prescribing (V300), but above all an enthusiasm to take on new roles and change practice in the light of research evidence.

In 2004 the Nursing and Midwifery Council (NMC) decided to establish a third part of the nursing register specifically for health visitors, school nurses and occupational health nurses as it took the view that these public health-focused nursing disciplines have distinct features that differ significantly from general nursing and midwifery. A nurse who successfully completes an appropriate NMC-approved programme of study is entered onto the third part of the register as a specialist community public health nurse. Specialist community public health nursing aims:

... to reduce health inequalities by working with individuals, families, and communities promoting health, preventing ill health and in the protection of health. The emphasis is on partnership working that cuts across disciplinary, professional and organisational boundaries that impact on organised social and political policy to influence the determinants of health and promote the health of whole populations. (NMC 2008)

School nurses are recognized for their ability to network and act as effective links between education, health and social care and through this they make health services more accessible to pupils, parents, carers and staff (DfES, DH 2006b). Their two key responsibilities are:

- to assess, protect and promote the health and well-being of school-aged children and young people
- to offer advice, care and treatment to individuals and groups of children, young people and the adults who care for them (DfES, DH 2006b: 8).

The DfES and DH (2006b: 8) outline the services that school nurses can offer:

- As the first point of contact for children, young people and parents or carers needing health advice or information. This involves assessing individual needs, offering care and treatment, and referring on to other services as necessary. Many school nurses provide 'drop-in' sessions in schools for this purpose.
- Supporting children and young people with ongoing or specific health needs. This may include children with complex health needs or a learning and/or physical disability. Activities could include direct care and treatment, promotion of self-care, supporting parents and carers, referral to other specialists and coordination of a range of services.
- Initiating and supporting activities for promoting health across the school and community. These public health activities include contributing to PSHE delivery, working with the school to achieve the Healthy School Standard or advising on whole school programmes to address particular issues, e.g. sexual health, healthy eating. School nurses may also work in the wider community to improve children's health. Activities of this sort are likely to develop with the expansion of children's centres and the extended schools programme.

School nurses are the only public health professionals to straddle health and education, with knowledge of both, and they always work in an interagency environment. All recent documents advise that a whole school approach to public health works best, and so an effective school nurse attends his/her schools several times a week and is well known to staff and pupils. In all parts of the UK there are versions of the WHO health-promoting schools approach (Stewart-Brown 2006) in operation. This initiative, launched in 1995, is guided by the Ottawa Charter for Health Promotion (WHO 1986), and aims to strengthen health promotion and education activities at local, national, regional and global levels, to improve the health of the whole school community. Both the Healthy Schools Programme (Department for Children, Schools and Families England, Welsh Assembly Government) and Health Promoting Schools (Scottish Government, Northern Ireland Assembly) are overarching schemes which give direction for schools on all aspects of health and well-being. These are used by school nurses, Healthy Schools coordinators and PSHE teachers, alongside National Institute for Health and Clinical Excellence (NICE) guidance and policy documents already mentioned, to develop school policies around medicines, healthy eating, sex education, bullying, asthma, health and safety, etc.

The school nurse meets with class teachers in the summer term or at the beginning of the new school year, to plan his/her involvement in PSHE lessons, offering expertise in health. Health promotion sessions may include: hand washing; hygiene; healthy eating; nutrition and obesity; puberty; sex education including breastfeeding, conception, contraception, abortion, sexually transmitted infections, same sex relationships; lifestyle; stress; emotional well-being; bullying; behaviour; homophobia; accident prevention; testicular cancer; sun safety, etc. (Ball and Pike 2005). Some school nurses have done courses to help them deliver health education in the classroom.

The clinical side of the role may include running enuresis clinics, organizing and giving immunizations, nurse prescribing, first aid updating for staff, liaising with the special education needs teacher regarding health issues, dealing with medicines in school, pregnancy testing, *Chlamydia* testing and helping school staff to deal with sick children in the medical room. Some health boards and PCTs continue with screening programmes for height and weight monitoring, vision and hearing, although this is usually performed by healthcare assistants, directed by the school nurse.

Children may attend school with only a vague description of their health problem, and the school nurse must liaise with parents, community paediatricians, specialist clinical nurses, GPs and hospital consultants to draw up a care plan. Children with disabilities in mainstream schools usually have a support assistant with whom the school nurse must develop a good working relationship to deal with any health problems. Nurses in special schools attend to severely disabled children with complex needs and must maintain close communication with parents/carers and school staff. These children may need to be given routine or as-required medication during the school day. Teachers are usually reluctant to give medicines and so if there is no nurse available, the child may have to miss school.

Most school nurses run 'drop-in' clinics once a week at their secondary school, where young people can self-refer for a wide variety of reasons, both physical and emotional. A few school nurses have additional training to deliver tier 1 and tier 2 CAMHS interventions. Some drop-ins are specifically for parents, especially in primary and infant schools. Other school nurses organize smoking cessation groups, where they may prescribe nicotine replacement therapy, as well as use behaviour change strategies.

Safeguarding and child protection is a large part of the role and school nurses are involved with case conferences, report writing and planning meetings with social workers, regarding health aspects of care (Ball and Pike 2005). This is very often a problem of neglect of vulnerable children, and much time is spent organizing and arranging for them to attend appointments at CAMHS, speech therapy, dentist, immunization, eye clinic, hospital outpatients, etc. Some parents need considerable support to make sure that children are bathed regularly, their hair is combed for head lice, and they attend school wearing clean clothes and warm clothes in winter.

School nurses often work in partnership with Looked After Children's nurses, and in some areas they undertake statutory annual health assessments, which inform social services care plans. When young people are excluded from school, they have to attend a pupil referral unit (PRU). This is run by the education authority, and the pupils have individual learning plans to deal with their behaviour. Some education authorities also run 'medical PRUs' where young people who refuse to attend school because of anxiety go to try to deal with their problems. School nurses need to be creative to engage these 'hard to reach' young people. They may have missed significant amounts of school, and their health knowledge is often sparse, and not founded upon fact. Their lifestyles may mean that they are at greater risk of unplanned pregnancy, sexually transmitted infections, smoking, alcohol and drug taking, and poor nutrition.

Schools in England have been told to extend their school day to offer extracurricular activities and guidance to children, young people and families. These extended schools will offer further scope for school nurses to develop their public health role, such as offering parenting support and guidance, or sexual health clinics. It should also give more scope for wider community engagement on public health issues such as road safety, traffic pollution, air quality, housing, etc.

School nursing: challenges and opportunities

There is continuing failure of employing authorities in both education and health to recognize the potential value that proactive modern postgraduate qualified school nurses (specialist community public health nurses) can give to the health and welfare outcomes of school-aged children and young people, both at school and at home, if they were employed in sufficient numbers to lead the health agenda in schools and given authority to do so (see Chapter 23 for further information). They need mobile phones so that they are contactable, and laptops so that they can best use and retrieve client records and school data. Qualified school nurses should be part of the peripatetic team in school, alongside Connexions advisers, social workers and education welfare officers. In many areas, however, they work in isolation, and are unaware of the direction of the children's service agenda in their area, as they are just too busy (Ball and Pike 2005).

In some areas, adult trained community staff nurses with no training or experience of working with children or young people, or of public health nursing, are being employed as 'school nurses'. Consequently many 'school nurses' are ill-equipped to deal with the hustle and bustle of school, have no confidence in contributing to the curriculum and are unable to work with teenagers. They do not have the skills to assess the health status of the school within the wider community, and they revert to task-based 'screening'. The result is that school staff fail to see the value of their input, and do not respect the profession. There is a dearth of outcomes data, owing to lack of interest by researchers, and lack of commissioning by health departments. It is a mainly female, part-time term time only workforce, which means that boys do not have access to men to discuss their health issues. However, nurses are trusted by young people because they listen to their concerns in a non-judgemental way and help them to plan strategies to deal with their problems, and the fact that nurses are happy to talk about sex and relationship education (SRE). They understand that the role of a nurse is different from that of a teacher. Case studies 16.1 and 16.2 stimulate the reader to reflect upon some of the challenges faced by school nurses.

School nursing is not an equitable service across the UK; some areas have seen investment in the service and an up-skilling of staff, whereas other areas have removed posts and employed lower skilled staff, bearing no relationship to health needs. School nurses have taken over the role of the 'school doctor' in many parts of the UK, without remuneration following the patient. Overall the management of children's health and well-being is aimless, and lots of different staff have been employed by different agencies to deal with the bits which have become a problem, but this piecemeal approach

---

Case study 16.2

Marsha decided to become a school staff nurse as the hours fitted around her growing family. She hadn't worked in the community before, nor had she had experience of working with children. However, she impressed at interview with her enthusiasm, and the team were very pleased to have her, as they were considerably understaffed.

She was given a caseload of five primary schools of 240 children each, one secondary school of 1000 pupils, and a mentor to show her the ropes. She worked four days a week term time only. The catchment area was socially disadvantaged, and all schools had high health needs; the free school meals entitlement averaged 40%.

Marsha was very willing to be a good school nurse, but was unsure how to go about this. Her mentor was often very busy, and there was no one else available to help her. She arranged height and weight checks on the 5-year-old entrants, but the school staff did not seem to need her services, even though it was obvious to Marsha that there were many vulnerable children. She quickly became caught up in the never-ending safeguarding issues, and needed to write reports and attend case conferences regularly. She had never done any work like this before, and found it distressing and daunting, particularly when she was required to make a decision on the panel at case conferences about whether or not a child should go onto the child protection register. Unfortunately, a few months after she started the job, she sustained a health problem which meant that she was off sick for several months. On her return to work after the summer holidays, she found that she was stressed and panicky, and unable to perform effectively. She was withdrawn with colleagues, needed to take odd days off sick, and was defensive with her (new) team leader.

Her team leader decided to do annual performance assessments with all staff as a way of approaching these problems without being seen to single out this failing nurse.

It transpired that Marsha had missed out on basic child protection training, and had only accessed specialized training. She had received no mentoring or in-house training about school health priorities, and did not understand the relevance of policy documents to her work. She had never appreciated that public health work was different from clinical work, which was why she was confused about the remit of her job. She had never learnt anything about health education or promotion, and did not know about the national curriculum in schools. It was frankly unreasonable to expect her to be effective at all. Her team leader decided to make time to work with her a couple of days a month in her schools, and a plan of learning was drawn up incorporating regular meetings with the team leader to discuss policies, public health and clinical supervision, as well as short courses and reading. Marsha perceived that her manager had no confidence in her work, and had to be reassured that she would become more confident as she became more competent.

Discussion points

1. Are 'transferable skills' the same as 'competencies'? Should nurses transferring from one area of nursing to another undergo a short period of mandatory training? What responsibility do you have to skill yourself when undertaking a new role? How would you have approached this new job?

2. What do you consider to be the point of annual performance assessment reviews? Think about occasions when you have been offered these. Were they useful opportunities to consider your career progression and future training needs? Did you feel an equal partner in the negotiation, or were you just relieved that your manager found nothing wrong with your work? What responsibility do you have if your manager delays initiating annual reviews?

lacks leadership and direction, and is not under-pinned by public health values. For example, counsellors (often without relevant qualifications) are employed to deal with social and emotional issues; educational welfare officers chase up children with regular absence from school. 'Brain gym' and other schemes with no evidence base of effectiveness are seen as a panacea for stress and behaviour; office staff are expected to supervise medicines in school with no knowledge, or training; teachers are spending time making phone calls to hospital departments and GPs; and special education needs teachers write statements without knowledge of health services which could be beneficial to the particular child.

There are 'bought in' childhood obesity programmes which are not related to the school curriculum, nor the Healthy Schools scheme, nor the school nurse. The National Child Measurement Programme in England to weigh and measure all 5-year-olds and 11-year-olds is not evidence based and there is no intervention aligned to this programme; it is not related to any of the health or education policy documents. No one is monitoring the outcome when health services are redesigned, or flagging up gaps in the services to children and young people. PCTs (England) do not take school nurses into account as part of the public health workforce, and community health trusts (Scotland) are expecting their community health nurses to know everything about improving public health and delivering optimum clinical outcomes from cradle to grave; which has never been achieved before.

PCTs (England), community health partnerships (Scotland), local health boards (Wales) and local health and social care groups (Northern Ireland) must recognize the unique opportunity to influence the health outcomes of school-aged children who are obliged to be in education for 11 years, and employ one full-time *qualified* school nurse per secondary school and its cluster of primaries, according to assessed health need. School nurses must be supported to understand and develop their public health function in line with the Every Child Matters agenda in England and other relevant policy documents in all four countries, and proactively develop their role. Children only get 'one shot' at childhood, and we need to ensure their optimum mental and physical health throughout their school years.

SUMMARY

- Modern school nursing is supported by all four governments' strategic guidance, but as this is not statutory, it remains to be seen how far this will translate into training places and jobs.
- The value of specifically trained public health nurses is not well understood by decision-makers and planners, who assume that all 'nurses' can deliver public health outcomes.
- There is a general lack of operational leadership of the public health agenda for school-aged children, and school nurses are ideally placed to take up this mantle.

DISCUSSION

1. How do you know that you are effective in your role? What criteria are you measuring your outcomes against? Have you planned your work to deliver these outcomes? How would you explain to another health professional what you achieve for school-aged children?

2. What do you understand by 'public health'? Do you ensure that public health principles underpin the way you approach your work? How do you develop the principles of the Ottawa Charter for health promotion to incorporate them into work with school-aged children?

3. Do you have the competency and skill to lead the health component of the Health Promoting Schools (or Healthy Schools) agenda in the schools where you work? Are you monitoring adherence to health policies in your schools? Are you liaising with local public health staff to increase emphasis on aspects of this agenda which impact specifically on the schools where you work? Are you using data to direct your interventions? Do you need to develop yourself professionally to meet the challenges ahead?

References

Allen D, Carnwell R, Griffiths L, et al 2004 Review of primary care and community nursing in Wales: summary and recommendations. Welsh Assembly Government, Cardiff

Barnekow V, Buijs G, Clift S, et al 2004 Health-promoting schools: a resource for developing indicators: being well, doing well. Scottish Health Promoting Schools Unit. Online: http://www.healthpromotingschools. co.uk/aboutus/index.asp

Ball J, Pike G 2005 School nursing: results from a census survey of RCN school nurse in 2005. Royal College of Nursing, London

Children Act 2004 HM Government, London

Department for Children, Schools and Families 2007 The children's plan: building brighter futures. HMSO, London

Department for Education and Skills 2003 Every child matters. HMSO, London

Department for Education and Skills 2004 Healthy living blueprint for schools. HMSO, London

Department for Education and Skills, Department of Health 2006a The school nurse practice development resource pack. HMSO, London

Department for Education and Skills, Department of Health 2006b Looking for a school nurse. HMSO, London

Department of Education 1944 Education Act. HMSO, London

Department of Education 1981 Education Act. HMSO, London

Department of Education 1993 Education Act. HMSO, London

Department of Health 2004a National Service Framework for children, young people and maternity services. HMSO, London

Department of Health; 2004b Choosing health. HMSO, London

Department of Health; Department of Health, Social Services and Public Safety; Scottish Executive; Welsh Assembly Government 2006 Modernising nursing careers. HMSO, London

Department of Health, Social Services and Public Safety 2003 Community health nursing: current practice and possible futures. DHSSPS, Belfast

Harris B 1995 The health of the school child: a history of the school medical service in England and Wales. Open University Press, London

Irvine F, Kenkre J 2004 A re-examination of the review of health visiting and school nursing. Welsh Assembly Government, Cardiff

National PSHE CPD Programme 2008 VT education and skills. Online: http://www.pshe-cpd.com

Nursing and Midwifery Council 2004 Standards of proficiency for specialist community public health nurses. NMC, London

Nursing and Midwifery Council 2008 What does a SCPHN do? Online: http://www.nmc-uk.org/aArticle. aspx?ArticleID=2737

Scottish Executive 2006a Getting it right for every child: implementation plan. HMSO, Edinburgh

Scottish Executive 2006b Visible, accessible and integrated care: report of the review of nursing in the community in Scotland. HMSO, Edinburgh

Scottish Executive 2007 Delivering a healthy future: an action framework for children and young people's health in Scotland. HMSO, Edinburgh

Stewart-Brown S 2006 What is the evidence on school health promotion in improving health or preventing disease and, specifically, what is the effectiveness of the health promoting schools approach? Copenhagen: WHO Health Evidence Network report. Online: http://www.euro. who.int/document/e88185.pdf

Welsh Assembly Government 2007 One Wales. HMSO, Cardiff

World Health Organization 1986 Ottawa Charter for Health Promotion. Online: http://www. who.int/hpr/NPH/docs/ottawa_ charter_hp.pdf

World Health Organization 1998 HEALTH21: the health for all policy framework for the WHO European Region. Online: http://www.euro.who.int/ InformationSources/Publications/ Catalogue/20010911_38

Recommended reading

DeBell D (ed.) 2007 Public health practice and the school-age population. Edward Arnold, London

An invaluable text for students; an analysis of the key issues facing practitioners is offered in relation to the needs of school-aged children in contemporary Britain today. This book is an essential reference text for school and community nurses.

Selekman J (ed.) 2005 School nursing: a comprehensive text. FA Davies, Philadelphia

This text highlights the role of the school nurse in coordinating a comprehensive school health programme. The text illustrates the vital role of the school nurse in the clinical management of child healthcare. A practical resource grounded in evidence-based practice, this will be a valuable resource for students undertaking school nursing educational programmes as well as school nurse practitioners.

Specialist community public health nurse: occupational health nursing

Bashyr Aziz

KEY ISSUES

- The historical background to occupational health nursing
- The development of occupational health nursing
- A competency framework for occupational health nursing
- Emerging challenges for occupational health nurses

Introduction

There have been occupational health nurses in the United Kingdom ever since 1878, when the wife of a mustard factory owner asked a local district nurse to go in and look after the health of the workers in her husband's manufacturing plant (Charley 1954). Since then, factory nurses, industrial nurses and then occupational health nurses have been employed by different types of organizations to carry out a variety of roles to ensure as far as possible that workers remained productive and free from work-related injury or illness.

Unlike many other community nurses, occupational health nurses in the United Kingdom have not had a framework for practice or their roles and functions spelt out clearly by a single higher authority, nor has the law ever made it mandatory for any organization to employ occupational health nurses. This has had both negative and positive effects on occupational health nursing. A negative impact has been that employers have frequently found it expedient to downsize or even do away with occupa-

tional health provision when it has become necessary to cut costs. A positive impact has been that occupational health nurses have been able to be creative and entrepreneurial, and adaptive to the needs of changing patterns of work in order to ensure that their role remained relevant in a rapidly changing world of work.

Although occupational health nursing education in the United Kingdom originated within the public health arena (Charley 1954), for many years occupational health nursing has been seen as being outside public health; it was only in 2004, when the Nursing and Midwifery Council (NMC) created the specialist community public health nursing (SCPHN) part of its register and placed occupational health firmly within that alongside health visiting and school nursing (NMC 2004a) that occupational health nurses again started to explore the vast contribution they could make in public health.

The roles and functions of occupational health nurses have had to change and adapt to the changing nature of work in the United Kingdom and other Western industrialized countries. The power and influence of occupational health nurses has waxed and waned over the decades, usually in step with the power and influence of trade unions. In recent years, following the appointment in 2005 of a national director for health at work, and the publication of her review of the health of Britain's working population in March 2008 (Black 2008), occupational health nurses have begun to feel that they are at the start of a new, exciting and challenging phase in their contribution to a strong and healthy economy.

Background

Early influences

The fact that some types of work can be harmful to health has been known for a very long time. Agricola (1494–1555), an official town physician in Bohemia, and Paracelsus (1493–1541), a physician in Austria, both made observations about the high risk of injury and disease associated with mining. Agricola made the interesting observation that in the mining areas, he had met women who had married seven husbands, all of whom had died prematurely from diseases related to mining. However, it is Bernardino Ramazzini (1633–1714), a physician in Italy, who is generally referred to as the father of occupational health. His book about the dangers to health of different types of work, *De Morbis Artificum*, is still a fascinating read, available in translation as *Diseases of Workers* (1993), and it contains advice to occupational health practitioners which is still relevant, and sadly often not followed. First published in 1715, Ramazzini's book also describes conditions which seem more modern, such as stress and repetitive strain injury.

Despite the understanding of the harmful effects of some types of work, there was not great regard paid to occupational health in the United Kingdom until the First World War. Prior to this there was either general indifference, or a fatalistic attitude to the harmful effects of some types of work. Dirty jobs such as mining had to be done, and it was inevitable that the poor people who did such jobs eventually ended up with illness or injury caused by their work.

It is likely that the US Declaration of Independence in 1776, based on the premise 'that all men are created equal, that they are endowed by their Creator with certain unalienable rights, that among these are life, liberty, and the pursuit of happiness', and the motto adopted by the French Revolution, promising *liberté, égalité, fraternité*, played some part in influencing employers and governments to consider the health of workers. It is also significant, that following the Russian Revolution in 1917, the Bolshevik party formulated a health policy with the principle that health services should be free to all

and should concentrate particularly on prevention (Schilling 1981).

The industrial revolution

It was only after the start of the industrial revolution, towards the end of the 16th century, when cotton textiles and then other manufacturing factories began spreading through Europe and North America, that people with influence in government and some enlightened employers started taking a close interest in the health of workers (Schilling 1981). Industrialization had a profound effect on community health, with family life being disrupted as men moved away from their families in rural areas to work in industrial areas. Severe overcrowding and poor sanitation caused epidemics, and there was a rise in malnutrition, alcoholism and prostitution. There was also poverty and unemployment resulting from fluctuations in the economy.

Thomas Percival (1740–1804), a Manchester physician, when investigating an epidemic of typhus, went beyond his remit and produced a report on hours of work and conditions of young persons. This influenced Sir Robert Peel, a mill owner and member of parliament, to produce the Health and Morals of Apprentices Act of 1802. This led to more acts of parliament which, over the ensuing years, reduced the working hours of women and children, prohibited the employment of children under 14, and provided for education, hygiene and sanitation in the workplace.

Charles Turner Thackrah (1795–1833), a Leeds physician who is renowned for the work he did in persuading the government to record occupations in the recording of deaths and calculations of mortality, is also recognized as a great pioneer in occupational medicine. His text, *The Effects of the Principal Arts, Trades and Professions and of Civic States and Habits of Living on Health and Longevity* (1832) is still often quoted. He also was instrumental in setting up the first medical school outside the capital cities of London and Edinburgh: all remarkable achievements, considering that he died of pulmonary tuberculosis at the age of 38.

The health of working women

For many years after the first laws to address health at work were enacted in the early 1800s, the health of women at work was largely ignored. This was partly because there were very few women employed in the occupations perceived as being dangerous, and the working roles that women did undertake, such as domestic service, nursing and teaching, were not covered by the legislation. It was during the First World War, when women were thrust into factories as many men went off to fight on the front, that the health of women at work began to come into focus. During the war, about 50 000 workers, most of them women, were employed in the munitions factories to manually fill shells with trinitrotoluene (TNT), a highly toxic substance. The work was very hard, with a high risk of explosion, and the Ministry of Munitions described the work as 'particularly suitable for women, as they were not seen as minding its unskilled, monotonous and dead-end nature – it suited their temperament' (Ineson and Thom 1985: 90). Exposure to TNT caused many symptoms in the women, including a yellow staining of the skin, leading them to be referred to as canaries, and although neither factory doctors nor trade unions did anything to help at the time because the war effort and the need to get the shells to the front took precedence over any health issues, this did lead, at the end of the war, to the first in-depth examination of the impact of work on women's health.

The role of trade unions

The large number of trade unions which were created in the latter half of the 1800s were concerned primarily with reducing hours of work and raising wage levels in their early years (Schilling 1981). It was a lot later that they started taking an interest in workers' health and safety. During the 20th century, trade unions became more directly involved in health and safety in many countries. Thomas Morison Legge (1863–1932) was appointed as the first Medical Inspector of Factories, and a few years before his death he became Medical Adviser to the Trades Union Congress, where he wrote his classic text, *Industrial Maladies*, published after his death in 1934.

Today, in Britain, it is obligatory for workers to be represented in the workplace in safety committees through safety representatives. Through this role, and by working closely with occupational health nurses, trade unions have continued to have an important influence on the work of occupational health nurses. Currently, the Trades Union Congress in the United Kingdom (http://www.tuc.org.uk/), the European Trade Union Confederation, with headquarters in Brussels (http://www.etuc.org/), and the International Labour Organization (ILO), based in Geneva (http://www.ilo.org), all play an important part in ensuring that occupational health and safety remains high on governments' agenda.

The ILO, through its *Promotional Framework for Occupational Safety and Health Convention 2006* (ILO 2008), is urging all member countries to 'promote continuous improvement of occupational safety and health to prevent occupational injuries, diseases and deaths' (Article 2). There is some discussion in government about whether the United Kingdom should finally make it an obligation on all employers to provide occupational health services for their workers (see Chapter 8 for further information on workplace health).

The birth of industrial nursing

It was after the NMC established the third part of the NMC register for specialist community public health nurses in 2004 that occupational health nursing was formally recognized as being a specialty within public health. However, the roots of occupational health nursing as a public health specialty go back to a meeting attended in 1932 by thirty industrial nurses at the College of Nursing (later to become the RCN), where a resolution was passed, that industrial nurses should be encouraged to join the public health section of the college, and that special training should be arranged for new entrants to the service. The first course was held in 1934, and a Miss D.A. Pemberton was the only student that year to graduate with a certificate in industrial nursing (Charley 1954: 106).

In September 1950, a United Nations committee made up of representatives from the World Health Organization (WHO) and the ILO met in Geneva to report on different aspects of health in relation to work. The committee also wrote down a definition of the aims of occupational health, which remains relevant today (Box 17.1). Following the United Nations declaration, in 1952, the Royal College of Nursing (RCN) decided to change the name of its Certificate in Industrial Nursing to the Occupational Health Nursing Certificate (Charley 1954).

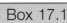

Box 17.1

Aims of occupational health (Slaney 2000)

Occupational health should aim at:

1. The promotion and maintenance of the highest degree of physical, mental and social well-being of workers in all occupations.
2. The prevention among workers of departures from health caused by their working conditions.
3. The protection of workers in their employment from risks resulting from factors adverse to health.
4. The placing and maintenance of the worker in an environment adapted to his or her physiological and psychological equipment.

An important milestone was the Health and Safety at Work etc Act 1974, which established the Health and Safety Executive (HSE), and within that, the Employment Medical Advisory Service (EMAS). Within the 14 regional branches of EMAS, there were occupational health nurses in the role of employment nursing advisers (ENAs), headed by a powerful and influential chief employment nursing adviser, also an occupational health nurse. For many years, ENAs played a very important part, providing an important link between occupational health nurses in the workplace and their employers on one side, and the research, advisory and enforcement officers in local government and the HSE on the other side. Sadly, in recent years, the government has started severely downsizing the HSE and dismantling EMAS.

The development of occupational health nursing

Practice

Most nurses in the community, whether they are employed in the NHS or by the independent sector, have their roles and functions through the Department of Health, or one of its many branches, such as NHS Management. Standards of care are set by the National Institute for Health and Clinical Excel-lence (NICE), and their adherence to clinical governance and quality are audited by the Care Quality Commission. Occupational health nurses, like all other nurses, whatever their field of practice are regulated by the NMC, and responsible to their professional code of practice (NMC 2004b). The roles and functions, and day-to-day activities of occupational health nurses, however, are informed by many different agencies, and often are dependent on the nature of their employers' undertakings. Many occupational health nurses working in industry can feel quite disconnected from activities directly governed by the Department of Health or the NHS. For their activities and decisions, they are as likely to be held accountable under employment law and their employers' policies and protocols, and answerable to employment tribunals, the Health and Safety Executive or the Department for Work and Pensions (DWP), as they are to nursing and health regulatory bodies.

The fact that the role and functions of occupational health nursing have been so ill defined, until recently, can seem bizarre to other community nurses. However, there are good reasons for this. In the first place, although occupational health nursing has been around as a profession for 150 years and as an educational qualification for over 75 years, there has never been a statutory requirement for occupational health nurses in any industry in the United Kingdom, although there are some regulations which stipulate input from doctors qualified in occupational health. Second, the professional requirements and day-to-day duties of an occupational health nurse are as likely as not to be set by the nurse's employer. While the fundamental principles, outlined by the ILO (1985) remain the same, the job of an occupational health nurse can vary from one organization to another. A nurse working in a manufacturing plant has little in common with a nurse working for a foundry, or local government, or bank, or hospital.

The lack of a clear framework for practice has had both benefits and drawbacks. The lack of a framework has enabled occupational health nurses to respond rapidly to the changing nature of work. As large national industries have given way to smaller ones, and the manufacturing base has largely been replaced by service industry, the health needs of workers have changed, and occupational health nurses have adapted to these changes in a way that would have been impossible had their role been written on slabs of stone.

Because the provision of occupational health nursing has not been a statutory requirement, it has been easy for employers to cut down on occupational health services when the economic climate has demanded a tightening of belts. This has meant that only occupational health nurses who have been able to demonstrate clearly their cost-effectiveness have been able to remain in post. Occupational health nurses like to claim that their contribution to the workplace results in less time being lost from work through sickness absence or ill-health retirement, and that it saves money that would have been spent on dealing with litigation and fines. It has not always been easy to substantiate such claims, and while this has resulted in some job insecurity for occupational health nurses, it has also meant that they have had to learn how to make a strong business case, and become adept at marketing their services to employers, employees and trade unions.

In effect, although occupational health nurses do complain, at the times when occupational health departments are under threat, that their work is made harder by the fact that there is no statutory requirement for the provision of occupational health services to all workers, they should also acknowledge that because of this lack of a statutory requirement, occupational health nurses in the United Kingdom have acquired more autonomy and a higher profile than their counterparts in the Scandinavian countries, North America and some European countries such as Greece and Italy, where statutory requirements have resulted in occupational health departments being dominated by occupational physicians, with nurses playing a secondary role.

As large factories and manufacturing plants give way to smaller organizations, there are fewer occupational health nurses employed directly to provide services for one employer or location. Occupational health nurses are increasingly likely to work as independent consultants, working for themselves and providing a service covering geographical areas or types of work, or as occupational health nurses for companies selling occupational health services across regions or nationally.

Many of the routine, repetitive tasks carried out by occupational health nurses in the past, such as audiometry, spirometry or vision tests (required by law for people working in areas with high noise levels, with dusts or other sensitizing chemicals, or with high use of computers respectively), are increasingly likely to be handed over to occupational health technicians. This helps to free up the nurses to become more involved in preventive and health-promoting activities.

Education

Over the years since the first certificate in industrial nursing was offered by the RCN in 1934, courses in occupational health nursing were developed at certificate and then diploma level in a number of regions, starting with Birmingham, Sheffield, Glasgow and Wolverhampton. However, many nurses working in occupational health services chose to undertake training that was not necessarily aimed at nurses, and there are occupational health nurses with a wide range of qualifications accredited by bodies such as the Institution of Occupational Safety and Health (IOSH) or the International Institute of Risk and Safety Management (IIRSM), or with qualifications in ergonomics, occupational hygiene or safety management.

Since the creation of the third part of the NMC register for specialist community public health nurses (SCPHNs), nurses have been able to register an occupational health qualification by completing an NMC-accredited course in occupational health nursing at degree or postgraduate diploma level. Some nurses were allowed to register as SCPHNs without completing an accredited course, by presenting evidence of SCPHN competencies, but only for a limited period. However, because of the lack of statutory requirements or competency standards, there are many nurses working as occupational health nurses without being registered with the NMC as SCPHNs. There are, and will continue to be for the foreseeable future, courses leading to a diploma, degree or even a Masters in occupational health which are not accredited by the NMC, which nurses can undertake in order to gain an occupational health qualification which will not enable them to register their qualification with the NMC. In the end, it will be employers and the market that will decide whether nurses should continue to work as occupational health nurses without being on the NMC's SCPHN register. The Association of Occupational Health Nurse Educators (AOHNE) keeps an up-to-date list of occupational health nursing courses, which can be accessed at its website: http://www.aohne.org.uk.

Occupational and public health

Although occupational health nursing education had its origins in the public health section of the College of Nursing (see above), in the following 50 years or so, occupational health nurses did not identify themselves as being part of the public health nursing community. In fact, they often felt closer professionally to people in their own organizations and in agencies who were involved with safety management, human resources and occupational hygiene. The only healthcare professionals with whom they were likely to communicate were general practitioners or consultant physicians and surgeons, and more often than not, that was in relation to an employee's work-related illness or injury. There were good reasons for this. First of all, many of the directives that informed the role and functions of the occupational health nurse emanated, not from the Department of Health, but from health and safety legislation and employment law. Second, because United Kingdom law has never made occupational health nursing mandatory in the workplace, nurses in the workplace have had to market their services and prove their worth to employers and employees, rather than the wider public or society in general.

However, there were a number of factors that gradually brought occupational health nursing firmly back into the public health arena, culminating in the recognition by the NMC in 2004 that occupational health nursing is very much a part of the community public health nursing profession.

The first influence was the series of inquiries into inequalities in health, starting with the Black Report (Department of Health and Social Services 1980). Although the Registrar General's office had recorded cause and occupation in relation to all deaths since the middle of the 19th century, it was only with the Black Report, which the government had apparently tried to sweep under the carpet by printing only 260 copies for restricted distribution, that data were produced which demonstrated clear correlations between occupational class and mortality. In effect, what the Black Report did was to show that the work people did had an influence on the health and welfare of the workers, their families and the societies they lived in, and that lifestyles, nutrition, levels of exercise, alcohol intake and many other factors affecting families, societies and whole regions were influenced by work. The message to occupational health nurses was that it was not only the limited area of workplace hazards and what workers did during the 8 hours at work that they should address, but also the much wider influences of work upon public health (see Chapter 23 for further information).

The Black Report was followed by a number of follow-up inquiries, with the most recent being the Acheson Report (1998). Although Acheson found a substantial improvement in health in general, he still found a wide gap in health between different occupational groups, and among his recommendations are that to reduce inequalities in health, there should be 'policies which improve the opportunities for work and which ameliorate the health consequences of unemployment'. Acheson also recommends the assessment of 'the impact of employment policies on health and inequalities in health' (Acheson 1998: 121).

Another factor that made occupational health nurses and their employers look wider than the workplace was the decision in the case of *Walker* v. *Northumberland County Council* (1995). Although this case was settled out of court, the significant factor is that this was the first time that it was recognized that an employer had a duty to protect workers from stress, or as Mr Justice Colman put it, 'there is no logical reason why risk of psychiatric damage should be excluded from the scope of an employer's duty'. Until that point, employers could legitimately ask their nurses to focus on diseases and injuries that could clearly be attributed to work. Following *Walker* v. *Northumberland*, illness or injury which could be multifactorial also needed to be taken into consideration.

The first time that the Department of Health seems to have recognized the workplace as a forum for health improvement is *The Health of the Nation* White Paper (Department of Health 1992), which under a Conservative government identified the prevention of accidents as one of its key areas and acknowledged that the workplace, where most people spent around a quarter of their time, should play a part in improving the health of the nation. The following Labour government re-emphasized the public health role of occupational health in its own White Paper *Saving Lives: Our Healthier Nation* (Department of Health 1999). Government responded with a strategy statement (Department of the Environment, Transport and the Regions 2000) and this was followed with recommendations by the Occupational Health Advisory Committee (Health and Safety Commission (HSC) 2000). Occupational health nursing very firmly started returning to its public health roots at this point, and its position as a community public health nursing specialism was confirmed by a Department of Health document addressed at occupational health nurses and their employers, in both the public and private sectors (Department of Health 2003).

In recognition that occupational health operates away from the mainstream health services, and that workplace health interventions are likely to require input from different departments and agencies, a cross-government programme, Health, Work, Well-being, sponsored by the Department for Work and Pensions, the Department of Health, the Health and Safety Executive, the Scottish Office and the Welsh Assembly, was set up in 2005 (http://www.workingforhealth.gov.uk). Having largely ignored the workplace as a health-promoting environment for many years, the government was beginning to realize that occupational health could play an important part in reducing health inequalities and improving the health and well-being of the working age population.

A competency framework for occupational health nursing

Evolving roles and functions

It is significant that while the aims of an occupational health service were defined by the WHO in 1950, and there was a more detailed discussion of the role and functions of occupational health services in the ILO's convention and recommendations of 1985 (ILO 1985), it was only in 1993 that these were translated into particular functions specific to occupational health nursing. This was done, not by the Department of Health, nor by a nursing professional or regulatory body, but by the Health and Safety Executive. The main functions specific to occupational health nursing were identified as:

- health supervision of workers
- surveillance of the working environment
- accident prevention

- prevention of work-related ill health
- treatment of illness and injury at work
- organization of first aid
- promotion of health and prevention of ill health
- counselling
- rehabilitation and resettlement into work
- provision of records and reports
- liaison and cooperation with internal and external agencies
- administration of the health unit
- research, including surveys (Dorward 1993).

While all these functions remain relevant to varying degrees, the role of occupational health nurses has undergone massive change as the nature of work in the United Kingdom has changed. In the past few decades, as heavy manufacturing industry such as coal mining, car manufacture and textiles has given way to service industries; and as huge, national and multinational companies such as British Coal, British Leyland and British Rail have given way to smaller and medium size enterprises (SMEs), occupational health has shifted more towards health promotion and prevention of injuries, rather than its traditional role of dealing with illness and injury. This shift has also taken the focus away from occupational physicians, who have had an essential role in the diagnosis of occupational disease, the provision of advice in relation to ill-health retirement and rehabilitation, and the provision of advice as appointed doctors for certain hazardous types of work.

In the new world of work in the UK and other Western economies, the primary focus for occupational health is in the following three areas, as defined by ILO/WHO in 1995:

- the maintenance and promotion of workers' health and working capacity
- the improvement of the working environment and work to become conducive to safety and health
- the development of work organization and working cultures in a direction which supports health and safety at work (ILO 1995).

These areas are far more about prevention, rather than treatment, and a psychosocial and holistic approach that occupational health nurses are so much better equipped to deliver.

Standards of proficiency and essential skills

It is clear that when the NMC created the SCPHN register in 2004, they lacked understanding of the role of the occupational health nurse. This became clear when they made a decision, later revoked, that over a period of some years, occupational health nursing, health visiting and school nursing (and family health nursing in Scotland) would all converge into one qualification with common standards of proficiency. This became especially embarrassing, as in the following years, the government established that major steps were needed in order to improve the health of the working age population, a role for which occupational health nurses were best equipped.

Following the publication of SCPHN proficiencies by the NMC (2004a), the RCN developed its integrated career and competency framework for occupational health nursing (RCN 2005) with the aim of both supporting the NMC proficiencies, but also emphasizing the specialist nature and divergence of occupational health nursing from other nurses on the SCPHN register. The RCN framework also mapped occupational health nursing competencies against the *Knowledge and Skills Framework* (Department of Health 2004) introduced following the NHS Agenda for Change.

The 15 or so higher education institutions in the UK that offer courses accredited by the NMC, leading to registration as SCPHN, and the additional half a dozen institutions offering occupational health courses for nurses that do not lead to SCPHN, all aim to develop nurses worthy of the title of 'occupational health nurse'. Their curricula differ widely, however, and although the NMC would prefer only nurses on its SCPHN register to be able to be employed as occupational health nurses, this is unlikely to happen while the demand for nurses looking after the health of workers remains high.

It is difficult to obtain accurate information about numbers, but following a request under the Freedom of Information Act, it was estimated by the NMC in 2005 that of 6189 nurses with a recordable qualification in occupational health nursing prior to the creation of the SCPHN register, 5999 were transferred to the SCPHN register (along with 27 000 health visitors, 1000 school nurses and 34 family health nurses). There are likely to be around 1000

further nurses working as occupational health nurses, of whom a couple of hundred have occupational health qualifications ranging from diploma to Masters degrees. These qualifications, though not recognized by the NMC for the SCPHN register, are widely recognized and highly valued by employers and other professional bodies.

With such a diversity of education and definitions for occupational health nursing in the United Kingdom, it is not easy to define a framework for practice for occupational health that will remain relevant in all different types of work and in the changing world of work, taking into consideration changes in demography, patterns of work and government policy. The Association of Occupational Health Educators, representing all teachers of occupational health nursing in the United Kingdom within and outside the NMC-accreditation framework, issued a list of essential skills for occupational health nurses. These are listed in full in Box 17.2.

Box 17.2

Essential skills for occupational health nurses

1. Using health needs assessment to identify the positive and negative effects of work on health, and health on work.
2. Contributing to the public health agenda by recognizing the impact that workplace hazards can have on the health of individuals, their families and the wider community.
3. Understanding, evaluating and applying relevant legislation relating to employment and health and safety law, in order to ensure compliance.
4. Working at a strategic level with employers, employees and their representatives to achieve optimum organizational health and productivity.
5. In collaboration with organizations, statutory and voluntary agencies, advising on the adaptation of the workplace to meet the needs of vulnerable people.
6. Using the workplace as a health-promoting environment in order to reduce health inequalities.

Case study 17.1

As a senior staff nurse in a chest clinic in the industrial heartland of England, Yasmin became increasingly aware that many of the patients she saw were suffering from diseases caused by exposure to harmful substances in their places of work. It caused her concern that by the time these patients first saw a chest physician, their work-related disease had usually got to a stage where it could not be cured, but only managed. Many of the patients she saw had had to give up a career, physical activities or hobbies because of their respiratory disease. For some of her patients, their disease had a significant impact on their family and social life, and on their self-esteem.

Yasmin was convinced that most of the illnesses she saw could have been avoided by effective health education and promotion, and the provision of information and training in the workplace. She felt that the prevention of work-related respiratory disease would have been so much more beneficial than clinicians' efforts to control the consequences of exposure to harmful working conditions.

With her experience in the chest clinic, her interest in workplace health and her interest in academic study, Yasmin had no difficulty in obtaining funding to undertake a degree course leading to a qualification in specialist practice in public health in occupational health nursing. Undertaking the course as a part-time student over 2 years, Yasmin was able to spend time in a variety of occupational health services on placement.

After gaining her degree, Yasmin has gone to work for a company that provides occupational health services to a number of small engineering and manufacturing companies in the Black Country. She visits her different clients, providing health education, advice and training to managers and the workforce; she also provides health surveillance, including spirometry, to organizations where there is a likelihood of exposure to substances hazardous to health.

Yasmin has recently spoken about the prevention of work-related asthma at a conference for occupational health nurses, and she has received accreditation from the British Lung Foundation to teach spirometry and lung function tests to occupational health nurses and technicians. Yasmin is confident that as a result of her work, there will be a decrease in work-related respiratory disease and consequent incapacity in the Black Country.

On her wall at work, Yasmin proudly displays the following quotation:

'He who cures a disease may be the skillfullest, but he that prevents it is the safest.'
(Thomas Fuller 1608–1661)

Discussion points

1. How would you make an assessment of the health needs of the working age population in your locality?
2. What steps could you take to work in collaboration with other health and social services specialists to improve the health and well-being of the working population in your area?

Emerging challenges for occupational health nurses

The world of work is changing rapidly in the first decade of the 21st century. People are living and working longer; there is an increase in chronic illness such as diabetes and obesity; computerization and mechanization, and the decline in heavy industry has meant fewer accidents, but an increase in work-related stress and musculoskeletal disorders; there is an influx of workers from the new member countries in eastern Europe. All these factors are creating new challenges for occupational health nurses, some of which are explored hereunder.

Worklessness

Despite the decline of dirty, heavy and very hazardous industry in the United Kingdom, the level of time lost through sickness absence has remained very high. It is estimated that in 2006, 175 million working days were lost to UK industry, and the annual cost to industry of sickness absence, worklessness and ill health is estimated to be as high as £100 billion, which is greater than the annual budget for the NHS and equivalent to the entire gross domestic product of Portugal (Black 2008).

Out of around 2.5 million people of working age on incapacity benefit, the Department of Work and Pensions (DWP) feels that around a million could be coerced, or in the government's words empowered and supported, to return to work (DWP 2006), especially as a review of research has shown that being at work is a lot better for health than being unemployed (Waddell and Burton 2006).

Occupational health nurses have not, in the past, been involved with worklessness, as by definition, their role has been with people in occupations, at work. However, with new initiatives from government to get people off incapacity benefit and into

233

work, occupational health nurses will play a major part on many fronts. First, they will become involved in ensuring that a meaningful risk assessment is carried out so that any adaptations required are put into place, as required under the Disability Discrimination Act 1995, to ensure that the returning worker does not pose a risk to himself or other workers; and then they will work with the organization, other healthcare workers and voluntary agencies to ensure that workers with chronic disease and long-term conditions are supported at work without spending too much time in clinics or Accident and Emergency.

Obesity

The environment and lifestyles in the United Kingdom have become increasingly obesogenic. People are leading more sedentary lives and eating less healthily and this had led to over two-thirds of men and half of women being overweight. It is estimated that if current trends continue, then levels of overweight or obesity in working people will rise to 90% in men and 80% in women by 2050 (Department of Health and Department of Children, Schools and Families 2008), and of course, with obesity are associated a large number of health issues, including diabetes, back pain and heart disease. NICE has produced a guideline for employers (NICE 2008) aimed at encouraging physical activity in the workplace. Here again is a new challenge for occupational health nurses. This NICE guideline is unusual in that it is targeted at employers, rather than the NHS or other healthcare agencies. It is occupational health nurses, in the main, who will put the guideline into effect. The guideline will also increase the impetus for occupational health nurses to work more closely with school nurses in order to address the problems of obesity and lack of physical activity early, before an obese school child becomes an obese worker.

Collaborative working

While occupational health nurses in industry have always worked in close collaboration with hygienists, safety specialists, personnel advisers and ergonomists in their own organizations, they have not been very good at working with other healthcare workers

in the community. However, with the ageing working population, and the likely increase in workers with chronic disease, there will be greater need for contact with social services, school nurses, community psychiatric nurses, and doctors and nurses involved in the care of patients with chronic physical and mental illness (see Chapter 21 for further information on partnership working in health and social care).

Regulation

Ever since the SCPHN register was created by the NMC, many occupational health nurses have had a perception that the NMC does not understand the role and functions of occupational health nurses. The NMC has responded positively to this perception to some degree, by back-tracking on earlier plans to merge all the specialist areas within the SCPHN register. However, as the role of occupational health nursing expands with some of the other challenges, many occupational health nurses are likely to be looking for more informed discussions about the regulation of occupational health education and practice. There is still a perception among some occupational health nurse managers and employers that the NMC standards and proficiencies for occupational health nursing are not likely to provide nurses with the skills in occupational health required by their work.

One possible impact of dissatisfaction with the NMC's regulatory framework for occupational health nursing could be that employers will increasingly seek to employ level one nurses (with a qualification in adult general or mental health nursing), who have additional qualifications in occupational health, but not necessarily an SCPHN registration. This will reduce the value to occupational health nurses and their employers of registration on the third part of the NMC register, and lead to an increase in occupational health nurses who are not on the SCPHN register from the current level of around one in seven.

Migrant workers

In previous decades, when there was an influx of workers from the Indian subcontinent and Africa, occupational health nurses had to make adjustments to deal with high levels of diseases such as tuberculosis or HIV/AIDS. Now, with an influx of workers from countries in eastern Europe newly admitted to the European Union, there had been a perception that because the migrants were european and ethnically similar to the indigenous UK population, there would not be major occupational health adjustments. However, in some working areas, occupational health nurses are having to address issues such as cultural differences in risk behaviours, language and health behaviours, and in areas such as healthcare, the fact that in some eastern European countries, the prevalence of blood-borne viruses such as hepatitis B and C is a lot higher than in the UK.

Conclusion

The nature of occupational health nursing has undergone many changes, in order to adapt to the evolving nature of work in the United Kingdom. As heavy industry and highly hazardous workplaces have declined, the occupational health nurse has shifted increasingly into a health-promoting and preventative role. An increase in disease and ill health related to poor lifestyle choices, along with an increase in the ageing population at work, means that occupational health nurses have to emerge from their relative isolation, and work in greater partnership and collaboration with other health and social care providers.

SUMMARY

- Occupational health nursing is a dynamic profession, having to keep up with a changing world of work.
- In the UK, there is no legal obligation on employers to provide occupational health nursing services.
- As the nature of work in the UK changes, occupational health nursing is becoming increasingly about health promotion and prevention of ill health.

DISCUSSION POINTS

1. Should the United Kingdom, like some other industrialized countries, make it mandatory for employers to provide occupational health services to their workforce?
2. Should nurses with occupational health qualifications that do not lead to SCPHN registration be permitted to work as occupational health nurses?
3. Does occupational health nursing require statutory principles and a framework for practice as required for health visiting?

References

Acheson D 1998 Independent Inquiry into Inequalities in Health. TSO, London:

Black C 2008 Working for a healthier tomorrow: review of the health of Britain's working age population. TSO, London

Charley IH 1954 The birth of industrial nursing: its history and development in Great Britain. Baillière, Tindall and Cox, London

Department of the Environment, Transport and the Regions 2000 Revitalising health and safety: strategy statement. DETR, London

Department of Health 1992 The health of the nation: a strategy for health in England. Cm1986. HMSO, London

Department of Health 1999 Saving lives: our healthier nation. Cm 4386,

July 1999. The Stationery Office, London

Department of Health 2000 The NHS Plan: a plan for investment, a plan for reform. Cm 4818-I July 2000. The Stationery Office, London

Department of Health 2003 Taking a public health approach in the workplace: a guide for occupational health nurses. Department of Health (in association with the RCN Society for Occupational Health Nursing and the Association of Occupational Health Nurse Practitioners (UK)), London

Department of Health 2004 Knowledge and skills framework. HMSO, London

Department of Health and Department of Children, Schools and Families

2008 Healthy weight, healthy lives: a cross-government strategy for England. DH Publications, London

Department of Health and Social Services 1980 Inequalities in health: report of a research working group. DHSS, London

Disability Discrimination Act 1995 c 50

DWP 2006 A new deal for welfare: empowering people to work. Cm 6730. The Stationery Office, London

Dorward AL 1993 Managers' perceptions of the role and continuing education needs of occupational health nurses. Research Paper 34. Health and Safety Executive, Sudbury

HSC 2000 Occupational Health Advisory Committee report and recommendations on improving access to occupational health support. Health and Safety Commission, London

ILO 1985 Convention and Recommendations. ILO, Geneva

ILO 1995 Report of the Joint ILO/WHO Committee on Occupational Health, Twelfth Session. ILO, Geneva

ILO 2008 Promotional framework for occupational safety and health convention. ILO, Geneva

Ineson A, Thom D 1985 TNT poisoning and the employment of women workers in the First World War. In: Weindling P (ed) The social history of occupational health. Croom Helm, London: 89–107

NICE 2008 Workplace health promotion: how to encourage employees to be physically active. NICE, London

Nursing and Midwifery Council 2004a Standards of proficiency for specialist community public health nurses. NMC, London

Nursing and Midwifery Council 2004b NMC code of practice. NMC, London

Ramazzini B 1993 Diseases of workers. (Translated from the Latin text DeMorbis Artificum of 1713 by Wilmer Cave Wright.) OH&S Press, Thunder Bay

RCN 2005 Competencies: an integrated career and competency framework for occupational health nursing. RCN, London

Schilling RSF (ed.) 1981 Occupational health practice, 2nd edn. Butterworths, London. (Although this title is in its fourth edition, it is the second edition that provides the best historical perspective on occupational health.)

Slaney BM 2000 Nursing at work. Slaney, Bushey

Waddell G, Burton AK 2006 Is work good for your health and well-being? The Stationery Office, London

Recommended reading/resources

RCN Society for Occupational Health Nursing (SOHN)
The RCN has a number of members identified as occupational health nurses. SOHN has a number of regional branches which hold regular seminars and study days. It also has a quarterly electronic newsletter, and it holds an annual national conference, usually in late November or early December. Website: www. rcn.org.uk.

Association of Occupational Health Nurse Practitioners (UK)
Set up in 1992, AOHNP is a professional organization for occupational health nurses with the aim of raising the profile of occupational health nursing practice. Website: www.aohnp.co.uk.

Association of Occupational Health Nurse Educators (AOHNE)

Information regarding occupational health nursing education at UK institutions of higher education is provided at the AOHNE website: www.aohne.org.uk.

Discussion list
Occupational health nursing has an international discussion list with over 700 subscribers, almost half of whom are in the United Kingdom. Website: www.jiscmail.ac.uk/lists/occ-health. html.

18

Community mental health nursing

Ben Hannigan

KEY ISSUES

- The emergence of community mental healthcare and community mental health nursing
- The interprofessional and interagency context
- Policy, practice and contemporary debate

Introduction

In the United Kingdom (UK) nurses are the largest of the professional groups with responsibility to provide specialist mental healthcare (Department of Health 2006a). Reflecting global trends, the focus of mental health service provision since the 1950s has shifted away from institutions towards care in the community. In this context community mental health nurses (CMHNs) have come to play vital roles as providers of care to individuals and families.

This chapter begins with a brief overview of the emergence of community care in the UK, and the first appearance of CMHNs. I then analyse the development of the CMHN as a key professional in the provision of services to people with severe mental health problems, set in the context of the interagency and interprofessional community mental health team (CMHT). Since the beginning of the 1990s mental healthcare has been subject to growing public, policy and professional scrutiny. I review these developments, which have included the challenge that care in the community has failed, before bringing the chapter up-to-date with an analysis of current policy and practice in the field. Here I pay particular attention to the impact of mental health modernization (including the emergence of new

roles for workers, and the appearance of new types of functional specialist team providing home-based care to differentiated groups of service users). I also consider recent professional reviews of mental health nursing in the UK.

Community mental health nursing: from the post-war years to the 1990s

Growth in numbers, growth in specialization

A complex set of ideological, economic, social and political factors combined together to bring forward the era of community mental healthcare in the UK from the second half of the last century onwards (Rogers and Pilgrim 2001). With origins clearly linked to the process of deinstitutionalization for people with long-term mental illnesses, pioneering community mental health nursing services appeared in the mid 1950s from hospital bases in Surrey and Devon (Hunter 1974). In the decades following, repeated nationwide surveys pointed to a spectacular growth in CMHN numbers. While only a handful of mental health nurses were plying their trade in people's homes by the end of the 1950s, 7000 were doing so in England and Wales some 40 years later (Brooker and White 1997).

The remarkable rise in CMHN numbers was paralleled by a growth in specialization. Survey data generated in 1990 revealed that one in seven was, at that time, specializing in a therapeutic approach (most commonly family therapy, behaviour therapy or counselling). Just over 40% also reported specializing with a particular client group, of whom almost 60% were working with older people (White 1993). These trends were confirmed in the most recent national survey of the workforce, completed in 1996 (Brooker and White 1997). Larger numbers than in 1990 reported working with people with severe mental illnesses, while fewer described themselves as specializing in the care of older people, or in the care of children and adolescents. Respondents in 1996 also reported working specifically with people with substance misuse problems, with mentally disordered offenders, with people with eating disorders and with the homeless. Therapeutic specialization was also found to have increased, with counselling and 'psychosocial interventions' (discussed in more detail below) the most commonly cited approaches used.

Primary care drift

Surveys of the UK's CMHN workforce in 1990 and 1996 took place at critical junctures. Findings from the first study revealed that CMHNs were moving closer to colleagues based in primary care. In the 5 years to 1990 referrals to CMHNs from general medical practitioners (GPs) had increased to the extent that over a third of referrals were reported to have originated from this source. Compared to clients referred by psychiatrists, people referred to CMHNs by GPs were less likely to have had previous admissions to hospital, to be experiencing 'chronic mental illness' or to have a diagnosis of schizophrenia. White also found that, among CMHNs working in England at the start of the 1990s, around one-quarter had no clients on their caseloads with a diagnosis of schizophrenia (White 1993).

These were controversial findings. Working autonomously and receiving independent referrals from GPs helped further community mental health nursing's claims to professional status (Godin 1996). Many commentators also saw in White's 1990 data clear evidence of a worrying drift away from the provision of care to the most needy service users: people with severe, enduring, mental health problems. For example, Gournay described the apparent lack of CMHN focus on this group as 'scandalous' (Gournay 1994). Drawing on findings generated from a randomized controlled trial of CMHNs using

counselling interventions to people with common mental disorders in primary care, Gournay also reported that the benefits to clients from seeing CMHNs were no greater than the benefits of receiving GP-only treatment (Gournay and Brooking 1994). For the sternest critics of community mental health nursing in the early and mid 1990s, therefore, CMHNs were not only seeing too many of the wrong sort of clients – the 'worried well' – but were also using clinical interventions with this group which did not seem to generate any positive health outcome. At this juncture readers are encouraged to consider discussion point 1 given in the 'Discussion points' section which appears at the end of this chapter.

Mental health as a priority for health and social care development

Professional concerns in the early and mid 1990s of a possible loss of CMHN focus resonated with policy makers' concerns that the post-war community care experiment was not working as intended. From the beginning of the last decade onwards mental healthcare emerged as a UK health and social policy priority. Specific actions initiated in the years up to the mid 1990s to facilitate the delivery of more effective and integrated services to people with severe mental health problems living in the community are summarized in Box 18.1.

Box 18.1

Actions initiated in the years up to the mid 1990s to facilitate the delivery of effective and integrated services

- The establishment of interagency and interprofessional community mental health teams (CMHTs)
- The introduction of the care programme approach (CPA)
- The delivery of evidence-based psychosocial interventions to individuals and their families
- A renewed emphasis on education for the workforce

Interagency and interprofessional community mental health teams

By the 1990s, interagency and interprofessional community mental health teams (CMHTs) had become the accepted model for organizing specialist services at the local level, and were described as such in policy guidance of that period. Most CMHNs, having previously worked in single-profession teams, soon found themselves grouped together with psychiatrists, mental health social workers, occupational therapists, clinical psychologists and others (Brooker and White 1997).

CMHTs were set up in the belief that they are the best way to deliver flexible and accessible local mental health services. Their appearance was not met with universal support, however. In an influential early critique Galvin and McCarthy argued that CMHTs are prone to inadequate planning and poor management (Galvin and McCarthy 1994). While broadly supportive of the CMHT model, Onyett and colleagues noted the challenges facing CMHTs and those who manage them, including the tensions for practitioners between being members of both a team and a profession (Onyett et al 1997). Some professionals, including those traditionally enjoying high levels of autonomy, also struggled to adjust to the more managed environment encountered in the typical interprofessional team setting. In addition, CMHTs were soon found to be struggling to reconcile conflicting policy priorities. While teams were clearly directed in central government guidance to focus their collective energies on meeting the needs of the severely mentally ill, they simultaneously found themselves being pulled towards ongoing work with people with distressing, but more transient, problems in primary care settings (Hannigan 1999). Interprofessional team working is the focus of discussion point 2 appearing at the end of this chapter (for further information on interprofessional working see Chapter 21).

The care programme approach

Mental health services in the community are typically provided by members of multiple occupational groups, working in different agencies and physically located in workplaces which are geographically dispersed. These factors combine to make the organization of services for individuals and families a highly

---

Box 18.2

Key elements of the care programme approach (Department of Health 2006b)

1. Systematic arrangements for assessing the health and social needs of people accepted into specialist mental health services
2. The formation of a care plan which identifies the health and social care required from a variety of providers
3. The appointment of a key worker [now termed care coordinator] to keep in close touch with service users and to monitor and coordinate care
4. Regular review and, where necessary, agreed changes to the care plan

---

complex task. Widespread recognition of the difficulties associated with care coordination led to the appearance of the care programme approach (CPA), which was first launched in England at the start of the 1990s. The four key elements of the CPA, as these have been summarized in successive documents, are described in Box 18.2.

While members of any occupational group have been able to fulfil the care coordinator role, the task of negotiating and overseeing interprofessional plans of care soon became a central component of the day-to-day work of CMHNs.

Evidence-based interventions

At the same time as doubt was being cast on the value of CMHNs delivering counselling-style interventions to people with problems such as mild to moderate depression and anxiety (Gournay and Brooking 1994), evidence was also emerging of the value of training nurses to provide behavioural family therapy to people with severe mental illnesses and their carers (Brooker et al 1994). It has since become customary to pool together a range of clinical and social approaches to working with people with severe and disabling mental health problems under the broad title of psychosocial interventions (PSIs). The term PSI referred initially to family interventions alone, but has more recently assumed a much wider meaning (Brooker 2001). Box 18.3 draws on Brooker's work to outline the main components of a PSI approach.

Box 18.3

Key components of psychosocial interventions for people with severe mental health problems (Brooker 2001)

- Outcome-oriented assessment
- Behavioural family work
- Psychological management strategies
- Case management
- Early intervention
- Psychopharmacology

The theory and research base underpinning the individual elements of PSIs is well established. For example, the concept of expressed emotion which underpins a range of family interventions aimed at people with schizophrenia and their carers was first developed in the 1950s (Pharoah et al 2006). Similarly, the psychological management strategies emphasized in PSIs invariably include the use of cognitive behavioural techniques, an approach which has been developing over a number of decades (Jones et al 2004).

Education for the workforce

Beyond the necessity of being registered on the appropriate part of the Nursing and Midwifery Council Register, no mandatory education requirement has ever existed for UK mental health nurses aiming to practise in the community. However, since the early 1970s optional university-based courses have been available, with established programmes continuing to this day in many parts of the country. Important new evidence-based PSI courses also started to appear from the early 1990s, aimed at nurses and others wishing to develop their skills in working with people with schizophrenia and other severe mental disorders. With their origins in courses developed in London and Manchester, programmes of this type (often badged as Thorn courses, after the funding given to early schemes by the Sir Jules Thorn Charitable Trust) emerged, their curricula including training in evidence-based assessment and care management, psychological interventions and in family work (O'Carroll et al 2004).

Contemporary policy and practice

Mental health services under New Labour: a decade of rapid change

Mental healthcare remains a key policy and practice priority. Shortly after the 1997 election, notification of the New Labour government's early intentions came with the publication of *Modernising Mental Health Services: Safe, Sound and Supportive* (Department of Health 1998). This drew attention to the stigma and misunderstanding which many people with mental health difficulties experience. The document also noted that poverty and social exclusion play a powerful part in precipitating and worsening mental ill health. The government also referred in this publication to its plans for a review of the Mental Health Act 1983 in England and Wales, and restated its intention to 'address the responsibility on individual patients to comply with their programmes of care' (Department of Health 1998: 40).

The pace of change in mental health policy and practice in the last decade has been rapid (Hannigan and Allen 2006). *Modernising Mental Health Services* – which included the controversial claim that community mental healthcare in the UK had failed (see discussion point 3 below) – was soon followed in England by the launch of *A National Service Framework* (NSF) *for Mental Health* (Department of Health 1999). Similar documents have appeared elsewhere in the UK. The devolved administration in Wales, for example, produced a strategy for the mental healthcare of adults (National Assembly for Wales 2001) followed by both an original and a revised (Welsh Assembly Government 2005) NSF for the provision of services to working age adults. In Scotland, mental healthcare has been made a policy priority most recently through the construction of *Delivering for Mental Health* (Scottish Executive 2006a), while in Northern Ireland mental health has been identified as a key area for development in the wide-ranging *Investing for Health* (Department of Health, Social Services and Public Safety 2002).

National frameworks, guidelines and reviews

National frameworks are important documents which usually set out targets and timescales for the improvement of services. For example, England's Mental Health NSF of 1999 contained seven standards associated with five areas. These are summarized in Box 18.4.

The framework also set out a series of fundamental values which should underpin the provision of mental health services, and established a set of guiding principles. These are summarized in Box 18.5.

Under its programme of modernizing services, policy makers have also continued to promote the use of evidence in practice. A key part of this process has been the production of national clinical guidelines, which in England and Wales has been pursued through the work of the National Institute for Health and Clinical Excellence (NICE). Devolution has proved significant here, too. For example, in Scotland the responsibility to generate guidelines

for practice falls to NHS Quality Improvement Scotland. This body advises health service organizations on the suitability in the Scottish context of NICE guidance developed specifically for use south of the border.

NICE in England and Wales has a rolling programme of reviews, and thus far has produced guidance on the care of people with a wide range of mental health problems. Box 18.6 details some of these documents, and includes details of the website from where copies can be downloaded.

The NICE document on the care of people with schizophrenia, a revised version of which is expected in 2009, is being formally reviewed as part of NICE's commitment to updating its guidance and provides clear recommendations on the types of service which CMHNs (and other members of the health and social care workforce) should be providing. This guidance reaffirms the value of PSI approaches and includes various recommendations, which are summarized in Box 18.7. Readers are also encouraged to consider the issues raised in discussion point 4 below on the relationships between national-level guidelines and everyday practice.

In contemporary community mental health settings CMHNs continue to fulfil important roles as care coordinators under locally implemented care programme approach arrangements. In the years following its introduction in England, anecdotal evidence accumulated that the CPA was burdensome

Box 18.4

Key areas identified for service development in England's NSF for Mental Health (Department of Health 1999)

- The promotion of mental health and action to tackle the discrimination experienced by people with mental health problems
- Mental health in primary care settings and access to specialist services
- The provision of care to people with severe mental illnesses
- Services for informal carers
- The reduction of suicide

Box 18.5

Guiding principles in England's NSF for Mental Health (Department of Health 1999)

- Service user involvement
- The provision of high-quality and effective care
- Non-discriminatory practice
- Accessible services
- Services that are safe
- Offering choice and independence
- Well-coordinated care
- Staff support
- Continuity of care
- Accountability

Box 18.6

National Institute for Health and Clinical Excellence (NICE) guidelines relevant to mental health nursing practice in the community

- Schizophrenia (National Institute for Clinical Excellence 2002)
- Bipolar disorder (National Institute for Health and Clinical Excellence 2006)
- Dementia (National Institute for Health and Clinical Excellence/Social Care Institute for Excellence 2006)
- Anxiety (National Institute for Health and Clinical Excellence 2007a)
- Depression (National Institute for Health and Clinical Excellence 2007b)

For further information on the work of NICE in the field of mental health, go to: http://guidance.nice.org.uk/topic/behavioural.

> ## Box 18.7
>
> **Key points from the National Institute for Health and Clinical Excellence (NICE) guidelines for the treatment and management of schizophrenia in primary and secondary care (NICE 2002)**
>
> - Early intervention for people suspected of having a first episode of schizophrenia-related crisis
> - Early treatment with modern antipsychotic medications
> - The use of dedicated crisis resolution and home treatment services where necessary
> - Cognitive behavioural and family interventions
> - The provision of services aimed at meeting the physical health needs of people with schizophrenia

to operate, placing a heavy administrative load on workers. Recent research has added to this perception, with one in-depth study revealing that fulfilling the care coordinator role limits the time and space available to CMHNs to provide evidence-based therapeutic interventions (Simpson 2005). As one element in its programme of reviewing standards for mental healthcare, the operation of the CPA has recently been subjected to consultation and review, with the aim of affirming best practice in this area (Department of Health 2006b).

New teams in the community

The use of evidence to inform practice (now organized through the use of NICE guidelines and their equivalents outside England and Wales), and the importance of effective care coordination, are two examples of enduring mental health policy and practice themes. A third important area – and one where significant developments have taken place in recent years – is in the organization of teams.

Beginning with developments in England following the appearance of the Mental Health NSF (Department of Health 1999), a gradual shift has taken place towards the establishment of multidisciplinary teams in the community with an emphasis on specific functions (Peck 2003). Unlike locality CMHTs, teams of this type make no attempt to provide comprehensive mental healthcare, but instead offer closely specified interventions to

defined groups. England's *Mental Health Policy Implementation Guide* (Department of Health 2001) contains information on the characteristics of a number of teams of this type, which are summarized in Box 18.8.

Mental health nurses play important roles as managers and practitioners in teams of this type, and readers at this juncture may wish to consider discussion point 5 below. While these new services offer staff the opportunity to provide effective, targeted care to closely defined groups, a proliferation of specialist teams also makes for a more fragmented system and potentially increases the number of barriers to effective working across organizational interfaces (Hannigan and Allen 2006). New teams also need new staff, who may be difficult to recruit in conditions where the workforce is relatively static. The requirement to provide new types of community mental health service also has implications for occupational roles and responsibilities. This, too, is an area where rapid change has occurred in recent years.

New ways of working

Roles and responsibilities in the mental health field are developing rapidly, with consequences for CMHNs and the work they do. A recent trend has been to clarify the values, knowledge and skills needed for practice in the mental health field irrespective of occupational identity. For example, influential recent work by England's Department of Health has led to the development of the *Ten Essential Shared Capabilities* (ESCs) document (Department of Health 2004), which is intended to capture the common capabilities that all mental health workers are expected to achieve during their initial preparation for practice. The ten ESCs, which mental health nursing education programmes are now beginning to reflect, are summarized in Box 18.9.

Beginning with a review of the work of psychiatrists in the context of the interprofessional team (Department of Health 2005), new attention is also being paid to the specific roles of all members of the mental health workforce. *Mental Health: New Ways of Working for Everyone* (Department of Health 2007) summarizes many of the new nursing roles which have developed in recent years, including the positions of modern matron and consultant and the emergence of nurses as prescribers of psychiatric medications. As is noted in this document, review

Box 18.8

New types of team providing specialist services in the community (Department of Health 2001)

Crisis resolution/home treatment teams

Teams of this type are intended for people with mental health problems experiencing acute psychiatric crisis 'of such severity that, without the involvement of a crisis resolution/home treatment team, hospitalization would be necessary'.

Teams are expected to:

- gatekeep services, and offer rapid assessment and referral
- provide immediate multidisciplinary home-based care and treatment 24 hours a day, 7 days a week where appropriate
- provide services to people experiencing acute, severe mental health difficulties in the least restrictive environment possible
- remain involved in the care of the individual until the crisis has resolved and the service user has been transferred for ongoing care
- be actively involved in discharge planning in cases where people are admitted to hospital, and provide intensive care at home to enable early discharge
- work with service users to improve their resilience to crisis.

Assertive outreach services

Services of this type are designed for people with:

1. A severe and persistent mental disorder (e.g. schizophrenia, major affective disorders) associated with a high level of disability
2. A history of high use of inpatient or intensive home-based care (for example, more than two admissions or more than 6 months' inpatient care in the past 2 years)
3. Difficulty in maintaining lasting and consenting contact with services
4. Multiple, complex needs including a number of the following:
   - History of violence or persistent offending
   - Significant risk of persistent self-harm or neglect

- Poor response to previous treatment
- Dual diagnosis of substance misuse and serious mental illness
- Detained under Mental Health Act (1983) on at least one occasion in the past 2 years
- Unstable accommodation or homelessness. (Department of Health 2001)

Teams are expected to:

- improve engagement
- reduce hospital admissions
- reduce length of stay in hospital
- increase stability in the lives of service users and their carers/family
- improve social functioning
- be cost-effective.

Early intervention in psychosis

Early intervention services are intended for the under-35s with a first presentation of psychotic symptoms, and for the under-35s during the first 3 years of psychotic illness.

Teams are expected to:

- reduce the stigma associated with psychosis and improve awareness of the symptoms of psychosis and the need for early assessment
- reduce the length of time young people are undiagnosed and untreated
- develop meaningful engagement, provide evidence-based interventions and promote recovery
- increase stability in the lives of service users and help develop personal fulfilment
- provide a user-centred service that integrates child, adolescent and adult mental health services and works in partnership with primary care, education, social services, youth and other services
- at the end of the treatment period, ensure that the care is transferred thoughtfully and effectively.

---

of the legal framework for mental health services in England and Wales is leading to additional roles for mental health nurses in two distinct areas (see discussion point 6 below). First, nurses will have opportunities to fulfil the role of approved mental health professionals (AMHPs). The work of AMHPs is intended to be similar to the work currently undertaken by approved social workers (ASWs), who in England and Wales have specific legal responsibilities to make applications for people to be treated for mental disorder on a compulsory basis. Second, it is envisaged that nurses will be able to fulfil the position of responsible clinician, and after completion of an appropriate competency-based

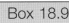

Box 18.9

The ten essential shared capabilities (Department of Health 2004)

- Working in partnership
- Respecting diversity
- Practising ethically
- Challenging inequality
- Promoting recovery
- Identifying people's needs and strengths
- Providing service user centred care
- Making a difference
- Promoting safety and positive risk taking
- Personal development and learning

Box 18.10

The principles of a Recovery Approach

The Recovery Approach is based around a number of principles that stress the importance of:
- working in partnership with service users (and/or carers) to identify realistic life goals and enabling them to achieve them
- stressing the value of social inclusion (clear evidence exists which demonstrates that inclusion has a strong link with positive mental health outcomes)
- stressing the need for professionals to be optimistic about the possibility of positive individual change

Reproduced from Department of Health (2006a).

---

training take the lead professional role in overseeing the care and treatment of people being treated under sections of a new Mental Health Act.

Reviews of mental health nursing

New policies, actual and proposed new legal frameworks and new ways of working together create considerable occupational uncertainty. It is in this specific context that important recent reviews have taken place of the work of mental health nurses. In England, the country's Chief Nursing Officer commissioned a review in 2005 with the aim of answering the question, 'How can mental health nursing best contribute to the care of service users in the future?' The product of this process, *From Values to Action* (Department of Health 2006a), appeared in 2006 along with a number of supporting documents including a literature review (the outputs from which are available as downloadable documents at: http://www.nursing.manchester.ac.uk/projects/mentalhealthreview/).

Underpinning *From Values to Action* is the idea that mental health nurses should, in all practice contexts, incorporate the principles of recovery in their work with service users. Considerable interest has emerged in recent years in the idea of 'recovery', with the principles of a 'Recovery Approach' (as these are summarized in *From Values to Action*) given in Box 18.10.

From Values to Action is a comprehensive review, and alongside its endorsement of the principles of recovery is a series of recommendations grouped under three broad themes, as is summarized in Box 18.11.

Box 18.11

From Values to Action: recommendations (Department of Health 2006a)

Putting values into practice

1. Applying Recovery Approach values
2. Promoting equality in care
3. Providing evidence-based care

Improving outcomes for service users

4. Meeting the greatest need
5. Strengthening relationships with service users and carers
6. Holistic assessments and managing risk effectively
7. Improving physical well-being
8. Providing psychological therapies
9. Increasing social inclusion
10. Recognizing spiritual needs
11. Responding to the needs of people with substance misuse problems
12. Improving inpatient care

A positive, modern profession

13. Developing new roles and skills
14. Strengthening pre-registration education
15. Working effectively in multidisciplinary teams
16. Supporting continued professional development
17. Improving recruitment and retention

The final discussion point below invites readers to reflect on the relationships between national reviews (exemplified by *From Values to Action*) and everyday roles.

Conclusion

Mental health services, and mental health nursing, are changing rapidly. New types of team and new roles for nurses are appearing, with further developments in train. This chapter's professional case study (Case study 18.1), for example, gives a flavour of the type of clinical and service development opportunity increasingly available to nurses working in this field.

Internally, mental health nursing continues to be characterized by vigorous and healthy debate. Hot topics (which are likely to include the future status of mental health nursing as a distinct branch within the family of nursing and midwifery) are aired in a variety of places and in a variety of formats. The reader is referred to the Recommended reading section below for more information. Here, a selection of some of the live issues occupying community mental health nursing is given.

Not surprisingly in the context of rapid policy-driven changes in occupational roles, there continues to be a sustained debate over the content of mental health nurses' work. This chapter has included an outline of the increase in interest over the last 15 or so years in psychosocial interventions for people with severe mental health problems. For some, this concern with the pursuit of 'psychotechnologies' – such as behavioural family interventions and cognitive behavioural approaches – is largely at odds with what the 'proper focus' of mental health nursing should be (see, for example, Barker et al 1999). Rather than concentrating solely on the acquisition of evidence-based skills, Barker has argued eloquently for a very different basis for mental health nursing practice. This approach is one that is primarily concerned with the relationship between nurse and service user, and is characterized by an attention to the lived experience of mental ill health rather than to the treatment of mental illness per se (Barker 2001). There is also considerable debate over the expansion of mental health nursing into particular spheres of activity. The introduction of nurse prescribing, for example, has provoked both supportive (Gournay and Gray 2001) and more cautious (Cutcliffe 2002) professional responses.

Case study 18.1

Having spent 4 years working as a staff nurse in a psychiatric hospital, Aled applied for a job working as a community nurse in one of his employing NHS trust's locality community mental health teams. After a year of practising in this team and providing care for adults of working age with mental health problems, the opportunity arose for Aled to apply for a place on a postgraduate diploma in Community Health Studies at his local university. During his next 2 years of part-time study Aled became particularly interested in relapse prevention strategies for people with severe mental health problems. Having completed his diploma, Aled elected to progress to his MSc dissertation, and with the support of his manager and the trust's professional head of mental health nursing, decided to focus on the development of plans to improve the delivery of relapse prevention services. Aled reviewed the literature on early warning signs in psychosis, and studied the process of service change in large organizations like the NHS. Alongside completing his dissertation Aled worked with a stakeholder group comprising his manager, other nurses, the team's consultant psychiatrist, a CMHT clinical psychologist and representatives drawn from the local service user community. Together they developed a strategy to improve the routine provision of relapse prevention services. Implementation of this strategy was negotiated with all team members, with Aled and his psychologist colleague drawing on their skills and knowledge to train CMHT staff in relapse work. Two years on, practice in the team has changed substantially as a result of this initiative and service users and carers give favourable evaluations of participating in relapse work. Aled also draws on these experiences and on his specialist knowledge when he teaches pre-registration student nurses at his local university.

Discussion points

1. What specialist skills, knowledge or interest do you have that could be used to develop local enhanced services?
2. What knowledge do you have of the process of change in inter-professional and interagency health and social care settings?

SUMMARY

- Over recent decades in the UK, care for people with mental health problems has increasingly been provided in community settings.
- It is usual to date the origins of community mental health nursing in the UK to developments which took place from the mid 1950s onwards.
- The community mental health nursing workforce has grown considerably over the last 50 years, with the result that CMHNs now play a major part in the provision of care to people experiencing a wide range of mental health problems.
- Recent policy has urged CMHNs to concentrate on meeting the needs of people identified as experiencing severe and long-term mental health problems. Reflecting this refocusing, increasing interest has been shown in recent years in new ways of educating practitioners to work with this group of people.
- Other recent policy initiatives have grouped together CMHNs and other mental health professional groups in multiagency and multidisciplinary community mental health teams.
- Recent initiatives with an impact on the work of CMHNs include the emergence of new types of team in the community, including those providing crisis resolution/home treatment, assertive outreach and early intervention services.
- Rapid developments in mental health services continue to have implications for the work of CMHNs.

DISCUSSION POINTS

1. Meeting mental health need in primary care settings

Levels of mental health problems in the general population remain high, with depression and anxiety being particularly prevalent.
- In the locality you work in:
  - how are the mental health needs of people presenting in primary care settings currently met?
  - what are the specific roles played by CMHNs and other community nurses in identifying, assessing and providing care for people with common mental health problems such as depression and anxiety?
  - with reference to the available evidence, are these needs being met in an effective and efficient way?
  - what opportunities exist for the improvement of services?

2. Working in interprofessional teams

Mental health nurses usually work as members of interprofessional and interagency teams.
- In the locality you work in:
  - how are community mental health services currently organized?
  - based on your local knowledge and observations, are professional and agency roles and responsibilities clear?
  - if you are not a mental health nurse, would you know how to get in touch with your local community mental health services?
  - if you are a mental health nurse, how well do you and your mental health colleagues communicate with staff based in primary care settings?

3. Has community mental healthcare failed?

In the late 1990s the UK government declared that mental healthcare in the community had failed.
- To what extent do you agree or disagree with this sentiment?
- Why?

4. Guidelines for practice

NICE documents are intended to provide authoritative guidance for the provision of effective local services. However, the processes by which high-level guidance becomes translated into everyday practice are complex.

DISCUSSION POINTS—cont'd

- In the locality you work in (and if you want with reference to just one current mental health guidance document produced by NICE):
  - to what extent do mental health services reflect NICE guidance?
  - what are the factors helping and hindering the local implementation of national-level policies and guidance?

5. New teams in the community

In recent years new types of mental health team have appeared, providing specific services to particular groups of users.
- In the locality you work in:
  - what types of community-based teams providing mental health services now exist?
  - what are the roles of nurses, and the roles of members of other occupational groups, in these teams?
  - based on your knowledge and observations, how well are these different teams integrated?

6. Possible roles for mental health nurses under a new Mental Health Act for England and Wales

Mental health law in different parts of the UK is (or has been) under review, and in England and Wales new roles for nurses are being actively considered.
- What are your views on mental health nurses fulfilling the role of 'approved mental health professional'?
- What are your views on mental health nurses fulfilling the role of 'responsible clinician'?

7. Reviews of mental health nursing

In recent years mental health nursing has been subjected to professional reviews, leading to the production of documents such as England's *From Values to Action* (Department of Health 2006a) and Scotland's *Rights, Relationships and Recovery* (Scottish Executive 2006b).
- What has been the impact of these reviews on the work of mental health nurses?

References

Barker P 2001 The Tidal Model: developing an empowering, person-centred approach to recovery within psychiatric and mental health nursing. Journal of Psychiatric and Mental Health Nursing 3(3): 233–240

Barker P, Jackson S, Stevenson C 1999 What are psychiatric nurses needed for? Developing a theory of essential nursing practice. Journal of Psychiatric and Mental Health Nursing 6(4): 273–282

Brooker C 2001 A decade of evidence-based training for work with people with serious mental health problems: progress in the development of psychosocial interventions. Journal of Mental Health 10(1): 17–31

Brooker C, White E 1997 The fourth quinquennial national community mental health nursing census of England and Wales, Manchester and Keele. Universities of Manchester and Keele

Brooker C, Falloon I, Butterworth A, et al 1994 The outcome of training community psychiatric nurses to deliver psychosocial intervention. British Journal of Psychiatry 165: 222–230

Cutcliffe J 2002 The beguiling effects of nurse-prescribing in mental health nursing: re-examining the debate. Journal of Psychiatric and Mental Health Nursing 9(3): 369–375

Department of Health 1998 Modernising mental health services: safe, sound and supportive, Department of Health, London

Department of Health 1999 A national service framework for mental health. Department of Health, London

Department of Health 2001 The mental health policy implementation guide. Department of Health, London

Department of Health 2004 The ten essential shared capabilities. A framework for the whole of the mental health workforce. Department of Health, London

Department of Health 2005 New ways of working for psychiatrists: enhancing effective, person-centred services through new ways of working in multidisciplinary and multi-agency contexts. Final report 'but not the end of the story'. Department of Health, London

Department of Health 2006a From values to action: the Chief Nursing Officer's review of mental health nursing, Department of Health, London

Department of Health 2006b Reviewing the care programme approach. Department of Health, London

Department of Health 2007 Mental health: new ways of working for everyone. Developing and sustaining a capable and flexible workforce. Department of Health, London

Department of Health, Social Services and Public Safety 2002 Investing for health. Department of Health, Social Services and Public Safety, Belfast

Galvin SW, McCarthy S 1994 Multi-disciplinary community teams: clinging to the wreckage. Journal of Mental Health 3(2): 157–166

Godin P 1996 The development of community psychiatric nursing:

a professional project? Journal of Advanced Nursing 23(5): 925–934

Gournay K 1994 Redirecting the emphasis to serious mental illness. Nursing Times 90(25): 40–41

Gournay K, Brooking J 1994 Community psychiatric nurses in primary health care. British Journal of Psychiatry 165: 231–238

Gournay K, Gray R 2001 Should mental health nurses prescribe? Maudsley discussion paper number 11. Institute of Psychiatry, London

Hannigan B 1999 Joint working in community mental health: prospects and challenges. Health and Social Care in the Community 7(1): 25–31

Hannigan B, Allen D 2006 Complexity and change in the United Kingdom's system of mental health care. Social Theory and Health 4(3): 244–263

Hunter P 1974 Community psychiatric nursing in Britain: an historical review. International Journal of Nursing Studies 11(4): 223–233

Jones C, Cormac I, Silveira da Mota Neto JI, Campbell C 2004 Cognitive behaviour therapy for schizophrenia. Cochrane Database of Systematic Reviews

National Assembly for Wales 2001 Adult mental health services for Wales: equity, empowerment, effectiveness, efficiency. National Assembly for Wales, Cardiff

National Institute for Clinical Excellence 2002 Schizophrenia: core interventions in the treatment and management of schizophrenia in primary and secondary care. National Institute for Clinical Excellence, London

National Institute for Health and Clinical Excellence 2006 Bipolar disorder: the management of bipolar disorder in adults, children and adolescents, in primary and secondary care. National Institute for Health and Clinical Excellence, London

National Institute for Health and Clinical Excellence 2007a Anxiety (amended): management of anxiety (panic disorder, with or without agoraphobia, and generalised anxiety disorder) in adults in primary, secondary and community care. National Institute for Health and Clinical Excellence, London

National Institute for Health and Clinical Excellence 2007b Depression (amended): management of depression in primary and secondary care. National Institute for Health and Clinical Excellence, London

National Institute for Health and Clinical Excellence/Social Care Institute for Excellence 2006 Dementia: supporting people with dementia and their carers in health and social care. National Institute for Health and Clinical Excellence/ Social Care Institute for Excellence, London

O'Carroll M, Rayner L, Young N 2004 Education and training in psychosocial interventions: a survey of Thorn Initiative course leaders. Journal of Psychiatric and Mental Health Nursing 11(5): 602–607

Onyett S, Standen R, Peck E 1997 The challenge of managing community mental health teams. Health and Social Care in the Community 5(1): 40–47

Peck E 2003 Working in multidisciplinary community teams. In: Hannigan B, Coffey M (eds) The handbook of community mental health nursing. Routledge, London

Pharoah F, Mari J, Rathbone J, Wong W 2006 Family intervention for schizophrenia. Cochrane Database of Systematic Reviews

Rogers A, Pilgrim D 2001 Mental health policy in Britain, 2nd edn. Palgrave, Basingstoke

Scottish Executive 2006a Delivering for mental health. Scottish Executive, Edinburgh

Scottish Executive 2006b Rights, relationships and recovery: the report of the national review of mental health nursing in Scotland. Scottish Executive, Edinburgh

Simpson A 2005 Community psychiatric nurses and the care coordinator role: squeezed to provide 'limited nursing'. Journal of Advanced Nursing 52(6): 689–699

Welsh Assembly Government 2005 Raising the standard: the revised adult mental health national service framework and an action plan for Wales. Welsh Assembly Government, Cardiff

White E 1993 Community psychiatric nursing 1980 to 1990: a review of organization, education and practice. In: Brooker C, White E (eds) Community psychiatric nursing: a research perspective, volume 2. Chapman and Hall, London

Recommended reading

Books

Callaghan P, Waldock H (eds) 2006 Oxford handbook of mental health nursing. Oxford University Press, Oxford

This pocket-sized text gives practical and up-to-date advice on all aspects of mental health nursing care.

Hannigan B, Coffey M (eds) 2003 The handbook of community mental health nursing. Routledge, London

This book brings together authoritative contributions from leading mental health researchers, educators and practitioners to provide a comprehensive text for community mental health nurses in training and practice.

Repper J, Perkins R 2003 Social inclusion and recovery: a model for mental health practice. Baillière Tindall, Edinburgh

This book addresses the ways in which practitioners can help people with mental health problems, in the context of service user accounts of their knowledge of the types of assistance found to be valuable.

Journals

Journal of Psychiatric and Mental Health Nursing

This is the UK's leading research-led mental health nursing journal.

Internet

The online psychiatric nursing discussion list can be accessed at: www.jiscmail.ac.uk/lists/psychiatric-nursing.html. This is a lively forum for the exchange of news and views, and includes contributions from nurses all around the world.

19

Community learning disability nursing

Ruth Wyn Williams and David Coyle

KEY ISSUES

- The values and principles underpinning community learning disability nursing
- Role of the community learning disability nurse
- Evidence-based practice
- Influences and opportunities for community learning disability nursing

Introduction

The aim of this chapter is to provide the reader with an overview of the role and context of community learning disability nurses (CLDNs), identifying key issues in contemporary learning disabilities nursing practice. The value base and principles underpinning CLDNs are reviewed in light of current legislation and policy. The role of the community nurse is discussed considering professional guidelines and the interdisciplinary challenges arising from policies originating from the United Kingdom Central Council for Nursing, Midwifery and Health Visiting (UKCC; 1998), and the Nursing and Midwifery Council (NMC; 2007), as well as the Scottish Executive (SE; 2000), Department of Health (DH; 2001) and the Welsh Assembly Government (WAG; 2007). The chapter concludes with examining the potential and the challenges for the role in an ever-changing environment and the continual push for the nurse to work in partnership with service users and their families to attain good health and good lives. The pace and rate of development within CLDN practice since the publication of the previous edition necessitates a full discourse on the role and context for practice today and in the future.

The values and principles that underpin community learning disability nursing

Much is often made of the role that values have in learning disability practice (DH 2007). It appears that only CLDNs rely on an articulated theory that places the person at the centre of nursing interventions. Were this the case, CLDNs would indeed be exceptional. All nursing branches have at their core a set of beliefs that inform and influence their interactions with the client or patient. Nurses and public health workers are not so different, though in the case of learning disabilities; the history and social legacy of the client group may well be. Additionally, the work of CLDNs does not support a homogeneous population. The 210 000 people with severe learning disabilities and 1.2 million people with moderate or mild learning disabilities (DH 2001) they support are heterogeneous with resulting complexity for organizing services.

It is not the intention of this section to retrace historical lineage of learning disability nursing. Students may find such accounts in other works (Gates 2006), and in the substantial output of Mitchell (2000). It is of significance though to reflect that CLDNs have, over the past three decades, shaped and focused their practice responding to changing cultural, social and moral drivers. CLDNs have responded with flair and innovation to meet the progressively changing needs of people with learning disability and continue to do so. They have achieved this without losing their health promotion role for the client group. While we must see how history informs today's practice, we must equally look to the future, free from the past's constraints (Jukes and Bollard 2003).

The principle upon which modern learning disability services are founded is a social model of impairment (Swain et al 2003) and also upon the principles of person-centred planning (Sanderson et al 1997, Sanderson 2003). This approach can be seen to be at the heart of current legislative and social policy in all the home nations: *Valuing People* (DH 2001), *The Same as You?* (SE 2000), *Statement on Policy and Practice for Adults with a Learning Disability* (WAG 2007), *Equal Lives* (Department of Health, Social Services and Public Safety (DHSSPS) 2005). The challenge for services today is in tackling exclusion and stigma and improving quality of life and participation for people with disabilities.

The increased legislative basis of rights in society from the Human Rights Act (1998), Disability Discrimination Act (1995), individual service plans (Duffy 2005) and the Mental Capacity Act (2005) has shifted the balance of power from professionals to the individuals, user groups and organizations that represent their needs, wishes and rights.

A social model of impairment

It is known that health inequalities and high morbidity of preventable disease are prevalent in people with learning disabilities (Cooper et al 2004). An understanding of the social model helps the CLDN recognize needs and aspirations of a population excluded from mainstream health, culture and politics as it acknowledges the connections between social activity and health across the domains of health promotion and maintenance.

The principles of ordinary life as embodied in influential papers such as the seminal five service accomplishments (O'Brien 1987) laid the foundation of today's services. Person-centred approaches now form the foundation principle of support. Indeed, John O'Brien (2004) stated that in order to achieve the keystone objectives of *Valuing People* (DH 2001), person-centred planning as proposed by Sanderson et al (1997) has to exist. The one could not function without the other.

The social model of impairment does not deny the problem of disability but locates it within wider society. An individual's limitation in any aspect of daily living or health maintenance is not the central problem. This is to say that the social model does not undermine nursing and health roles. On the contrary, it brings into sharp focus the action required to address inequalities in health and develop strategies to identify and support the client with health promotion, health gain and towards inclusion and citizenship. It is most important that this approach should not be confused with a social model of provision (Swain et al 2003) where health need may be overlooked with detrimental consequences for the person with learning disabilities (Northway et al 2006).

For the CLDN the social model provides a focus for partnership and intervention. Rather than trying to fix the person, the emphasis is on supporting access and inclusion to healthier lifestyles and developing opportunities for the individual to be a part of healthier communities. Rather than trying to make the person adapt, for example learn to read sufficiently well to access and understand health promotion literature, literature instead is adapted to be accessible to the person, resulting in the possibility of health gain. By responding in this way, a more active personalized approach to health gain might be achieved and dependence and passivity within the individual avoided.

Social policy such as *Our Health, Our Care, Our Say* (DH 2006) and direction from within learning disability nursing itself, such as *Shaping the Future* (Northway et al 2006) demand that practitioners avoid an individual model and instead work in partnership toward a more social model approach while retaining and supporting the client's journey towards health (Aldridge 2004). Succinctly put, the Department of Health summarizes the role of the learning disability nurse within healthcare:

> ... *the main objective for the NHS is to 'enable people with learning disabilities to access a health service designed around their individual needs, with fast and convenient care delivered to a high standard, and with additional support where necessary'. (DH 2001: 23)*

Rights

The aim of nursing is the promotion and attainment of healthy lifestyles in which the people themselves have greater choice over their lives and are integrated into their local communities (O'Brien 1987, Duffy 2005). The Disability Discrimination Act

1995, although taking 10 years for full implementation, is making an impact on the access to health and communities for people with learning disabilities. In combination with the Mental Capacity Act 2005 and the existing Human Rights Act 1998, people with learning disabilities have never had their rights acknowledged and protected to their current extent.

Initiatives within the UK such as 'In Control' (Duffy 2005) provide people who have learning disabilities with real power through financial decision-making and choice to buy individually designed services that cannot be delivered through traditional health and social care providers. The person's aspirations as the focus of service response are the basis of a rights culture that the modern learning disability nurse works within. In identifying health need and developing effective individualized packages of care, the CLDN can forge and facilitate working partnerships that empower the service user or client to experience a healthier life.

The Disability Rights Commission (DRC; 2006) (now the Equality and Human Rights Commission) has highlighted the inequality for people with learning disabilities in getting access to physical health services. They point to a number of failings on the part of primary care trusts (PCTs) in adequately providing for this client group. They are concerned that PCTs are not being advised on the unique needs that this group has. They recommend that each PCT has a strategic health facilitator role to champion the needs of people with a learning disability and to provide expert clinical advice to ensure equal access to the primary care services.

This is a clear example of how a rights-based culture now informs and directs services afforded to people with a learning disability. Rather than lamenting the high rates of clinical morbidity and low rates of uptake in preventative screening, the rights-based approach states that it is unacceptable for the current inequity to continue and demands action to redress the imbalance. The following section outlines the contexts in which CLDNs practise, the challenges they face and some approaches that may assist in supporting people with a learning disability.

The role of the community learning disability nurse

Current policy and practice are moving away from a paternalistic model to featuring choice as a central theme (Leadbeater et al 2008). The essential foundation of practice for the CLDN and others involved in supporting people with learning disability is person centredness (DH 2007). Fagan and Plant (2003) state that empowering people with a learning disability to identify and meet their health and social needs is the greatest challenge learning disability practitioners have. To be able to work in partnership identifying what is important to and for the person with the challenges and potential for conflict inherent is equally challenging.

In the last 8 years (2000–2008), learning disability services and practitioners in health and social care have seen profound changes. Some of these drivers have been people with disabilities themselves demanding better treatment, human rights awareness and a greater understanding of disability rights. However, in spite of the great progress in promoting the rights of people with learning disabilities, the uncovering of poor, abusive or negligent practice still arises and is a grave cause for concern (Commission for Healthcare Audit and Inspection 2007). We might on the other hand suggest that because of a greater expectation of rights for vulnerable people, the systems to protect individuals and expose unacceptable care are more robust and effective in safeguarding people with learning disability.

Learning disability health and social care policy can be identified as a concurrent policy, in that NHS and Social Services provide the same function throughout the UK. As such, CLDNs are expected to work to local (as well as individualized) levels, but also be cognizant of national policies, a task made harder by some service innovations such as 'In Control' (Duffy 2005) being scaled up by government without proper testing and evaluation (Leadbeater et al 2008).

The intentions for policy are clear. The principles of rights, independence, choice and inclusion (DH 2001) are clearly stated within *Valuing People*. Five areas that are central to learning disability services

Activity box 19.1

- Consider how closely the practice of the team you work within adheres to the principles stated by the UKCC (1998) (Box 19.1).
- How person centred are the statements?

> ## Box 19.1
>
> ### UKCC guidelines for practice 1998
>
> - Accountability
> - Autonomy
> - Consent
> - Interdisciplinary working
> - Evidence-based practice
> - Advocacy
> - Relationships
> - Confidentiality
> - Risk management

in Northern Ireland are identified: citizenship, social inclusion, empowerment, working together and individual support (DHSSPS 2005). Wales has developed the *Statement on Policy and Practice for Adults with a Learning Disability* (WAG 2007: 12) stating:

> *All people with a learning disability are full citizens, equal in status and value to other citizens of the same age. They have the same rights to:*
>
> - *live healthy, productive and independent lives with appropriate and responsive treatment and support to develop their maximum potential*
> - *be individuals and decide everyday issues and life-defining matters for themselves joining in all decision-making which affects their lives, with appropriate and responsive advice and support where necessary*
> - *live their lives within their community, maintaining the social and family ties and connections which are important to them*
> - *have the support of the communities of which they are a part and access to general and specialist services that are responsive to their individual needs, circumstances and preferences.*

These rights should determine the value base upon which all practitioners in learning disability should base their practice on in Wales. Joint working among these professionals is central in these policies as one aspect that could improve the service pro-

vided. The clear person-centred vision in these policies can only be achieved through integration of services and CLDNs have the potential to be at the heart of this.

In practice, CLDNs may work across a range of settings, including working in care management, though 'good practice' (DH 2007) warns that for CLDNs working in social care, to be most effective, the learning disability nurse should have a health focus.

To consider the tasks undertaken by CLDNs we may use Aldridge's (2004) Ecology of Health Model, which was developed for supporting people with learning disabilities based on ordinary life principles. The model is a three-dimensional concept aiming to articulate the roles and contexts in which a person with learning disabilities can be supported to achieve a valued and healthy life. Matousova-Done and Gates (2006) cite Aldridge (2004) in stating the model is an:

> *… ever-changing state of individually defined optimal functioning and well-being, determined by the interplay between the individual's internal physiology and psychology and their external environment. (Aldridge 2004: 172)*

Using the Ecology of Health Model headings as a framework for discussion, the role of the community learning disability nurse will be explored:

- an assessment role
- a teaching and developmental role
- a therapeutic role
- a healthcare role
- a network and supportive role.

The appropriate identification and assessment of need

Assessment is an essential aspect of the CLDN role. It enables the practitioner to obtain information about a client's health needs and wishes, prior to intervention. The client and carer are central in the assessment process, which often begins with an exploration of health need from a broad perspective. Assessment tools utilized by the CLDN will need to address areas such as health status and screening. This initial assessment often leads to more in-depth exploration of specific areas.

Promoting and maintaining health: a teaching and developmental role

When promoting the health of people with a learning disability several different approaches can be used. These are: medical, behavioural, educational, empowerment and social change. Barr (2006) reports that any of these approaches could be utilized by the CLDN, depending on the needs of the individual and the other people involved. Central to the *Valuing People* (DH 2001) initiative, and the appropriate strategies formulated in Wales and Scotland, the role of health promotion is paramount. The creation of health action plans (HAPs) (DH 2002) and health partnership boards where every person with a learning disability will have a HAP by 2005 was meant to ensure that individual susceptibility to illness and poor health among people with learning disabilities would be identified and addressed. The fact that people with learning disabilities are still proportionally more unhealthy with a higher mortality than the general population is an indication that much work has still to be done (Mencap 2007).

The CLDN has clear roles in identifying health need, coordinating and promoting health with and for people with a learning disability. In many ways the roles outlined for nurses supporting people with a learning disability by the UKCC (1998) are still relevant for today's services.

A therapeutic role

The ability of the health professional to understand a person's concerns or complaint is central to meeting health need, yet due to a CLDN's difficulty in overcoming the impairments of receptive and expressive communication in an individual with learning disabil-

---

Activity box 19.2

Health facilitation, whoever does it and whatever way, in whatever setting is about ensuring healthier lives and better health for people with learning disabilities.

(Department of Health Guidance 2002, section 2, p. 12)

- Consider the statement above in relation to CLDNs and accountability. Would the statement be true for all branches of nursing?

---

ities, delays in gaining appropriate interventions may arise (Barr et al 2001). Professionals' uncertainty regarding consent and best interests has been identified as an area needing improvement (Hardy et al 2006). Research shows that even though it is known that people with a learning disability have poorer health, they still receive poorer access to health services across primary and secondary mainstream services and that those with greater need are often the most neglected (Elliott et al 2003).

The phenomenon of diagnostic overshadowing (Hardy et al 2006) has become widely accepted. Physical or behavioural manifestations are attributed to the learning disability, rather than as some diagnostically significant symptom, e.g. incontinence being indicative of developmental function, rather than of a potential urinary tract infection. The government is so concerned that the health of people with learning disabilities is significantly poorer and their uptake of regular screening so much lower than that of the general population, they have made many recommendations to ensure PCTs fulfil their responsibilities under health action plans and partnership boards (Valuing People Support Team (VPST) 2007). The CLDN is well placed therefore to use health promotion activities to highlight and address these issues. The CLDN's role is an enabling one which ultimately aims to enable people to improve their own health in therapeutic partnerships (Thompson and Cobb 2004).

Disability nurses have skills and knowledge that enable them to undertake specialist practice across a range of need (Slevin et al 2008). Some CLDNs have specialized in supporting people whose behaviour challenges. Others have skilled expertise in managing and supporting epilepsy, mental health issues or with children and young people with sleep disorders.

Aldridge (2004) identifies the following areas for legitimate intervention under the therapeutic role. The nurse may engage in activities that reduce or lessen the impact of a medical condition for the individual. Where the condition is life threatening or limiting, the nurse engages in a palliative function. Therapeutic action may be in the form of monitoring illness or the deterioration of that condition. A CLDN working with an individual with an affective disorder might under this section use cognitive behavioural interventions to identify triggers for negative thoughts as well as develop strategies with the client for when they experience distress. A CLDN working with someone with diabetes may help the person to understand their condition and also provide them with support to ensure appropriate blood tests are carried out.

A healthcare role

Barriers impacting on many of the general population have a greater negative effect on a person with a learning disability. Most people with learning disabilities do not drive and may be reliant on another to assist them to attend a health centre. People with a learning disability are also known to experience difficulties in obtaining work, which can lead to low income, inadequate housing conditions and poverty. Such poverty is a large part of the everyday lives of learning disabled individuals, and is associated with powerlessness, exclusion and an inability to participate in society (Naidoo and Wills 1998). Circumstances such as these can have a detrimental effect on both the mental and physical health of people with a learning disability.

Activities such as health education, primary, secondary and tertiary prevention of health loss (Ewles and Simnett 2003) can form the basis of healthcare intervention for CLDNs. The CLDN's role in promoting healthy lifestyles is clear. A fundamental aspect of health promotion is to improve access for the person with learning disability to health by working directly with the person, advising families and advocating appropriate health interventions with professionals across all disciplines. This may include providing information in an accessible medium on how to look after their health (Hardy et al 2006), how to access appropriate health services, or on factors in the wider environment that are detrimental to health (VPST 2007). The CLDN should be a source of appropriate and often specialist information to support professionals in providing adequate healthcare. Given the often appalling consequences of poor healthcare delivered to people with learning disabilities (Mencap 2007), this role is crucial.

Partnerships of care: a network and supportive role

Partnership and collaboration among professions and teams are used in a wide range of contexts and are enthusiastically encouraged as a way forward for services (DH 2001). Throughout the UK, CLDNs work in a variety of interprofessional settings affected by legislation and policy. Services for people with learning disability have been and remain predominantly within social care. However, literature and recent reports (Barr 2006, Cooper et al 2004, Elliott et al 2003, Melville et al 2006) have identified that the health needs of people with a learning disability are still not being met. One approach offered that might help to bridge the gap between health and social care is by improving joint working practices between professionals. However, there is little evidence to support the notion of joint working. Tope and Thomas (2006) explain that people with complex health and social care may require the skills from a range of professionals associated with different agencies to work together. They further suggest that:

> … policy makers and strategists have made it crystal clear that the creation of an interprofessional workforce is critical for the health and welfare of future generations and to ignore their advice would, at the very least, be foolhardy. (Tope and Thomas 2006: 4)

The financial arrangements for each country in the UK differ and are always an issue of debate. The review of *Valuing People* (DH 2001, 2007) has shown that the ambitious goals of *Valuing People* have not been wholly achieved (Harbridge 2007). The fierce spending review at the end of 2007 meant that for many people with learning disabilities, access to funds, inequity of eligibility criteria and overall cut in total monies will impact enormously on those in receipt of services. Harbridge (2007: 1) stated that without:

> … ring-fenced funding and incentives for local authorities…Valuing People will remain a distant dream for many people.

One intention of social policy generally can be described as attempting to reduce social exclusion (Peckham and Meerabeau 2007). This can be clearly identified in social policy relating to learning disability. Hannigan and Burnard (2000) advocate reviewing the policies that advocate joint working by suggesting that nurses need to understand and have clear awareness of policy if they are going to appreciate the context in which they work (see Chapter 21 for further information on the political influence on partnership working in health and social care).

Challenges facing CLDNs: evidence-based practice

The evidence base for learning disability is:

> ... not fit for purpose in terms of its extent, quantity or quality. (Griffiths et al 2007: ii)

This damning statement from the King's Fund appears to cast a doubt over the use and effectiveness of learning disability nursing research. However, the review makes clear some of the challenges that lie ahead for learning disability nursing and its use and generation of research. When thinking about evidence-based practice, we need to be clear about what this means. For instance, do we mean knowledge transfer, research utilization, best practice or critical appraisal of available evidence? Or do we mean evidence in the Cochrane hierarchy of type one and type two evidence, whose main contributors will originate from the world of biosciences and medicine? Importantly the hierarchy of evidence would appear to exclude information and evidence from the perspective of the user, their carers and possibly the CLDN. Griffiths et al (2007) have been roundly criticized by Caan and Toocaram (2008) for the bias expressed by the review. They claim that the review amounts to a 'cursory and superficial' (p. 78) account, missing on many contributions to best practice.

What constitutes evidence may not be clear, though the role of the learning disability nurse is more so. The King's Fund (Griffiths et al 2007) states that theory and knowledge do not derive from learning disability nursing but that the field utilizes evidence from a range of disciplines across diverse settings. While it appears true that the basis for practice in learning disability is in the main:

inspirational, theoretical or opinion based rather than evidence based (Slevin et al 2008: 59)

this does not dismiss the interventions of the CLDN. There are good examples of sound practice to be found within the UK where CLDNs have led innovation and contributed to real change. The Department of Health (DH 2007) has attempted to show evidence-based practice from learning disabilities nursing, though readers might use some of the networks for practitioners such as the Foundation of Nursing Studies (see resources listed below). The implications for CLDNs from recent reviews may appear stark. Nurses need to articulate their practice base, recognizing that it might draw on diverse fields and unexpected places.

Influences and opportunities for community learning disability nursing

While CLDNs have evolved their practice and responded to the changing landscape of social and health policy, they have never lost the focus of their work, that of supporting people with learning disabilities. They are the only group of nurses and professionals with such focus. While some critics might argue that CLDNs leave their nursing roots behind, others recognize the opportunities for health improvement and health gain possible when strong and articulate advocates with specialist knowledge and competencies facilitate on behalf of people with learning disabilities (see Chapter 23 for further information).

Changes in legislation and in organizing the care arena mean that CLDNs will continue to evolve their roles and function in new settings and face new challenges. Below are some changes that may impact in a beneficial way on the working world of the CLDN and of people with learning disabilities.

- The impact of the Mental Capacity Act 2005 is yet to be fully realized, with the code of practice only months old. What is clear is that decisions taken by CLDNs and those people whom they manage will need to be conversant with capacity, best interest and daily decision-making issues.
- Prescribing in England and Wales has grown enormously in the past 8 years. Increasingly the

Activity box 19.3

- Consider your use of evidence in clinical practice. Is it evidence-based practice? Knowledge transfer in practice? Is it dissemination of best practices?
- Why might it be important to think about evidence in practice through these lenses?
- How might the perspective of the client or service user differ in terms of their wants, needs and aspirations when one thinks of evidence?

number of nurses successfully undertaking the independent prescribing course has grown. The potential role for CLDNs to operate independently of patient group protocols is an exciting prospect.

- *Valuing People* (DH 2001) identified the role of the 'health facilitator'. Although the document did not identify community learning disability nurses as the natural candidate, given the continued inequality of health for this population, it might be time to respond by ensuring CLDNs champion people with learning disabilities at all levels.

- The creation of nurse consultants in 1998 heralded a new age for nursing. Over the past 7 years the role of these practitioners has expanded and their influence in establishing and maintaining excellent services through evidence-based practice has grown (Northway et al 2006). The consultant nurse network has continued to grow and extend the remit of specialist practice within the UK (see Chapter 22 for further information on the nurse consultant role).

- The move of the present government to increase the individualization agenda in scaling up initiatives such as 'In Control' (Duffy 2005) will gather pace. Social care will face a process of increased person-centred delivery with a concomitant disaggregation of traditional service provision. How this will impact on CLDNs will need to be seen.

- Finally, the further development of good person-centred planning combined with self-directed services will challenge the role and practice of all practitioners as the recipients of

services will further assert their growing influence and confidence. This will be in general a good thing, both for people with learning disabilities in terms of health gain, but also for CLDNs as they will no doubt be well placed to respond with flair and innovation to meet this final challenge.

Conclusion

This chapter has provided an overview of some of the issues that have shaped community learning disability nursing and outlined factors that continue to challenge this area of nursing. Issues relating to professional practice and skilled implementation of care have been discussed in the light of the nurses' role, and collaborative practice has been critically evaluated. A brief account such as this cannot be seen as exhaustive; it is simply intended to be a starting point for discussion and reflection. The issues raised within this chapter are pertinent to all disciplines involved with the care and support of people with a learning disability. Through discussion, the ever developing role of the CLDN can be articulated. Learning disability nurses have a value base that promotes the interests of the person with a learning disability as the focus, enabling them to live fuller, healthier and more autonomous lives. CLDN practice is framed within the health context and nurses in this field are rightly proud of their contribution to improvements over the years. Working within teaching, developmental, therapeutic, healthcare and supportive roles (Aldridge 2004), CLDNs can maintain and develop their clinical credence within a wider public health focus.

SUMMARY

- Learning disability nurses work in partnership with and for people with learning disabilities, their families and friends and in close collaboration with other professionals.
- The ever developing role of the CLDN can be articulated and can be evidenced.
- Learning disability nurses have a value base that promotes the interests of the person with a learning disability that is being used by other branches of nursing.
- CLDN practice is framed within the public health context and continues to make an

invaluable contribution to the health of people with learning disabilities.
- CLDNs' knowledge and practice base is diverse and by working within teaching, developmental, therapeutic, healthcare and supportive roles, the health and well-being of people with learning disabilities can be enhanced.
- The focus for CLDNs in a more personalized and self-directed health and social care agenda is strong.

DISCUSSION POINTS

1. Consider ways in which the CLDN can support social inclusion.
2. Guidance from government still suggests that healthcare professionals should engage in interprofessional work. How might collaboration be improved within:

- your team
- the family and friends of the persons you support
- the wider community?

3. In what ways can nurses develop research to support the role of the CLDN?

References

Aldridge J 2004 Intellectual disability nursing: a model for practice. In: Turnbull J (ed.) Learning disability nursing. Blackwell, Oxford

Barr O 2006 The evolving role of community nurses for people with learning disabilities: changes over an 11-year period. Journal of Clinical Nursing 15: 72–82

Barr O, Gilgunn J, Kane T, Moore G 2001 Health screening for people with learning disabilities by a community learning disability nursing service in Northern Ireland. Journal of Advanced Nursing 29(6): 1482–1491

Caan W, Toocaram J 2008 Learning disability is bigger than a cursory review. British Journal of Nursing 17(2): 78–79

Commission for Healthcare Audit and Inspection 2007 Investigation into services for people with learning disabilities provided by Sutton and Merton Primary Care Trust. Healthcare Commission, London

Cooper SA, Melville C, Morrison J 2004 People with intellectual disabilities: their health needs differ and need to be recognised and met. British Medical Journal 239: 414–415

Department of Health 2001 Valuing people. A new strategy for learning disability for the 21st century. A White Paper. DH, London

Department of Health 2002 Action for health – health action plans and health facilitation. DH, London

Department of Health 2006 Our health, our care, our say: a new direction for community services. DH, London

Department of Health 2007 Good practice in learning disability nursing. DH, London

Department of Health, Social Services and Public Safety 2005 Equal lives: draft report of Learning Disability Committee. Department of Health, Social Services and Public Safety, Belfast

Disability Discrimination Act 1995 HMSO. Online: http://www.hmso.gov.uk/acts/acts1995/1995050.htm (accessed 12 Dec 2007)

Disability Rights Commission 2006 Report of the DRC Formal Inquiry Panel to the DRC's Formal Investigation into the inequalities in physical health experienced by people with mental health problems and people with learning disabilities. DRC, London

Duffy S 2005 Individual budgets: transforming the allocation of resources for care. Journal of Integrated Care 13(1): 8–16

Elliott J, Hatton C, Emerson E 2003 The health of people with intellectual disabilities in the UK: evidence and implications for the NHS. Journal of Integrated Care 11(3): 9–17

Ewles L, Simnett I 2003 Promoting health. A practical guide, 5th edn. Baillière Tindall, Edinburgh

Fagan N, Plant T 2003 Joint practitioners in health and social care. In: Jukes M, Bollard M Contemporary learning disability practice. Quay Books, MA Healthcare Ltd, Salisbury Wiltshire

Gates B (ed.) 2006 Care planning and delivery in intellectual disability nursing. Blackwell, Oxford

Griffiths P, Bennett J, Smith E 2007 The research base for learning disability nursing: a rapid scoping review. King's College London, London

Hannigan B, Burnard P 2000 Nursing politics and policy: a response to Clifford. Nurse Education Today 20(7): 519–523

Harbridge E 2007 The genie is out of the bottle – Government cannot afford to disappoint people again. Community Living 12(1): 1

Hardy S, Woodward P, Woolard P, Tait T 2006 Meeting the health needs of people with learning disabilities. Guidance for nursing staff. RCN Learning Disability Nursing Forum, Royal College of Nursing

Human Rights Act 1998 HMSO, London

Jukes M, Bollard M (eds) 2003 Contemporary learning disability practice. Quay Books, Salisbury

Leadbeater C, Bartlett J, Gallagher N 2008 Making it personal. Demos, London

Matousova-Done Z, Gates B 2006 The nature of care planning and delivery in intellectual disability nursing. In: Gates B (ed.) Care planning and delivery in intellectual disability nursing. Blackwell Publishing, Oxford

Melville CA, Cooper S-A, Morrison J, et al 2006 The outcomes of an intervention study to reduce the barriers experienced by people with intellectual disabilities accessing primary health care services. Journal of Intellectual Disability Research 50(1): 11–17

Mencap 2007 Death by indifference. Following up the Treat Me Right! Report. Mencap, London

Mental Capacity Act 2005 Office of Public Sector Information. Online:

http://www.opsi.gov.uk/ACTS/acts2005/ukpga_20050009_en_1

Mitchell D 2000 Parallel stigma? Nurses and people with learning disabilities. British Journal of Learning Disability 28(2): 78–81

Naidoo J, Wills J 1998 Practising health promotion: dilemmas and challenges. Baillière Tindall, London

Northway R, Hutchinson C, Kingdon A (eds) 2006 Shaping the future: a vision for learning disability nursing. UK Learning Disability Consultant Nurse Network

Nursing and Midwifery Council 2007 Covert administration of medicines – disguising medicine in food and drink. Online: http://www.nmc-uk.org/aFrameDisplay.aspx?DocumentID=3602&Keyword

O'Brien J 1987 A guide to lifestyle planning. In: Bellamy GT, Wilcox B (eds) The activities catalog. Paul H Brookes, London

O'Brien J 2004 If person centred planning did not exist, valuing people would require its invention. Journal of Applied Research in Intellectual Disabilities 17: 11–15

Peckham S, Meerabeau L 2007 Social policy for nurses and the helping professions. Open University Press, Maidenhead

Sanderson H 2003 Person centred planning. In: Gates B (ed.) Learning disabilities. towards inclusion. Churchill Livingstone, Edinburgh

Sanderson H, Kennedy J, Ritchie P, Goodwin G 1997 People plans and possibilities: exploring person-centred planning. SHS, Edinburgh

Scottish Executive 2000 The same as you? A review of the services for people with learning disabilities. Scottish Executive, Edinburgh

Slevin E, Truesdale-Kennedy M, McKonkey R, Barr O, Taggart L 2008 Community learning disability teams: developments, composition and good practice. A review of the literature. Journal of Intellectual Disabilities 12(1): 59–79

Swain J, French S, Cameron C 2003 Controversial issues in a disabling society. Open University Press, Basingstoke

Thompson J, Cobb J 2004 Person centred health action planning. Learning Disability Practice 7(5): 12–20

Tope R, Thomas E 2006 Europe's policy agenda: creating an interprofessional workforce. Paper 1. Creating and Interprofessional Workforce Programme. CAIPE, London. Online: http://www.caipe.org.uk (accessed 3 Dec 2007)

United Kingdom Central Council for Nursing, Midwifery and Health Visiting 1998 Guidelines for mental health and learning disabilities nursing. United Kingdom Central Council for Nursing, Midwifery and Health Visiting, London

Valuing People Support Team 2007 The commissioning specialist adult learning disability health services good practice guidance. Online: http://valuingpeople.gov.uk/dynamic/valuingpeople2.jsp (accessed 5 Nov 2007)

Welsh Assembly Government 2007 Statement on policy and practice for adults with a learning disability. Welsh Assembly Government. Online: http://new.wales.gov.uk/docrepos/40382/dhss/403821211/guidance/Contemporary_Policy_and_Pra1.pdf?lang=en

Recommended reading

Goward P, Grant G, Ramacharan P, Richardson M 2003 Learning disability: a life cycle approach to valuing people. Open University Press, Maidenhead

Thompson J, Pickering S (eds) 2001 Health needs of people with learning disability: the public health agenda. Baillière Tindall, London

Thompson J, Kilbane J, Sanderson H (eds) 2007 Person centred approaches for professionals. Open University Press, Maidenhead

Turnbull J (ed.) 2003 Learning disability nursing, Wiley, Blackwell Oxford

Online resources

Many online and web-based sites are available. These are useful links to documents and organizations.

Department of Health, accessed at http://www.dh.gov/uk

National Assembly for Wales, accessed at http://www.wales.gov.uk

Northern Ireland, accessed at http://www.dhssni.gov.uk

Scottish Health, accessed at http://www.scotland.gov.uk

National Network for Learning Disability Nurses, accessed at http://www.nnldn.org.uk/

General learning disability sites with excellent links, regularly updated: http://www.paradigm.org.uk, http://www.bild.org.uk

Excellent resource for nurses wishing to access health-based material: http://www.library.nhs.uk/learningdisabilities/

Care and treatment of offenders with learning disabilities: www.ldoffenders.co.uk (provides information on people with learning disabilities who have or are at risk of committing offences)

Valuing People Support Team resources pages: http://www.valuingpeople.gov.uk/dynamic/valuingpeople59.jsp

Mencap publications: http://www.mencap.org.uk/html/publications

Excellent health focused site: http://www.intellectualdisability.info/home.htm

People First (a national self-advocacy organization run by people with learning difficulties for people with learning difficulties): www.peoplefirstltd.com

Challenging Behaviour Foundation (provides guidance and information on supporting people with challenging behaviour, including fact sheets to download): www.thecbf.org.uk

The Down's Syndrome Association: www.downs-syndrome.org.uk

The National Society for Epilepsy: www.epilepsynseorg.uk

Chapter Twenty

Community children's nursing

Anna Sidey and David Widdas

KEY ISSUES

- The development of community children's nursing services in the United Kingdom
- The roles and responsibilities of community children's nurses alongside other nursing disciplines
- Family nursing as a framework for practice
- Integrated multiagency care pathways
- Transition to adult services

Introduction

Community children's nursing remains a relatively young discipline compared with more established branches of community nursing. As such, the corporate identity of services is still emerging. This lack of a traditional foundation can facilitate more imaginative and flexible approaches to identified care needs, but it can also cause confusion and misunderstanding for stakeholders and affect collaboration with other professional groups. In order to clarify the context of the current situation, this chapter begins with a brief overview of the development of community children's nursing services and then examines roles and responsibilities and the context of community children's nursing, as well as family nursing, integrated care pathways and the role of the key worker, followed by transitions to adult services and current challenges and opportunities for community children's nursing services. Case studies will be used to illustrate significant points and to challenge current thinking.

The development of community children's nursing

The formal existence of a community children's nursing service was first recorded in 1949 (Gillet 1954). While the development of services has been consistently supported in official reports and government directives since the 1950s, expansion of this provision remained slow until the early 1990s (Whiting 2005). The last decade has witnessed most growth and development in this discipline due to a number of reasons, which include:

- medical advances that have enabled infants and children to survive what were once fatal disorders
- the increased availability of medicines, therapies and technology to support associated care needs
- the government agenda that has pursued a shift from secondary care to primary care alongside a philosophy of increasing consumer expectations
- the recognition of community children's nursing as a discrete community specialist practitioner recordable qualification (United Kingdom Central Council 1994).

However, community children's nursing services are fragmented and anomalies continue to exist that give rise to confusion. For example, Box 20.1 illustrates ten different models of services in operation in the UK, as identified by Whiting (2005).

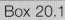

Box 20.1

Models of community children's nursing services

1. Hospital-based 'generalist' outreach services
2. Hospital-based services comprising a number of 'specialist' nurses
3. Community-based teams who are not specifically aligned with a single primary care trust
4. Primary care trust-based teams
5. Ambulatory care or assessment unit and hospital-at-home services
6. Services (including respite) for children with life-limiting illnesses including community, hospital- and hospice-based services
7. Continuing care teams
8. Specialist nurses based in tertiary referral centres
9. Services based in child development/Sure Start teams
10. Community neonatal services

Further to this, by 2004 in excess of 20% of UK regions did not have access to a service, with only a minimal number of existing services able to offer 24-hour access (Burr and Hughes 2005). Nationally, a 100% cover for the provision of palliative care is close to becoming a policy goal for the government and assemblies of the UK. However, a holistic, adequately staffed, nationwide community children's nursing service remains a distant vision (Craft and Killen 2007). (Current details of primary care trusts in the UK commissioning community children's nurses (CCNs) are available on the Royal College of Nursing website (www.rcn.org.uk).)

These variations have occurred essentially for the following reasons:

- Current standards regarding the care of sick children differ between hospital and community settings. For example, in 1991 the Department of Health stated that there should be at least two qualified children's nurses on duty 24 hours a day in all hospital children's departments and wards, a notion that was reinstated following the Beverley Allitt inquiry (Department of Health 1994). However, such a standard does not apply to the care of sick children in the community, despite being a recommendation following the review of

children's services by the House of Commons Health Committee (1997).

- There has been a lack of understanding and commitment by commissioning and purchasing authorities to meet the needs of sick children and their families in the community in some areas. The National Service Framework (NSF) for Children failed to provide the catalyst for commissioners to prioritize community children's nursing services (Department of Health 2004).
- An absence of a national strategy and corporate identity for community children's nurses continues to adversely influence professional recognition (Sidey and Widdas 2005).

Roles and responsibilities: the context of community children's nursing

At present, community children's nursing and the role of the CCN lacks a clear professional corporate identity, an issue not unique to this discipline. A corporate identity strengthens the culture and values of a service and provides a signpost for all staff. A stronger identity within community children's nursing would enhance interdependent working with other care providers. In order to facilitate this, the uniqueness of the CCN's role, alongside other nursing disciplines, needs to be established. A distinction between the titles that are often used synonymously within the literature (community children's nurse, clinical nurse specialist, specialist outreach nurse) follows.

Community children's nurses are registered children's nurses with a community specialist practitioner qualification. This role can be identified with models 1, 3, 4, 5, 6, 7 and 9 of Box 20.1. Based in either an acute or community setting, the CCN facilitates nursing care for a varied, yet defined, caseload of sick children in a range of community settings. The work of the CCN has been described as having seven broad areas (Box 20.2).

A clinical nurse specialist (CNS) may work independent of, or within, a community children's nursing team and concentrate on a disorder-specific subspecialty such as respiratory or community neonatal nursing. The CNS is a qualified children's nurse, usually with an increased level of expertise and further education and training in the defined

Box 20.2

The work of the community children's nurse (House of Commons Health Committee 1997)

1. Supporting the families of children with long-term nursing needs
2. Supporting children with a disability
3. Supporting families who are caring for a child during the terminal phase of his/her life
4. Neonatal and postnatal care, including the care of children with complex problems arising from prematurity and disorders presenting at birth
5. Supporting children undergoing planned surgery
6. Caring for children with acute nursing needs, which can reduce the need for and duration of hospital admission
7. Follow-up and support of children requiring emergency treatment which may assist the promotion of early discharge from hospital

subspecialty but not necessarily in community nursing. This role concurs with models 2, 8 and 10 presented in Box 20.1. Miller (1995) describes the role as clinical expert, resource consultant, educator, change agent, researcher, advocate and mentor.

Conversely the *specialist outreach nurse* (SON) provides care from either a secondary or tertiary healthcare setting and is often a member of a specialist multiprofessional team. This role links most closely with models 2, 6, 8 and 10 (Box 20.1). The SON is a registered children's nurse with further education and training in the specialty but not necessarily in community nursing. The philosophy underpinning practice is often one of 'shared care' either between primary and tertiary settings, between primary and secondary care, or between all three. This model is particularly well established in the care of children with malignant disease.

While some differences in these three roles are evident, they each aim to avoid admission to hospital, reduce the length of hospital stay and provide a high-quality, effective service (see Chapter 22 for further information on the range of nursing roles). This chapter is specifically concerned with the role and responsibilities of the CCN.

In the context of more established community nurses who work with children, such as specialist community public health nurses: health visitors (HVs) and school nurses (SNs), there are certain generic aspects that overlap with the CCN role. For example, health promotion and child protection clearly apply to the work of each of these three nurses but with varying degrees of emphasis. However, there are two distinguishing aspects to the CCN role that do not directly apply to other community nurses. First, all CCNs are registered children's nurses and second, the main focus of their work is either to provide direct 'hands on' care or to facilitate and coordinate this in a range of community settings. This second component requires the CCN to be able to perform complex nursing procedures, such as changing a tracheostomy tube in a fragile baby while being observed by parents and untrained carers, and then to teach these same skills to those who may be emotionally vulnerable and lack confidence. This, therefore, demands unyielding confidence and advanced competence in teaching complex tasks to enable parents and other carers to become experts in the child's care. Case studies 20.1 to 20.4 stimulate the reader to reflect upon the number of different health, social and voluntary personnel involved with families where children have complex health needs, highlighting some of the challenges faced by CCNs.

Ways of working: family nursing

The ability of parents to negotiate their degree of involvement in their child's home care is limited by a lack of alternatives (Kirk 2001). The dearth of community children's nursing services in the UK means that parents are often required to learn complex skills and assume 24-hour responsibility for their child, often without help and support or respite, in order to achieve home care. This involves parents performing highly technical procedures that have previously been considered the domain of professionals, and perhaps extended nursing practice, therefore adopting a 'neoprofessional' role. For example, this may entail administering intravenous therapy, providing tracheostomy and ventilation support and administering parenteral feeding.

The terms most often associated with the work of CCNs are 'partnership' working and 'family-centred care' by children's nurses skilled in child development and the recognition of the needs of the sick child. The concept of 'family nursing' is gaining increasing recognition in the UK for patients from all age groups (Scottish Executive 2006). Friedemann (1989) describes family nursing on three levels:

Case study 20.1 Roles and responsibilities

John is a young person of 11 years. He has had a complicated 7-year history of intractable constipation and recently had a colostomy performed as a result of this. He is reliant on oral medications. He receives support from an SON, CCN, HV and SN. The SON works within the gastroenterology team at a regional hospital in the Home Counties. She initially visited John in the children's ward following his operation and now assesses him in a nurse-led clinic in the outpatient setting following his discharge home. Here, she will see him approximately four times per year to oversee the effectiveness of his treatment and provide the link between hospital and community provision. Following his assessment and adjustment to his treatment in the clinic, she liaises with the local team of CCNs to advise his named nurse of his continuing care needs between clinic appointments. The CCN provides regular home visits to John and his family. The aim of these visits is to assess the effectiveness of his medication and make appropriate changes according to his symptoms, to teach John and his parents how to manage the colostomy and to act as a resource to the

HV and SN. The HV will eventually provide ongoing home visiting support to John and his family once they are independent in his care management and his condition stabilizes, using the CCN as a resource only. The HV will also organize a budget to provide regular supplies to the family and in the meantime, these continue to be supplied from the budget for the community children's nursing service. The SN works with the teachers to ensure that John has the necessary equipment, resources and support in school to enable him to attend without fear of being socially isolated. Each member of the team involved in John's care is dependent upon effective communication between all members to ensure continuity.

Questions

1. How might John's care be configured differently?

2. With the focus on new ways of working, how might services for children in the community be delivered differently in the future?

1. Individual: the nurse treats each individual in the family as an individual client.
2. Interpersonal: the nurse uses communication techniques with two or more individuals to address family processes such as decision-making, limit setting and defining family roles.
3. Family system nursing: the client becomes the whole family system and nursing goals are aimed at changes in the system.

Given the role expected of parents, it is necessary for the CCN to assess how the family works together as a team in meeting the complex demands made on them as a system and to identify their unique needs. This could be reframed into identifying both their personal and 'neoprofessional' needs. Evidence from both CCNs and families, as the recipients of services, supports this notion. For example, research commissioned by the English National Board for Nursing, Midwifery and Health Visiting identified 17 principles of CCN practice derived from interviews with families (Procter et al 1999; Box 20.3).

These principles identify the fundamental need for the CCN to work in the context of the family as a whole and to work with the family as a unit of care. Principles such as 'fostering family empowerment' and 'promoting the health of families' relate

both to family processes, using skills of 'listening and discovering', and to the client being the whole family system. This is further evidenced in the work of Carter (2000) whose study explored the role and skills used by CCNs caring for children with chronic illness. As a complement to the principles outlined in Box 20.3, CCNs themselves identified the need to have a deeply contextualized understanding of the child's and family's needs and the ability to work within an 'individual family's community'. This requires skilled negotiation and tremendous respect for the way families choose to live their lives (Carter 2000).

The need for continuity is imperative as the CCN works alongside the family while they develop their confidence and competence in providing highly skilled home care. The blurring of boundaries is an inevitable consequence, as parents become technical and intuitive experts in their child's care, often able to detect symptoms before professionals. This requires both professional maturity and flexibility on the part of the CCN in order to manage and develop appropriate relationship boundaries, which remain fluid as the home situation changes. These combined factors require skills that may be described as 'interpersonal' and 'intrapersonal' intelligence (Goleman 1995).

Case study 20.2 Family nursing as a framework for practice

Rashider is 3 years old. She has an undiagnosed degenerative disorder that causes spastic quadriparesis and episodes of severe spasms. She is fully dependent for all activities of daily living. She has feeding problems and requires a gastrostomy tube for overnight feeds and the administration of medication. She is cared for at home by her parents, both aged 26 years, and her grandparents. She has two brothers. Imran is 6 years old and attends the local school. He suffers from severe, uncontrolled eczema. Yusuf is 4 years old and is still at home. She also has a baby sister of 3 months. Her mother is the main carer and is showing signs of stress, appearing withdrawn and tearful. Her father works long hours for a local company. At present the following services are involved in this family's care:

Community children's nurse
School nurse
Pre-school counsellor
Consultant neurologist
General practitioner
Independent nurse for
  gastrostomy services

Health visitor
Geneticist
Community paediatrician
Asian liaison health worker
Dermatologist
Social worker

Respite care services from a local voluntary agency have been offered but refused by the family.

Questions

1. From this list of professionals, who could adopt a more central role in facilitating a family nursing approach, using the three levels of family nursing as a guide?

2. What might be the goals for this family?

Box 20.3

Guiding principles of community children's nursing practice

1. Promoting family-centred care rather than child-centred care
2. Maintaining or improving the quality of life of the family, rather than focusing on medical needs
3. Minimizing stressful events rather than giving routinized care
4. Fostering family empowerment rather than learned helplessness/dependency on professionals' solving abilities
5. Having an approach of partnership rather than the imposition of professional expertise
6. Appreciating the complexity of a problem rather than oversimplifying it
7. Solving or reframing problems rather than avoiding them
8. Recognizing the boundaries of one's own expertise and knowing where to turn for appropriate help, rather than trying to solve all problems independently
9. Establishing credibility with paediatric and primary healthcare colleagues through working together openly rather than having an insular approach
10. Having a flexible, organic, responsive role, rather than a formally directed set of functions
11. Having knowledge gained through experience rather than procedures
12. Having the knowledge to anticipate and plan for future directions in the care needs of the child, rather than reacting to crisis
13. Being available (light touch) for the family when the family wants it, rather than when it is most convenient to services
14. Promoting the health of families rather than focusing solely on tertiary interventions
15. Lightening the burden through manner of approach, rather than getting caught up in the anxieties of the situation and reinforcing the burden
16. Enabling children and families to lead ordinary lives, rather than this being regarded as secondary to biomedical interventions
17. Listening and discovering rather than imposing ready-made solutions from elsewhere

---

'Interpersonal intelligence is the ability to understand other people: what motivates them, how they work, how to work co-operatively with them' (Goleman 1995: 42). It includes the capacity to respond appropriately to the emotions, motivations and desires of other people. Intrapersonal intelligence, conversely, demands self-knowledge and looking inwards in order to access one's own feelings and to draw on them to guide behaviour. Both attributes are required in order to work with intelligence. This intelligence refers to the ability to 'be with' a situation while not needing one's own needs met or needing to have all the answers. Indeed, professionals who acknowledge their limitations have been shown to promote trust in the families they work with (Kirk 2001). It has been otherwise described as the 'emotional side of nursing' and refers to the non-technical skills or 'soft' skills, including empathy, compassion, facilitation, listening to and being with families. These skills are fundamental to the creation and maintenance of a supportive relationship with the child and family, an essential part of the CCN's role, and ability to nurse 'with' rather than 'of' the family (Carter 2000). However, there are challenges associated with this humanistic approach to practice, the most demanding of which is about creating the balance between personal and professional involvement. This phenomenon is not unique to CCNs' practice. Since there are no guidelines to define the balance between the personal and professional relationship, an individual management strategy is required. For example, such a strategy might include a personal reflective journal coupled with more formal clinical supervision in order to foster an explicit acknowledgement of this area of practice that is often difficult to discuss openly. As part of professional practice, CCNs have a responsibility to work with other practitioners to find ways to uncover and share their experiences and develop flexible approaches to managing relationship boundaries. The notion of interprofessional team supervision could provide a useful framework to take this forward. For example, within complex home care, agreements of care can offer a means of formulating roles and boundaries (Sidey and Widdas 2005).

Ways of working: integrated care pathways and the role of the key worker

It is clear that CCNs play a central role in the lives of families where there is a child with health and social needs and that a number of professionals and agencies are likely to be involved. This in itself requires great skill and negotiation on behalf of the CCN to effectively work within, and sometimes coordinate, complex packages of care. Practitioners no longer work in a professional vacuum. Most coor-

dinated care requires a multiagency response that demands a collaborative effort from all those concerned with the care of the child and family (Department of Health 2001a). Recent government policies for children's services have developed around their Green Paper *Every Child Matters* (Department for Education and Skills 2003). This document sets an agenda of integrated and coordinated service provision for all children across health, social care and education. The Children's National Service Framework considers this agenda from a health perspective. Within the field of palliative care the Association for Children with Life-threatening or Terminal Conditions and their Families (now called The Association for Children's Palliative Care; ACT) have produced the *Integrated Multiagency Care Pathways for Children with Life-threatening and Life-limiting Conditions* (ACT 2004). This pathway provides a framework for developing integrated children's services based upon the child and family's journey from diagnosis to death. The pathway has five standards:

1. breaking news
2. planning for going home
3. multiagency assessment of family's needs
4. multiagency care plan
5. end of life plan.

These are considered in terms of:

- child and young person
- family and carers
- environment.

This pathway is designed to:

- shift the focus away from organizational issues and re-focus on children and families
- promote the production of local integrated care pathways
- enable service re-design based upon key stages of the health and life journeys of children and their families.

For example, integrated multiagency care pathways could be used in three ways to enable:

- a child and family to understand the journey through palliative, life-changing and/or acute conditions
- commissioners to commission and evaluate services
- community children's nursing, education, social care and other care teams to structure their

activities around the five pathway standards above (D. Widdas, unpublished work, 2007).

Successful implementation of pathways can result in:

- new ways of working
- a flexible framework for care provision
- integrated service delivery
- greater family autonomy
- empowered and satisfied families
- reduction in family burden of care
- negotiated roles and role release/expansion
- care delivered by appropriate personnel at the appropriate time
- reduction in parental exploitation
- clarification of roles and expectations
- clarification of individual responsibility and accountability
- effective discharge planning
- increased range of care options
- pooled budgets
- reduced funding disputes
- planned and responsive respite care provision.

The nature of home care for children with complex healthcare needs is often constant and long term, requiring a vast number of professionals and agencies to be involved in supporting the family. It is not surprising that parents feel overwhelmed by a number of factors associated with this experience including:

- confusion around the roles and responsibilities of the different professionals
- the sheer number of visits from, and to, various professionals
- the need to coordinate the many services involved
- the need to act as advocate on behalf of their child.

These factors often require parents to act as their own key worker in an attempt to negotiate and meet their needs. Consequently, parents may experience symptoms such as exhaustion, burnout and stress-related illness, directly attributed to the sustained nature of caregiving and the lack of coordinated available support. The provision of a key worker to provide them with a single point of contact can help prevent this. A number of different terms may be used for this role, for example care 'coordinator', 'link worker' or 'family support worker'. The term 'key worker' (KW) is the most widely promoted and understood. The KW must be:

- acceptable to the family
- preferably chosen by them
- endorsed by all professionals and agencies involved as the main referral point and channel for discussion and communication.

The Care Co-ordination Network UK (CCNUK) promotes and supports key working for children and their families (CCNUK 2004). It has produced standards for key working (Box 20.4).

All professionals have a responsibility to act in the best interest of the child and their family and to ensure a coordinated programme of care. This requires teamwork and collaboration to break down professional barriers. Essential to this process is effective role negotiation and the clear articulation of individual responsibility and accountability for different aspects of care. Collaborative working, which may include selective joint visiting and shared care, assists in role clarification and the prevention of professional rivalry and overlap. The formal identification of a named KW is recommended for each family.

Clearly, the provision of an identified KW can assist in unravelling the complex variables impacting on the family and enhance interprofessional and multiagency case management. The KW should be a separate, statutorily recognized, valued and dedicated person to assist families in the coordination of care and services for their children and can be:

- 'designated' – the role is solely that of KW or
- 'non-designated' – those who key work a small number of families alongside their professional role (Greco et al 2004).

Where services exist, CCNs are often seen as the most appropriate practitioner to adopt such a role. Rarely, however, is this role formally acknowledged and identified within the CCN's work or caseload management. The implications of these combined facets are identified in Box 20.4. Home care for sick children that is coordinated using a multiagency care pathway with the support of an identified KW can result in an integrated service designed in the best interest of the whole family. If home is to remain the best and first choice as the place for essential care, then this must be negotiated and facilitated within such a framework.

Transition to adult services

Transition is defined as 'the purposeful, planned movement of adolescents and young adults with chronic physical and medical conditions from a child-centred to adult-orientated health care systems' (Blum et al 1993: 570). The life expectancy of children with chronic, life-limiting or life-threatening conditions has improved significantly. This increase, alongside the move from institutional to community-focused and family-centred care, has added to both the recognition and the importance of transitional services (Blum 1995). An unfortunate side effect, arising from the need to transfer care between different services, can be a loss of the skills more associated with children's care. There is increasing evidence of the link between good transition and better outcomes for young people (Department of Health 2006).

There are four groups of young people recognized as requiring planned transitional care and for whom CCNs may be providing or facilitating care. Some young people will span more than one group:

Box 20.4

Key worker standards

Organizational standards

1. Multiagency commitment at strategic and practice level
2. Multiagency management group
3. Agreed referral system and specific eligibility criteria for KW service
4. Joint policy for information sharing between agencies
5. Multiagency protocol for joint assessment, care plans and review
6. Communication strategy
7. KW manager who reports to multiagency management group
8. Ongoing resources to provide administrative support, induction, training and supervision for KWs
9. Job descriptions for KWs, managers and administrators
10. Agreed cover for KWs if absent
11. Links with agencies, for example housing, benefits, leisure, voluntary sector
12. Service monitoring, reviewing and evaluation

Practice standards

- Provide information
- Identify and address needs of all family members
- Provide emotional and practical support
- Assist families in dealing with agencies and act as advocate if required

How the KW is achieved

- Proactive, regular contact
- Family-centred approach
- Working across agencies
- Working with families' strengths, acting as advocate, enabling access to advocacy support as required
- Induction, ongoing training and development
- Professional, clinical and managerial supervision and peer support for KWs by committed and knowledgeable managers
- Formally protected time to undertake the KW role
- Explanation of the role of the KW to children and families and tailored information to guide them that is accurate, accessible, timely and appropriate
- Interagency care plan giving KW agreed power and credibility to access resources

The process of assessing, planning and reviewing key working

- Interagency assessment and care plan building on any other assessments undertaken
- Agreed system and timing for care plan and reviews in line with family's wishes
- Parents' and young people's preferences regarding assessment and reviews supported
- Support for children, young people and parents to participate in assessment and review process including those who do not use speech
- Ethnic and cultural needs supported to enable participation in assessment and review process
- Agreed system for record keeping
- Parent and/or young person held records

> ## Case study 20.3 The key worker
>
> Mandy has chronic lung disease. She was born prematurely at 28 weeks gestation and spent 3 months, with her parents, in a neonatal unit. Ventilation and intensive care were required for her first month of life. Gradually she was weaned off her ventilation but could not be weaned off continuous oxygen. A decision was made with the family to discharge Mandy. Their KW was the CCN who coordinated visits by professionals involved with the family and organized provision and funding for equipment and ongoing supplies. For the first two weeks the neonatal outreach nurse supported them at home. In the second week the neonatal nurse and the CCN undertook shared visits. Subsequently the CCN and parents assumed the responsibility for Mandy's care. The CCN's role initially focused on the assessment and support of her respiratory function. This role was gradually assumed by the parents. With the teaching and support from the CCN their confidence and competence developed and Mandy's nursing care became an extension to their usual caring role. Alongside this the HV commenced regular visits to monitor growth and development and support the establishment of a programme for meeting nutritional requirements. In the absence of an out-of-hours community children's nursing service the CCN arranged for the acute outreach service to be available if needed in partnership with the general practitioner (GP). During Mandy's first winter at home her parents observed a sudden deterioration in her respiratory function. They contacted their CCN who, together with the GP, commenced antibiotics and increased her level of oxygen. The outreach service supported and monitored the family overnight and during the weekend. Mandy's condition quickly returned to normal. This successful programme of management increased her parents' confidence and competence. By her first birthday the CCN and parents were able to wean Mandy off her continuous oxygen and the KW role was subsequently undertaken by her HV. At two years of age the CCN discharged Mandy and her family from his caseload.
>
> ### Questions
>
> 1. What support and resources would the CCN have required to effectively undertake the role of KW?
> 2. How might an integrated care pathway be successfully established to support the needs of preterm babies with ongoing healthcare problems?

- condition specific
- complex care
- palliative care
- learning disabilities.

Condition specific (cystic fibrosis (CF), diabetes, etc.) For these young people there is a clear transitional pathway to an established adult service but the focus of these services is often very different (Cooke 2007). In diabetes, children's diabetes nurses have a recommended caseload of 100 families. Anecdotal evidence suggests that within adult services caseloads may exceed 1000 individuals. Furthermore, the elderly overwhelmingly populate these services with a variety of complications from their condition. CCNs at tertiary centres report a lack of involvement in the transition process or children with CF (Cancelliere 2002).

Complex care Transition in complex care is extremely difficult. Young people with a learning disability and complex care needs have no clear referral paths in terms of nursing or medical support. The need for the development of specially commissioned local psychosocial disability teams to coordinate this aspect of care is recognized in *Bridging the Gaps* (Royal College of Paediatrics and Child Health 2003).

Palliative care Transition and palliative care should be considered together. With an increase in life expectancy, transition is an important part of the care process for some young people. The need for parallel planning is paramount. This should be aimed at following the planned transition of care but also at supporting end-stage care needs if required (Association for Children with Life-threatening or Terminal Conditions and their Families (ACT) 2001, 2003, Royal College of Paediatrics and Child Health 2003).

Learning disabilities The document *Valuing People* has put transition at the forefront of learning disability services (Department of Health 2001b). (See Chapter 19 for further information on caring for individuals with learning disabilities.)

The Transition Care Pathway produced by ACT (2007) comprehensively describes the necessary framework to facilitate effective and purposeful transition. The key points to this pathway are:

- recognizing the need to move on (plans for transition should be started by age 14 years)

Case study 20.4 Transition

Billy sustained severe brain injury at birth and was not expected to live beyond 6 months of age. Every year he had an episode of illness from which he was not expected to survive. He has a tracheostomy and is gastrostomy fed. In addition he suffers from severe seizures and profound communication difficulties. Billy lived with his mother and 7-year-old brother. At 18 years of age Billy's school placement was due to end. The learning disability team undertook a person-centred planning process to determine his wishes. Billy loved to be in water and disliked travelling. Both he and his mother wanted him to continue to live at home. During the day Billy wished to access activities outside the home and his mother felt unable to accompany him. No local respite or day centre provision was available to provide for his needs. A not-for-profit agency was commissioned to support Billy's care in a range of community settings. The staff were trained, by the CCNs, to safely support his care needs at home and in community venues, including staff at a swimming pool who agreed to provide their services. Eventually a room was found in a local respite centre as a daytime base. District nurses provided ongoing healthcare as needed. However, the completion of the transition process was significantly delayed.

Questions:

1. How should transition be planned when there is an uncertain prognosis?
2. Could this late transition have been avoided and how?

- the timing of transition should depend on the developmental stage of each young person
- every young person has a right to proactively plan for their future and planning should be based on their wishes
- young people and their parents need to be helped with transition from family-centred to young-person-centred care
- a KW designate should be identified from within adult services
- a reciprocal adult service should be available for their needs
- appropriate funding must be made available for any required overlap of service provision until a sustainable adult service is established
- the process of transition should be evaluated.

Challenges and opportunities for community children's nursing services

This chapter has outlined the central role that CCNs play in the delivery and coordination of care for sick children, young people and their families. However, in order to meet the future needs of these groups, CCNs need to develop their practice for the new world of integrated health, education and social care. This requires a clear corporate identity and strong professional leadership and without these key components community children's nursing risks being engulfed by those groups who have them. There has been specific reference to community children's nursing services through the radical restructuring of the NHS but limited outcomes. Consequently, reforms and the interpretation of policy documents for community children's nursing services provide both challenges and opportunities (Craft and Killen 2007, Department of Health 2004). As a minority service, CCNs have a responsibility to assert the need for appropriate provision for families and to work with other organizations. Care pathways provide the opportunity for this and for developing integrated frameworks for care provision. The independent review of palliative care services for children and young people provides clear evidence of the effectiveness of community children's nursing for children with both palliative and complex needs (Craft and Killen 2007). In addition, national service frameworks offer wider guidance on the provision of community children's nursing for children with a range of health care needs (Department of Health 2004, Welsh Assembly Government 2005). There is a clear mandate within policy to continue the expansion and development of community children's nursing but without concerted action from within the profession there remains a risk that CCNs will fail to fulfil their expected potential in the provision of education, management and care (see Chapter 23 for further information).

SUMMARY

- As parents learn complex skills and assume 24-hour responsibility for their child's care they adopt 'neoprofessional' roles and become experts themselves.
- The family as the unit of care remains central to community children's nursing practice.
- Managing the parent–professional relationship requires emotional maturity and intelligence on the part of the CCN in order to develop flexible boundaries in practice.

- Care should be planned and delivered using integrated multiagency care pathways with a named KW as the main referral point.
- A strong corporate identity aids interprofessional and multiagency working.
- The provision of flexible and innovative transition is an essential feature of healthcare provision.
- Effective professional leadership is the key to the development and enhancement of services.

DISCUSSION POINTS

1. Who provides professional leadership for children with healthcare needs and their families in community settings in your area?
2. Who assesses the parents' confidence and competence to undertake skilled nursing interventions at home?
3. What strategies are in place to meet the anticipated health and social needs of sick children and their families at home in your area of practice?

4. How is the KW role identified and evaluated in the delivery of multiagency care packages?
5. Consider what communication systems CCNs can access within primary care organizations.
6. Which care provider is the most appropriate to negotiate the level and content of respite palliative care?

References

Association for Children's Palliative Care (ACT) 2004 Integrated multiagency care pathways for children with life-threatening and life-limiting conditions. ACT, Bristol

Association for Children's Palliative Care (ACT) 2007 The transition care pathway. ACT, Bristol

Association for Children with Life-threatening or Terminal Conditions and their Families 2001 Palliative care for young people aged 13–24. ACT, Bristol

Association for Children with Life-threatening or Terminal Conditions and their Families (ACT) & Royal College of Paediatrics and Child Health 2003 A guide to the development of children's palliative care services, 2nd edn. ACT, Bristol

Blum R 1995 Transition to adult health care: setting the stage. Journal of Adolescent Health 17(1): 3–5

Blum R, Garell D, Hodgman CH, et al 1993 Transition from child-centred to adult-health care systems for adolescents with chronic conditions. Journal of Adolescent Health 14: 570–576

Burr S, Hughes J 2005 Role of the community children's nurse in influencing health care policies. In: Sidey A, Widdas D (eds) Textbook of community children's nursing, Chapter 4, 2nd edn. Elsevier, London

Cancelliere L 2002 An exploratory study into the experiences of Community Children's Nurses on the transition of adolescents with complex health care needs from child centred to adult focused health services. Unpublished dissertation. University College, Northampton.

Care Co-ordination Network UK 2004 Key worker standards. Online: http://www.ccnuk.org.uk

Carter B 2000 Ways of working: CCNs and chronic illness. Journal of Child Health Care 4(2): 66–72

Cooke E 2007 Transitional care for young people with diabetes: policy and practice. Paediatric Nursing 19(6): 19–22

Craft A, Killen S 2007 Palliative care services for children and young people in England. Department of Health, London

Department for Education and Skills (DfES) 2003 Every child matters. DfES, Nottingham

Department of Health 1991 The welfare of children and young people in hospital. HMSO, London

Department of Health 1994 The Clothier Report. HMSO, London

Department of Health 2001a The Bristol Royal Infirmary Inquiry: final report. The Stationery Office, London

Department of Health 2001b Valuing people: a new strategy for learning disability for the 21st century. The Stationery Office, London

Department of Health 2004 National service frameworks for children, young people and maternity services. DH, London

Department of Health 2006 Transition: getting it right for young people. DH, London

Friedemann M-L 1989 The concept of family nursing. Journal of Advanced Nursing 14: 211–216

Gillet JA 1954 Children's nursing unit. British Medical Journal 684: 1954

Goleman D 1995 Emotional intelligence. Why it can matter more than IQ. Bantam Books, New York

Greco V, Sloper P, Barton K 2004 Care coordination and keyworker services for disabled children in the UK. Social Policy Research Unit, University of York

House of Commons Health Committee 1997 Health services for children and young people in the community: home and school. Third report. The Stationery Office, London

Kirk S 2001 Negotiating lay and professional roles in the care of children with complex health care needs. Journal of Advanced Nursing 34(5): 593–602

Miller S 1995 The clinical nurse specialist: a way forward? Journal of Advanced Nursing 22: 494–501

Procter S, Biott C, Campbell S, Edward S, Redpath N, Moran M 1999 Preparation for the developing role of the community children's nurse. Researching professional education: Research Report Series, no. 11. English National Board for Nursing, Midwifery and Health Visiting, London

Royal College of Paediatrics and Child Health (RCPCH) 2003 Bridging the gaps: health care for adolescents. RCPCH, London

Scottish Executive 2006 The WHO Europe family health nursing pilot in Scotland. Final report. Scottish Executive, Edinburgh

Sidey A, Widdas D (eds) 2005 Textbook of community children's nursing, 2nd edn. Elsevier, London

United Kingdom Central Council (UKCC) 1994 The future of professional practice – the Council's standards for education and practice following registration. UKCC, London

Welsh Assembly Government (WAG) 2005 National service frameworks for children and young people and maternity services in Wales. WAG, Cardiff

Whiting M 2005 Historical overview of community children's nursing: 1888 to 2004. In: Sidey A, Widdas D (eds) Textbook of community children's nursing, Chapter 2, 2nd edn. Elsevier, London

Recommended reading

Association for Children with Life-threatening and Terminal Conditions and their Families (ACT) & Royal College of Paediatrics and Child Health 2003 A guide to the development of children's palliative care services. ACT, Bristol

Association for Children with Life-threatening and Terminal Conditions and their Families (ACT) 2004 Integrated multiagency care pathways for children with life-threatening and life-limiting conditions. ACT, Bristol

These complementary guides provide an overview of the measures that can help families and professionals meet the emotional, therapeutic, spiritual and physical needs of children.

Carling J 2005 Including me. Council for Disabled Children. Department for Education and Skills, London
A practical guide to managing complex health needs in schools and early years, including examples of good practice.

Leneham C, Morrison J, Stanley J 2004 The dignity of risk. Council for Disabled Children, London
A handbook for balancing and managing risk during care provision

by non-nurse careers. Provides examples of and advice on risk management strategies.*

Sidey A, Widdas D (eds) 2005. Textbook of community children's nursing, 2nd edn. Elsevier, London
An authoritative textbook, which provides an introduction to the major spheres in community children's nursing including historical perspectives, theory and clinical practice. The four sections of the book cover organizational facets, philosophical issues, dimensions of practice and the advancing picture of community children's nursing.

Section **Five**

Challenges for the future

This final section concentrates on current issues facing nurses and their public health roles and offers the reader an insight into alternative ways of working, innovative practice and challenges for the future. Nurses are encouraged not only to explore the concept of partnership working in health and social care, but also to consider patient and public involvement, and political and professional issues influencing the provision of care. The section concludes with a final chapter by the editors which raises issues for debate as to how nurses could strengthen their roles in public health.

The first chapter in this section introduces the concept of partnership working and highlights differences in the understanding of this term. It looks at the benefits and limitations of interprofessional working to professionals and service users. The following chapter outlines the emergence of a range of nursing roles in public health and community nursing practice. The final chapter in this section outlines a framework of engagement which summarizes nurses' current practice in public health and the philosophies on which they base their work. It acknowledges practice contexts and their influence on public health work and provides some recommendations that could maximize the nurse's role in promoting health. The reader is challenged to reflect critically on his or her practice in the light of the topic areas explored.

Partnership working in health and social care

Judy Cousins

KEY ISSUES

- Defining partnership working
- Exploring factors that promote and inhibit partnership working
- Promoting patient and public involvement

Introduction

A move towards integrated care and partnership working is evident throughout European health systems (Howarth et al 2006). The European Public Health Associates (EPHA; 2002) explain that a rise in chronic diseases accounts for this and state how a more integrated organization of health services is required in order to meet future user demands. Partnership working is a central feature of the Labour government's modernization agenda for health and social care services, being considered fundamental to safe, resource-effective professional practice (Dowling et al 2004). Farrell (2004) and Barr (2004) discuss benefits of partnership working to include improved communication and enhanced responsiveness, pooling together of expert knowledge, service users having fewer professionals to deal with, professionals gaining a greater understanding of each other's roles and responsibilities and a reduction in the duplication of services.

However, robust evidence to support these assumptions is scarce and what evidence does exist tends to focus on the process of partnership working rather than the outcome from the process (Dowling et al 2004). In addition, the Audit Commission (2005: 2) remind that 'working across organizational boundaries brings complexity and ambiguity that can generate confusion and weaken accountability for professionals'. Questions therefore exist on what the political and social drivers for partnership working are, what partnership working means, what messages from research exist to inform on the benefits and limitations of working collaboratively, for professionals and service users, and what knowledge is required by nurses in order to promote patient and public involvement. This chapter will explore these issues.

Partnership working: political and social drivers

For those examining health and social policy in the UK since 1997 it would be difficult to find legislation that failed to propose partnership working as a pivotal strategy in the quest to deliver safe and effective health and social care services (see, for example, Department of Health (DH) 2005, 2006, 2008, Northern Ireland Department of Health and Social Services (NIDHSS) 2004, Department of Health, Social Services and Public Safety (DHSSPS) 2005, Scottish Executive (SE) 2003, 2004, Welsh Assembly Government (WAG) 2001, 2005, 2007). Another significant driver for increased partnership working stems from the many non-accidental deaths of vulnerable children. The Department for Education and Skills (DfES; 2006) (which has recently been replaced by the Department for Children, Schools and Families) highlights how ineffective information sharing and a lack of collaborative working between agencies have acted as contributory factors in health and social care services failing to identify children facing extreme risk. Finally, the changing healthcare needs of an ageing society, and the drive to promote self-care and patient and public involvement in decision-making also figure significantly in the call for increased collaboration between professionals and between professionals and service users (DH 2008, WAG 2007).

Nursing policy from the four countries of the UK encourages practitioners to embrace partnership working initiatives (Box 21.1). This way of working is not new for public health and community nurses where informal collaborative working forms part of day-to-day practice. However, more formal partnerships are being called for in order to develop new ways of delivering services. *Modernising Nursing Careers* (DH et al 2006), for instance, refers to joint working practices as an essential element in the future planning of nursing services, particularly in primary care, where it is envisaged traditional working boundaries will become increasingly blurred in order to improve care delivery.

It is interesting to note how partnership, collaborative and joint working are often used synonymously, however these terms do not necessarily mean the same thing and this can be misleading and

---

Box 21.1

UK nursing policy

England

Department of Health (1999) *Making a difference: strengthening the nursing, midwifery and health visiting contribution to health and health care.* London: DH.

Department of Health (2002) *Liberating the talents: helping primary care trusts and nurses deliver the NHS Plan.* London: DH.

Department of Health (2004) *The Chief Nursing Officer's review of the nursing, midwifery and health visiting contribution to vulnerable children and young people.* London: DH.

Department of Health; Department of Health, Social Services and Public Safety; Scottish Executive; Welsh Assembly Government (2006) *Modernising nursing careers.* London: DH.

Northern Ireland

Department of Health, Social Services and Public Safety (2003) *From vision to action. Strengthening the nursing contribution to public health.* Belfast: DHSSPS.

Department of Health, Social Services and Public Safety (2005) *Realising the vision: nursing for public health.* Belfast: DHSSPS.

Northern Ireland Practice and Education Council (2005) *An exploration of nursing and midwifery roles In Northern Ireland's health and personal social services.* Belfast: NIPEC.

Department of Health, Social Services and Public Safety (2006) *Regional redesign of community nursing project.* Belfast: DHSSP.

Scotland

Scottish Executive Health Department (2001) *Nursing for health – a review of the contribution of nurses, midwives and health visitors to improving the public's health in Scotland.* Edinburgh: Scottish Executive.

Scottish Executive Health Department (2003) *Partnership for care.* Edinburgh: Scottish Executive.

Scottish Executive Health Department/Royal College of Nursing (2005) *Framework for developing nursing roles.* Edinburgh: Scottish Executive.

Scottish Executive Health Department (2006) *Rights, relationships and recovery – the review of mental health nursing in Scotland.* Edinburgh: Scottish Executive.

Wales

National Assembly for Wales (1999) *Realising the potential: a strategic framework for nursing, midwifery and health visiting in Wales into the 21st century.* Cardiff: NAfW.

National Assembly for Wales (2001) *Realising the potential briefing paper 2: aspiration, action, achievement – a framework for realising the potential of mental health nursing in Wales.* Cardiff: NAfW.

National Assembly for Wales (2002) *Realising the potential briefing paper 3: inclusion, partnership and innovation – a framework for realising the potential of learning disability nursing in Wales.* Cardiff: NAfW.

Welsh Assembly Government (2007) *Beyond 2007 – challenges and drivers for nurses, midwifes and specialist community public health nurses.* Cardiff: HMSO.

cause confusion. Gaining a greater understanding of the terminology used to describe different approaches to working with others will enable nurses to more clearly articulate the scope of their involvement when working closely with others.

Partnership working: myths and meanings

The range of terminology which describes different ways that health, social care professionals and service users interact has been described by Leathard (2003: 5) as a 'terminology quagmire'. Partnership and collaborative working appear as umbrella terms and these are often used synonymously; however, subtle differences between the two exist. The Audit Commission (1998) defines a partnership as a joint working agreement where partners cooperate to achieve a common goal but who are otherwise independent bodies, giving an impression of partnerships being more formal than collaborations. However, similar to partnerships, common to most interpretations of collaboration are shared purposes or goals and achieving outcomes that would not be possible if acting alone. According to Horwath and Morrison (2007), approaches to collaboration range from communication, to cooperation, coordination, coalition, and finally, integration. Arguably, these elements are also relevant to partnership working if accepting the Audit Commission's definition, yet Dowling et al (2004) consider a partnership as something that is beyond collaboration, defining this to include collaboration, along with cooperation and joint working.

Such confusion makes it difficult to articulate clear differences between these two terms. Carnwell and Carson (2004) provide a useful distinction when describing a partnership as what something *is* versus collaboration as what is *done*. As well as partnership being understood in relation to professional working practices, it is also a key term used to describe relationships between professionals and clients. In this context Bidmead and Cowley's (2005) concept analysis of partnership concludes that it is still an evolving theory but one which promotes mutual respect and empathy, enables choice and participation and is based upon honesty, equality and trust.

In relation to professional working practices, regardless of the term used, team working appears to be the vehicle used to facilitate partnership working, being considered the optimum way to share knowledge, skills, resources and experiences for the benefit of service users (Borrill et al 2002). As such, specialist community public health nurses, district nurses, community psychiatric nurses, practice nurses, community children's nurses, school nurses and learning disability nurses may already or soon find themselves working within multidisciplinary/agency or interprofessional/agency teams. Again, the terms 'multidisciplinary' and 'interprofessional' are often used interchangeably despite both having very different meanings.

Multidisciplinary/agency working

The Latin word 'multi' means 'many'; therefore multidisciplinary/agency working refers to two or more disciplines or agencies working with a patient, client or family. Crucially, however, these terms do not imply formal partnership or collaborative working between disciplines or agencies, as traditional divisions of professional knowledge and authority are retained in this way of working (Leathard 2003, Masterson 2002, Sheehan et al 2007). Multidisciplinary team members undertake independent assessments, and set goals and plan care in isolation (Batorowicz and Shepherd 2008). The multidisciplinary/agency team is composed of different professionals who work according to their particular scope of practice (Sheehan et al 2007). For example, primary care teams may be considered multidisciplinary, being composed of a range of practitioners such as GPs, practice nurses, district nurses, health visitors, etc. This form of working may be thought of as teams of practitioners from different backgrounds making 'different but complementary' contributions to healthcare (Leathard 2003: 5). Any collaboration between disciplines or agencies is invariably conducted on an informal basis.

Where working practices become more integrated, the term 'joint-working' is commonly used (Sloper 2004); for example, health visitors and learning disability nurses working together to deliver parenting programmes for parents with learning disabilities, occupational health and school nurses working collaboratively to prepare children for the transition to the workplace or district nurses and community psychiatric nurses planning joint initiatives to promote the mental health of the elderly.

Warmington et al (2004) discuss how multidisciplinary working results in practitioners working in isolation in the planning and delivery of services, leading to duplication of care. Yet Borrill et al (2002) state how this way of working is a prescription to put right the perceived short fallings of the NHS. It is unlikely, however, that Borrill et al's interpretation of multidisciplinary/agency working is similar to that proposed in this work, illustrating inherent difficulties evident when attempting to distinguish between concepts and approaches where different understandings exist.

Interprofessional/agency working

Borrill et al's (2002) understanding appears more akin to this work's interpretation of interprofessional/agency working. The prefix 'inter' means 'between' and implies interaction between two or more different groups (Leathard 2003). Therefore, interprofessional/agency working is taken to mean two or more agencies working together in planned and formal ways and not simply through informal networking (Warmington et al 2004). Goals and care plans are formulated following consultation from all team members and practitioners share and even relinquish their professional claims to specialized knowledge in circumstances where other professional disciplines can deliver service user requirements more efficiently (Batorowicz and Shepherd 2008, Masterson 2002). Interprofessional working is characterized by blurring of professional roles where shared problem solving is performed in planning care and interventions (Sheehan et al 2007). Interestingly, 'trans' interprets as 'across' and also implies professionals working across traditional role boundaries – but to an extent where professional boundaries begin to actually dissipate, resulting in professionals developing expertise in other practice areas (Batorowicz and Shepherd 2008). Sloper (2004) cautions against confusing 'interprofessional' with 'intraprofessional' – a term used to denote differing specialist disciplines arising from one professional group, such as in the case of community nursing involving health visitors, district nurses, community psychiatric nurses, practice nurses, school nurses, etc.

Accepting that confusion surrounds definitions of multidisciplinary, joint and interprofessional working, Jones and Thomas (2007) still believe that all relate to practitioners working closely with colleagues from other professions in ways that promote the blurring of boundaries. One of the major benefits perceived from partnership or collaborative working is the facility to reduce duplication of practice through the reorganization of services, where one discipline or profession takes responsibility for an aspect of care hitherto performed by all – so that role blurring occurs as the team becomes more integrated. 'Boundary blurring' is one of the more recent terms to emerge from healthcare policy and it is interesting how effective interprofessional working is often defined in terms of practitioners recognizing commonalities of practice and reorganizing service delivery to avoid duplication of practice. Indeed, Masterson (2002) notes the move towards the blurring of boundaries between professions as the tendency and drive for certain professional activities to merge occurs. However, while boundary blurring is a term receiving significant attention, it too appears to be an ill-defined concept that requires clarification.

Boundary blurring

Rushmer and Pallis (2003) explain how boundary blurring does not mean that one agency is able to deliver the entire expertise of another – if it did then there would be no need for the agency in the first place. What it means is that while professions each possess unique qualities specific to them, they also share commonalities of practice that one professional could perform for all. Examples such as nurses undertaking prescribing, previously considered the sole domain of the medical profession, is one way that professional boundaries have already blurred. Not that boundary blurring only applies to professionals; it also occurs following abdication of professional roles to unqualified staff (Goble 2003).

Dowling et al (2004) believe that existing divisions and demarcations between professions and professionals will need to be set aside in order to rise to the challenge to work differently and collaboratively in the interests of patient or clients. However, expecting practitioners to identify commonalities in working practices and relinquish aspects of their role is not as easy as it may seem. Boundary blurring may be threatening for professionals, nervous about losing their professional identity and status, and this factor may seriously hinder integrated partnership working. Support and guidance are key ingredients in the development of new roles and, crucially, professionals need to be explicitly clear regarding their understanding of shared

Activity box 21.1(a)

A specialist community public health nursing team of health visitors become concerned about the rising levels of childhood obesity in the locality. They decide that some forms of preventative interventions would be beneficial and believe that any action would be more effective if conducted in partnership with other health and social care professionals.

- What other professionals or agencies could the specialist community public health nursing team of health visitors work with in order to plan effective strategies to reduce childhood obesity?
- What barriers may impede such partnership initiatives?

commonalities of practice, to ensure they work according to their level of competence. In fact, it is clarity of roles and explicitness that Rushmer and Pallis (2003) believe will facilitate greater integrated working partnerships rather than role blurring, which after all implies vagueness and lack of clarity.

Ultimately, the many definitions that exist to describe the different ways professionals work together overlap, coincide, and lack clarity. However, Hudson (2000) notes that while the *what* remains vague, the *why* of partnership working is crystal clear. Partnership working is reported to improve communication, prevent duplication of service delivery, improve understanding of different professional roles, enhance role development and, most important of all, improve service delivery to users. As such, partnership working will undoubtedly remain centre stage in government plans to deliver quality health and social care services. However, research evidence to support these claims is scarce, and far from partnership working being considered a harmonious process, different organizational cultures and numerous professional tensions can contribute to this being viewed as a threat to professional autonomy (Warmington et al 2004).

Partnership working: messages from research

McLaughlin (2004) states that the concept of partnership working has become so central to government thinking that rather than asking if working in partnership is good or bad, questions instead centre on how to make partnerships work. This is some-

what naive according to Warmington et al (2004: 48), who remind that government policy 'perpetuates the notion of interagency working as a virtuous solution to joined-up social problems and underacknowledges interagency working as a site of tensions and contradictions'. Messages from research both corroborate and refute these opposing views.

Factors that promote and inhibit partnership working

A growing body of evidence informs on specific benefits experienced by practitioners from working collaboratively as well as factors that contribute to interprofessional working. For instance, Freeman and Peck's (2006) research explored the impact of partnership working in integrated specialist mental healthcare provision from the perspectives of frontline practitioners, service users, carers and service managers. Their findings revealed how staff involved in joint-working teams found opportunities to discuss clients' needs a valuable exercise, providing access to a range of perspectives hitherto not available. Co-location of teams reduced feelings of isolation and enhanced working relationships, and staff reported greater satisfaction and found their work to be more rewarding from having time and opportunities to work with previously difficult-to-engage clients in therapeutic ways.

Similarly, Hudson's (2007) findings revealed how interprofessional working between social workers, district nurses and housing officers facilitated the development of trust and respect between professionals as well as promoting clearer understandings of each other's roles and responsibilities, promoting the sharing of a common vision. The benefits of shared databases, access to IT resources and joint training also contributed to positive relationships. In addition, Larkin and Callaghan (2005) found statistically significant relationships between joint supervision, joint documentation and shared risk policies and increased awareness among professionals of interprofessional roles and responsibilities. Similar findings to the above have been reported by Molyneux (2001) and Shaw et al (2005) and together findings from these studies inform on a range of factors which promote interprofessional working (Box 21.2) and benefits experienced by practitioners as a result (Box 21.3).

However, if such working practices really are worthy solutions to the healthcare needs of society

Box 21.2

Factors that promote interprofessional practice

- Co-location
- Absence of a dominant agency
- Flexible and adaptable attitudes of staff
- Motivated, accessible, available and committed staff
- Effective IT resources
- Shared databases
- Joint training
- Joint supervision
- Joint documentation and risk policies
- Facilities for regular and effective communication between individuals
- Commitment of senior and front-line staff

Box 21.3

Benefits from interprofessional working

- Shared, common vision
- Increased trust and respect
- Sharing of knowledge
- Increased clarity on own and others' roles
- Increased support
- Reduced isolation
- Enhanced working relationships

as proposed by policy, evidence should reflect that partnership working results in better services and outcomes for users. Dowling et al (2004) state how the development of health and social care partnerships have been viewed as ends in themselves with an underlying assumption that improved outcomes for users would be a natural consequence of their formation. Little evidence informs on this but from that which does exist, a valuable insight is gained. For instance, parents in Carter et al's (2007) research appreciated professionals undertaking joint health assessments of children requiring healthcare, highlighting the strain felt by individuals from repeating information to different professionals. Continuity of staff within teams facilitated development of trusting relationships, which was also highly valued. Likewise, service users in Hudson's (2007) study reported how the speed of services had improved since the development of a joint agency initiative, while users in Freeman and Peck's (2006) work valued a specialist integrated mental health team's increased ability to

adapt to their changing needs. Therefore, joint assessments, continuity and adaptability are important principles to adhere to when developing partnership-working initiatives. However, these findings derive from just three contemporary studies, highlighting an urgent need for further research in this area.

Such findings certainly extol the virtues of partnership working. However, of equal relevance are factors that inhibit this, not least of which are issues associated with power and culture. The term partnership implies equality and neutrality between two or more disciplines or agencies; however, in relation to partnership working between health and social care professionals, this is not always evident. This was illustrated by Jones (2006) who reported how community psychiatric nurses, social workers, occupational therapists, a consultant psychiatrist, a senior house officer, a locality manager, a mental health purchaser and a psychologist approached the task of developing a care pathway for clients suffering from schizophrenia. Clinicians in minority groups experienced difficulties conveying their opinions and often acquiesced to majority views. Clinicians were also defensive when asked to define their interventions, and when this occurred, professionals felt threatened and a competitiveness to maintain professional identity became apparent. The need to conduct individual client assessments was used by all disciplines as a tactic to maintain separate approaches to care. This became a guarded professional ritual with no endorsement given to share assessment strategies, as these were perceived to work against professional roles. Therefore, despite policy informing on a need for boundaries to blur, evidence suggests professionals, when feeling threatened, cling to their boundaries as a strategy to maintain professional autonomy.

Oppressive behaviour faced by one professional group from another is not unusual in healthcare, and the influence of power should never be underestimated in its ability to hinder partnership working. This was illustrated by Lankshear (2003) whose research revealed how community psychiatric nurses, working with social workers and occupational therapists, were forced to accept referrals from GPs of people suffering from anxiety and depression rather than severe and enduring mental illness as planned. The community psychiatric nurses risked having funding withdrawn if they failed to abide by this requirement.

Evetts (2003) reminds that the medical profession has always been the most powerful of the health and social care professions and they have used their power to successfully dominate and maintain professional superiority. Evans (2003) suggests that a dominant medical discourse evident in contemporary Western society arises from the value attributed to scientific-based knowledge, and it is this that enables the medical profession to maintain control over influencing and delivering a medically orientated public health service. This can result in a series of contradictions and tensions for those involved in partnership working. More powerful groups juxtaposed with less powerful groups within what is considered an egalitarian structure, namely a team, is a major contradiction. Davies et al (2000) believe there is a need to expose how different professional groups legitimize the knowledge that empowers them and enables them to subjugate other groups. Until this is done, it is unlikely that partnership working initiatives will be the effective antidote thought of for all that is perceived wrong with the NHS. Indeed, consideration must be given to partnership working being a political quick-fix solution or crisis management strategy, doomed to failure while issues of professional domination exist.

While issues involving power illustrate tensions between professionals involved in partnerships, issues associated with organizational culture may help reveal tensions between professionals and service users. Davies et al (2000) describe culture as that which emerges from what is shared between individuals in an organization; which includes attitudes, beliefs, values and behavioural norms. Morrison (2000) referred to *adversarial*, *paternalistic* and *play fair* cultures and these help illustrate differing professional practices.

Adversarial Adversarial cultures are characterized by mistrust and professional vulnerabilities. Collaboration with other agencies is viewed with scepticism, with professionals believing that hidden agendas centring on exploitation of resources or infringement of professional territory are the primary aims of invitations to work collaboratively. This was evident in Jones' (2006) research discussed earlier, where professionals perhaps felt a need to continue their individualized approach to patient assessment as a strategy to maintain professional autonomy. Of note, where adversarial cultures exist, the needs and desires of service users get lost in the haze of the agencies' belief in the need to ensure self-preservation (Farrell 2004).

Paternalism Agencies which operate paternalistically engage with other agencies on their own terms as and when they deem appropriate. A sense of elitism is evident where the agency views itself as possessing unique expertise and there is a tendency to be dismissive of other agencies' contributions. The organizational culture is characterized by a top-down, power-coercive approach and organizational change is implemented in a prescriptive way with little or no consultation. In relation to users, Morrison (2000) states how professionals who adopt paternalistic approaches are more likely to refrain from involving users in healthcare decisions. Rutter et al (2004) found this in their study which explored professional perceptions of user involvement in mental health services. A concerning picture of patriarchal attitudes emerged where some managers viewed consultation with users a paper exercise, something that was important to be seen to do but not to act upon, while some nurses articulated how they resented the development of policies which aimed to involve users and placed no value on such an approach.

Where paternalistic attitudes exist they can work to disempower users. This was illustrated by Peck et al (2002) in a study which explored levels of mental health user involvement in the design and review of care plans. Involvement ranged between 49% and 60%, and where users were included in the planning of their care, 82% reported positive impacts on their quality of life, whereas of those not involved, only 12% reported such an outcome. Beresford and Branfield (2006) observe that where paternalistic conditions exist, tokenism is the strategy adopted, with no real effort given to working in partnership.

Play fair Morrison's (2000) play fair culture describes how collaboration with other agencies is valued and considered to be in service users' best interests. Users are actively consulted and their opinions on services sought as a means to ensure appropriateness. Organizations that subscribe to this philosophy seek feedback from service users to ascertain their views and experiences of services (DH 2006). However, for Poulton (1999), user consultation falls short of what she considers true user participation. Describing ranges of 'involvement' from information-giving, health education, consultation, consumer satisfaction, participation and empowerment, Poulton considers those levels below participation to be tokenistic attempts to involve users. Of note, some of the studies reviewed have portrayed information-giving and consultation as effective ways to promote patient and public involvement, e.g. Freeman and Peck (2006) and Carter et al (2007), and there is no doubt that both of these are necessary elements in any attempt to enable individuals to make choices and feel supported in doing so. However, Rutter et al's (2004) findings remind how consultation is open to abuse and can be used in tokenistic ways. A summary of barriers to interprofessional working are identified in Box 21.4.

Interestingly, research findings present two very different perspectives on partnership working. On the one hand, small teams of professionals who possess equal status appear to profit from interprofessional working, and where this occurs, benefits to service users also seem likely (see, for example, Carter et al 2007, Freeman and Peck 2006, Hudson 2007, Shaw et al 2005). On the other hand, larger and more diverse teams appear to be negatively affected from issues pertaining to power and culture, and where this is the case, little benefit is seen to be gained by either healthcare practitioners or service users (see, for example, Jones 2006).

Promoting patient and public involvement

The move to place patients and clients at the core of a modernized health service and include them in the planning and delivery of care has been a central objective of the government's plan for transforming health and social care over the past 10 years. *In the Public Interest* (NHS Executive et al 1998) predicted numerous benefits from improved patient and public involvement. These included better treatment and care outcomes, an increasing sense of control leading to improved self-esteem, a more pleasing experience of contact with healthcare services, and easier access to and a more responsive service, all of which result in a greater sense of confidence in health services. Despite this, little progress has been made in promoting patient and public involvement, especially in marginalized populations, who arguably would benefit the most from this approach. Lord Darzi's (DH 2008) report highlighted this and discussed the need for people to be able to exercise choice and be 'partners in decisions about their own care, shaping and directing it with high-quality information and support' (p. 40).

Fundamental questions still exist on what patient and public involvement means, and how increasing service user involvement influences their experiences of health and social care services. These are difficult questions to answer and depend in part upon how the concept of 'involvement' is perceived. Farrell (2004) defines this as the total involvement of clients or patients and their carers in their care and treatment. Many agree this standard is yet to be achieved for the majority of health and social care service users, who so frequently appear on the margins of any decision-making processes relating to their health. As already discussed, much patient and public involvement is considered tokenistic, and the main challenges associated with improving user involvement centre around issues of sharing power. However, this presents a difficulty when considering the tendency for health professionals to believe that their expertise is the only element necessary in order to make informed decisions on care (Pivik 2002). A willingness to cast aside 'expert-led' approaches to care may be an important first step in the move to promote patient and public involvement. This may require practitioners to embrace new philosophical approaches to care planning.

Arnstein's (1969) ladder metaphor describes power relationships between users and organizations. It provides a useful framework to examine factors that contribute to or inhibit the development of meaningful partnerships between users and professionals. Although criticized for undermining the potential of the user involvement process (see Tritter and McCallum 2006), Arnstein's framework offers useful distinctions on degrees of user involvement.

Each of the eight rungs of Arnstein's ladder represents the degree of power individuals possess in relation to influencing the care and services they receive. Anderson et al (2002) describe the lowest rungs, *manipulation* and *therapy*, as nonparticipatory where users have no say in their care planning and are informed on decisions relating to their care management. Information goes in one direction and user views are not sought. The third rung of Arnstein's ladder is *informing*, which is indicative that some important steps are being taken to legitimize participation. However, information still flows in one direction only, from professional to user, and limited channels for feedback exist. The fourth step, *consultation*, is usually performed via attitude surveys, neighbourhood meetings and public inquiries, and although this demonstrates an attempt to engage and take notice of user views, no guarantee of this is evident. Arnstein (1969) feels this is still a tokenistic attempt to involve users.

Ascending the ladder, the fifth step is called *placation*, where individuals are invited to participate within committees or become members of advisory bodies; however, McEvoy et al (2008) discuss how these invariably have no authority or power to effect change. The sixth step is *partnership*, and Arnstein (1969) describes this step as a higher level of tokenism; views are actively sought and this step does allow users an opportunity to advise and contribute to planning, but retains for those in authority the right to judge whether or not to act upon any infor-

mation given. Despite this, redistribution of power between those with and those without authority may occur in this step (McEvoy et al 2008). Personalized care planning resulting in 'packages of care' for patients as proposed by Lord Darzi in the *High Quality Care for All* review (DH 2008) may well contribute to more active partnerships between professionals and patients, particularly in relation to agreeing goals, choosing services and how and where to access these.

The final two rungs of Arnstein's ladder are termed *delegated power* and *citizen control* and these are the areas where power relationships between professionals and users become more diluted and where shared decision-making begins to occur or where users are given overall power of decision-making (Arnstein 1969). The plan to allocate personal budgets to some patients to provide them with greater control over the services they receive, and the providers from which they receive services, does illustrate moves by the government to delegate power and control to those requiring health services (DH 2008). This is a positive step in the move to develop active partnerships of care with healthcare users.

Nurses need to rise to the challenges associated with promoting and improving patient and public involvement in healthcare. Interestingly, Farrell (2004) reported how nurses are generally supportive of the principles of involvement but are reluctant to promote this when it conflicts with their professional ethic of protecting clients from negative experiences. Other barriers to increasing patient, client and public involvement are said to include negative perceptions of involvement, time, resource and organizational pressures, a lack of understanding of the nature of involvement, and a lack of training, skills and experience (McEvoy et al 2008: 6, Ridley and Jones 2002: 5). Entwistle et al (2002) also found health professionals less likely to encourage patient involvement where they perceived there to be only one feasible option relating to care planning, or if they thought users would fail to comprehend 'technical details' or if they themselves were not willing to compromise.

These tensions and dilemmas require urgent consideration and resolution to enable nursing interventions with users to evolve into more client-centred occurrences, where the need to promote patient/client involvement becomes a core consideration of professional practice.

Activity box 21.1(c)

Following joint discussions and determining 'what works', the following projects were developed:

1. Joint training was arranged for GPs, health visitors, school nurses and practice nurses to help practitioners identify overweight, at-risk and obese children, raise the issue with parents with confidence, offer standardized advice and know where and when to refer children and their families to more specialist services.
2. Working in partnership, midwives and health visitors developed a breastfeeding support group.
3. A walk-to-school scheme was developed, organized and run by local parents with support from the local health promotion unit.
4. Health visitors, dieticians, parents and Sure Start facilitators set up a local cooking club for mums with crèche facilities available for children.
5. School nurses, health visitors and teachers developed a weekly dance and movement club for toddlers and children.
6. Primary school teachers, school nurses and parents started a fruit fair at the local primary school.
7. Practice nurses and GPs invited personnel from the local health promotion unit to hold regular 'food fair' information sessions on health centre premises – this is run alongside a well-child clinic and helps to make information on healthy eating easily accessible.

• How would you evaluate the effectiveness of the planned activities?

practitioners deliver care or perform assessments previously the domain of another profession, they must demonstrate the necessary competence and skills to do so safely and effectively. This will be one of the major challenges facing those working in health and social care partnerships.

Appreciating the range of factors that enhance or hinder interprofessional working will better enable nurses to participate in partnership working with confidence. This will assist nurses to plan and lead on partnership working initiatives that aim to provide people with more choice, better information and more control, and in so doing 'will help to improve people's health and wellbeing, by organizing services around patients and not people around services' (DH 2008: 43).

SUMMARY

• Although difficult to define, formal ways of partnership working will undoubtedly remain centre stage in government plans to deliver quality health and social care services.
• To lead integrated teams, nurses in primary care need to appreciate the range of factors that inhibit or promote interprofessional working.
• A far greater emphasis will be placed on promoting patient and public involvement in the future and nurses need to consider ways that this can be accomplished.

Conclusion

The changing healthcare needs of the UK population call for professions in health and social care to embrace new ways to deliver services. Duplication of health and social care provision can no longer be tolerated in a fiscally challenged NHS. Expecting service users to engage with numerous professionals in pursuit of similar goals is unnecessary and unacceptable. New, more integrated ways of working are considered the way forward, and public health and community nurses working in public health and primary care environments need to prepare themselves to work within and across organizational boundaries. This will undoubtedly result in the blurring of professional roles. Crucially, where

DISCUSSION POINTS

1. What opportunities to develop interprofessional working exist in your work? What barriers would prevent this?
2. As a community nurse how could you promote greater involvement of marginalized populations?
3. Consider the competencies and skills you would require to enable you to practise within or lead interprofessional teams – what educational opportunities are available which will enable you to develop the knowledge and skills you require?

References

Anderson W, Florin D, Gillam S, Mountford L 2002 Every voice counts: involving patients and the public in primary care. King's Fund, London

Arnstein S 1969 A ladder of citizen participation. Journal of the American Institute of Planners 35: 216–224

Audit Commission 1998 A fruitful partnership: effective partnership working. Audit Commission, London

Audit Commission 2005 Governing partnerships: bridging the accountability gap. Audit Commission, London

Barr H 2004 Partnership, practice and participation. Journal of Interprofessional Care 18(1): 5–6

Batorowicz B, Shepherd TA 2008 Measuring the quality of transdisciplinary teams. Journal of Interprofessional Care 22(6): 612–620

Beresford P, Branfield F 2006 Developing inclusive partnerships: user-defined outcomes, networking, and knowledge – a case study. Health and Social Care in the Community 14(5): 436–444

Bidmead C, Cowley S 2005 A concept analysis of partnership with clients. Community Practitioner 78(6): 203–208

Borrill CS, Carletta J, Carter AJ, et al 2002 The effectiveness of health care teams in the National Health Service. Aston Centre for Health Service Organisation Research, University of Aston

Carnwell R, Carson A 2004 Understanding partnerships and collaboration. In: Carnwell R, Buchanan J (eds) Effective practice in health and social care: a partnership approach. Open University Press, Maidenhead

Carter B, Cummings J, Cooper L 2007 An exploration of best practice in multi-agency working and the experiences of families of children with complex health needs. What works well and what needs to be done to improve practice for the future? Journal of Clinical Nursing 16: 527–539

Davies HTO, Nutley SM, Mannion R 2000 Organisational culture and quality of health care. Quality in Health Care 9: 111–119

Department for Education and Skills 2006 Working together to safeguard children: a guide to inter-agency working to safeguard and promote the welfare of children. HMSO, London

Department of Health 2005 Creating a patient-led NHS: delivering the NHS improvement plan. DH, London

Department of Health 2006 Good practice for user involvement. Online: http://www.dh.gov.uk/PolicyAndGuidance/ResearchAndDevelopment/HealthInPartnership

Department of Health 2008 High quality care for all: NHS next stage review final report. The Stationery Office, London

Department of Health; Department of Health, Social Services and Public Safety; Scottish Executive; Welsh Assembly Government 2006 Modernising nursing careers. DH, London

Department of Health, Social Services and Public Safety 2005 Caring for people beyond tomorrow: a strategic framework for the development of primary health and social care. The Stationery Office, Belfast

Dowling B, Powell M, Glendinning C 2004 Conceptualising successful partnerships. Health and Social Care in the Community 12(4): 309–317

Entwistle V, Watt I, Bugge C, et al 2002 Exploring patient participation in decision-making. Health Services Research Unit, University of Aberdeen

European Public Health Associates 2002 Integrated care in an international perspective. EUPHA, Brussels

Evans D 2003 'Taking public health out of the ghetto': the policy and practice of multi-disciplinary public health in the United Kingdom. Social Science and Medicine 57(6): 959–967

Evetts J 2003 The sociological analysis of professionalism: occupational change in the modern world. International Sociology 18(2): 395–415

Farrell C 2004 Patient and public involvement in health: the evidence for policy implementation. Department of Health, London

Freeman T, Peck E 2006 Evaluating partnerships: a case study of integrated specialist mental health services. Health and Social Care in the Community 14(5): 408–417

Goble R 2003 Multi-professional education: global perspectives. In: Leathard A (ed.) Interprofessional collaboration: from policy to practice in health and social care. Routledge, London

Horwath J, Morrison T 2007 Collaboration, integration and change in children's services: critical issues and key ingredients. Child Abuse and Neglect 31(1): 55–69

Howarth M, Holland K, Grant MJ 2006 Education needs for integrated care: a literature review. Journal of Advanced Nursing 56(2): 144–156

Hudson B 2000 Inter-agency collaboration – a sceptical view. In: Brechin A, Brown H, Eby MA (eds) Critical practice in health and social care. the Open University/Sage, London

Hudson B 2007 Pessimism and optimism in inter-professional working: the Sedgefield Integrated Team. Journal of Interprofessional Care 21(1): 3–15

Jones A 2006 Multidisciplinary team working: collaboration and conflict. International Journal of Mental Health Nursing 15: 19–28

Jones N, Thomas P 2007 Inter-organizational collaboration and partnerships in health and social care: the role of social software. Public Policy and Administration 22(3): 289–302

Lankshear AJ 2003 Coping with conflict and confusing agendas in multidisciplinary community mental health teams. Journal of Psychiatric and Mental Health Nursing 10: 457–464

Larkin C, Callaghan P 2005 Professionals' perceptions of interprofessional working in community mental health teams. Journal of Interprofessional Care 19(4): 338–346

Leathard A (ed.) 2003 Interprofessional collaboration: from policy to practice in health and social care. Routledge, London

McEvoy R, Keenaghan C, Murray A 2008 Service user involvement in the Irish health service: a review of the evidence. Department of Health and Children, Health Service Executive, Belfast

McLaughlin H 2004 Partnerships: panacea or pretence? Journal of Interprofessional Care 18(2): 103–113

Masterson A 2002 Cross-boundary working: a macro-political analysis of the impact on professional roles. Journal of Clinical Nursing 11: 331–339

Molyneux J 2001 Interprofessional teamworking: what makes teams work well? Journal of Interprofessional Care 15(1): 29–35

Morrison T 2000 Working together to safeguard children: challenges and changes for inter-agency co-ordination in child protection. Journal of Interprofessional Care 14(4): 363–373

NHS Executive, NHS Confederation, Institute of Health Service Management 1998 In the public interest: developing a strategy for public participation in the NHS. NHS Executive, London

Northern Ireland Department of Health and Social Services 2004 A healthier future: a twenty year vision for health and wellbeing in Northern Ireland 2005–2025. The Stationery Office, Belfast

Peck E, Gulliver P, Towel D 2002 Information, consultation or control: user involvement in mental health services in England at the turn of the century. Journal of Mental Health 11(4): 441–451

Pivik JR 2002 Practical strategies for facilitating meaningful citizen involvement in health planning. Commission on the Future of Healthcare in Canada, Ottawa

Poulton B 1999 User involvement in identifying health needs and shaping and evaluating services: Is it being realised? Journal of Advanced Nursing 30(6): 1289–1296

Ridley J, Jones L 2002 Partners in change (Scotland). User and public involvement in health services: a review. Online: http://www.shstrust. org.uk/downloads/pinc_litreview.pdf

Rushmer R, Pallis G 2003 Inter-professional working: the wisdom of integrated working and the disaster of blurred boundaries. Public Money and Management 23(1): 59–66

Rutter D, Manley C, Weaver T, Crawford MJ, Fulop N 2004 Patients or partners? Case studies of user involvement in the planning and delivery of adult mental health services in London. Social Science and Medicine 58(10): 1973–1984

Scottish Executive 2003 Partnership for care. Scottish Executive, Edinburgh

Scottish Executive 2004 National Health Service Reform (Scotland) Act 2004. The Stationery Office, Edinburgh

Shaw A, De Lusignan S, Rowlands G 2005 Do primary care professionals work as a team: a qualitative study. Journal of Interprofessional Care 19(4): 396–405

Sheehan D, Robertson L, Ormond T 2007 Comparison of language used and patterns of communication in interprofessional and multidisciplinary teams. Journal of Interprofessional Care 21(1): 17–30

Sloper P 2004 Facilitators and barriers for co-ordinated multi-agency services. Child Care, Health and Development 30(6): 571–580

Tritter JQ, McCallum A 2006 The snakes and ladders of user involvement: moving beyond Arnstein. Health Policy 76(2): 156–168

Warmington P, Daniels H, Edwards A, et al 2004 Interagency collaboration: a review of the literature. Learning in and for Interagency Working Project, Bath

Welsh Assembly Government 2001 Improving health in Wales: a plan for the NHS and its partners. The Stationery Office, Cardiff

Welsh Assembly Government 2005 Designed for life: creating world class health and social care for Wales in the 21st century. The Stationery Office, Cardiff

Welsh Assembly Government 2007 Fulfilled lives, supportive communities: improving social services in Wales from 2008–2018. The Stationery Office, Cardiff

Recommended reading

Barrett G, Sellman D, Thomas J (eds) 2005 Interprofessional working in health and social care: professional perspectives. Palgrave Macmillan, Houndmills

This book examines the rationale underpinning interprofessional working and the conditions and skills required to facilitate effective joint working practices. It explores the concept of joint working from a range of professional perspectives and offers a valuable insight into factors that promote or inhibit interprofessional practice.

Carnwell R, Buchanan J (eds) 2004 Effective practice in health and social care: a partnership approach. Open University Press, London

This practical text defines partnership working and uses case studies to demonstrate partnership working initiatives used to promote inclusion of some of the most marginalized populations in society. An extremely useful resource for those planning partnership initiatives.

Leathard A (ed.) 2003 Interprofessional collaboration: from policy to practice in health and social care. Routledge, London

A key text, which offers a comprehensive overview of partnership working, from political, managerial and ethical perspectives. Theoretical partnership working models are reviewed and benefits and limitations of interprofessional education examined.

Alternative ways of working

Helen Beswick, Joanne Chambers, Julie Davidson,
Aileen Fraser, Celia Phipps, Kirsten Robson and Janet Vokes

KEY ISSUES

- Developing new advanced practice roles in the community
- Changes in policy and the impact on nursing
- How new nursing roles are evaluated and the need for the development of evaluation methods that reflect person-centred care as well as economic value

Introduction

In 2003, at the Chief Nursing Officer's (CNO) conference, John Reid, then Health Secretary, called on nurses to take their place on the front line both in delivering patient care and in running the NHS. The political drive for nurses to have an extended role in providing services started in 1990 with the introduction of the general practitioner (GP) contract. Nurses took on extended roles in chronic disease management and health promotion. This marked the early stages of a move to a more responsive, accountable and performance managed NHS with a focus on nursing as a key player in delivering more accessible, diverse services. The move to a market economy identifies patients as consumers with greater voice and choice (Department of Health 2000, 2006d). The new General Medical Services (GMS) contract of 2004 demonstrates this approach by focusing on payments for quality of care delivered by a practice rather than individual GPs and by opening the route for nurses to become partners within practices or specialist providers of nurse-led services (see Chapter 1 for further information on pressures for change in the NHS and Chapter 2 for

further information on the GMS contract).

The CNOs of the four countries in the UK have responded to this with a strategy for nursing (Department of Health 2006a) which includes:

- a shift from the traditional focus on acute care to highlighting the role of community nursing in nurse education
- different models of employment outside the NHS with nurses developing social enterprise models and being employed by organizations commissioned by primary care trusts to provide new services
- nursing roles developing to fit patient need.

These shifts are designed to produce a more patient-centred NHS but are also underpinned by the belief, unproven to date, that community services can be more cost-effective. More services are now offered closer to home and this trend will continue with increased community provision in the forms of intermediate care, community matrons and community hospitals. There is a focus on closer integration of health and social care and increased choice for patients in the form of direct payments, where people can purchase their own services. Patient voice will be given more power accompanied with requirements for action by statutory bodies (Department of Health 2006d).

In this chapter we have chosen to look at areas of development within nursing to illustrate how policy is working in practice. First we look at new advanced practice roles that have developed in community nursing such as nurse practitioners, consultant nurses and community matrons. Then we describe the development of new nurse-led services using walk-in centres as an example and concluding with changes to existing roles in relation to public health nursing for older people and how nurse prescribing has developed.

The nurse practitioner role

History

A nurse practitioner is defined by the Royal College of Nursing (RCN) as a registered nurse who has undertaken a specific course of study of at least first degree (Honours) level and who through this training is able to work autonomously, make clinical decisions, refer to other professionals, and instigate and evaluate treatment (Jones 1999).

Nurse practitioners have been established in North America for several decades but it was not until the 1980s that the role expanded in the United Kingdom. Nurse practitioner development in the UK was pioneered by Barbara Stilwell working in two general practices in Birmingham (Stilwell 1982) and by Barbara Burke-Masters working with homeless people in London (Burke-Masters 1986). During this time, the nurse practitioner was generally seen to be working within the primary care setting, but more recently, the role has been developed in a range of healthcare settings such as hospitals, mental healthcare and learning difficulties care.

Reasons for development of the nurse practitioner role

The reasons for the development of nurse practitioner roles within the NHS are varied but include issues of cost, the need to increase provision of care to improve access, difficulties associated with the availability of doctors and the skills and expertise of nurses (Horrocks et al 2002). The Cumberlege Report (Department of Health and Social Security (DHSS) 1986), the Tomlinson Report (1992) and the NHS Management Executive (1993) all supported the development of the nurse practitioner role in primary care.

Challenges of the nurse practitioner role

The development of the nurse practitioner role has enabled nurses to provide more holistic care to their patients. With the addition of nurse prescribing, the days of waiting outside doctors' doors are diminishing. However, change can be accompanied by tensions and challenges and this role continues to face both.

The United Kingdom Central Council for Nursing, Midwifery and Health Visiting (UKCC) did not recognize the title of nurse practitioner for those nurses who had undertaken appropriate training and no record of these nurses was made on the nursing register. However, the Nursing and Midwifery Council (NMC) has indicated that it will work towards regulating nurse practitioners in the future. This is of paramount importance in order that the title is recognized among the profession and also to protect the general public from individuals who call themselves a nurse practitioner but who have not completed appropriate training. In December 2005, it was agreed by the NMC that:

- advanced nursing practice competencies should be mapped against the Knowledge and Skills Framework
- nurses working at an advanced level should be registered on an additional sub-part of the nursing register. Before going ahead with this plan, the Department of Health must be consulted as it takes the lead on regulatory matters relating to healthcare across the United Kingdom. This work is ongoing
- nurses who believe that they are already working at an advanced level should be accommodated (NMC 2006).

The array of nurse titles within the NHS causes confusion, not only for service users but also among the nursing profession and other healthcare workers. Reveley and Walsh (2000) established that among six acute trusts, nurses were using 603 different titles.

Research on effectiveness

Particular interest has been shown as to whether nurse practitioners can provide front-line care, and by doing so, replace doctors. In a systematic review of all research relating to doctor–nurse substitution, Laurant et al (2007: 9) concluded that appropriately trained nurses can produce 'as high quality care as primary care doctors and achieve as good health outcomes for patients'. The review also suggests that nurse–doctor substitution has the potential to reduce doctors' workload but will only do so if doctors stop providing the care that has been transferred to nurses. The issue of cost savings is questionable, as nurse practitioners tend to have longer consultation rates and an increased recall rate compared to doctors.

Horrocks et al (2002) suggest that future research should focus around identifying the factors responsible in leading to high patient satisfaction with nurse practitioner consultations. This research should be extended to include more patient groups. Nurse practitioners have worked very successfully in areas of the country where there is poor access to general practitioners and also with patients who suffer from long-term conditions. This role enables patients to have more choice in how they access healthcare. The RCN states that the nurse practitioner is not a doctor substitute but is a complementary source of care to that offered by the medical profession as well as acting as primary care providers in their own right.

Consultant nurse/midwife role

History of the development of the consultant nurse/midwife (CN/M) role

Tony Blair launched the concept of the consultant nurse in 1998. This was picked up across the four nations of the UK in policy documents (Department of Health 1999, Scottish Executive 2001). There are currently 1200 of these posts across the UK and the majority are in England. The aim of this post was to provide a clinical pathway for senior nurses who did not want to progress through the managerial or academic pathways. This role aims to keep nurses by the bedside and to provide clinical leadership in facilitating the changes in nursing roles and the move to evidence-based practice. Clinical leadership is seen by many as central to the delivery of *The NHS Plan* (Department of Health 2000) and the reason for the development of this role was to ensure that there is a clinical role with the opportunity to influence strategy within the NHS at patient, staff and board level. Four key areas for these roles were defined:

- expert practice
- professional leadership and consultancy
- education and development
- practice and service development linked to research and evaluation.

All of these should be underpinned by a strong nursing foundation with education to Masters or Doctorate level and additional specialty-specific qualifications (Department of Health 1999).

Challenges to the CN/M role

Problems have emerged in terms of lack of:

- funding for roles
- clarity on the purpose and remit of the role
- mentorship
- succession planning (Booth et al 2006).

There have been reports of work overload coping with the demands of providing activity within each of the four domains and lack of support within organizations both for the role and for initiating change (Guest et al 2001). Consultant nurses should be spending half of their time in expert practice. This has led to debates on the nature of expert practice and the definition of 'clinical time'. Research into present roles has shown that this is an area where many consultant nurses struggle and a survey of consultant nurses in Scotland found that 4 of 13 nurses surveyed were not providing direct patient care (Booth et al 2006). It seems an important area for many reasons:

- to maintain expert clinical skills
- to support the development of other practice roles
- to provide improved services to patients
- to have a patient-focused understanding of how services are developed, delivered and evaluated to advocate for people who use the NHS.

Research on effectiveness

Many people describe this role as a creative and innovative one, which is making changes in the NHS to benefit patients (Sturdy 2004). Research supports this view in showing that the role has been influential in leadership roles and in developing innovative services (Guest et al 2001, Manley 2000). However, there has been no widespread formal role evaluation and some of the research that has been carried out has mainly been concerned with the role development experience (Booth et al 2006, Guest et al 2001).

There are difficulties in evaluation of outcomes but it is important, for this role specifically and for nursing generally, to attempt to measure the more intangible aspects of the role such as the impact of clinical leadership within an organization. Manley (2000) used an action research approach to evaluate the impact of the clinical leadership provided by the CN/M role on organizational culture and changes in practice. This work showed positive changes in terms of developing new roles, staff feeling more confident and a change to a culture of evidence-based practice. The reality of this role is that it is an exciting development for nursing. There are still very few of these posts in the community and the challenge for present and future consultant nurses lies in demonstrating that clinical leadership and improving the quality of services will facilitate the development of nursing for a future where nurses are at the forefront of creating new services and improving existing ones for and with patients.

Community matrons

The development of the community matron role

The NHS improvement plan (Department of Health 2005b) focuses on the care of patients with long-term conditions and states that a case management approach is the best way to improve quality of life and reduce unnecessary hospital admissions. Reducing unplanned hospital admissions is currently central to the commissioning plans of all primary care trusts. In addition, the NHS has been set a public service agreement to reduce unplanned bed day usage by 5% by 2008 (Department of Health 2006d). The professionals pivotal in the implementation of this are community matrons, 3000 of which were expected to be in post by 2008 (Department of Health 2005a).

The role of the community matron is to provide case management for the most vulnerable elderly people who may have one or more chronic diseases. These nurses care for patients at the top of the 'pyramid' developed by Kaiser Permanente, an American health company (Department of Health 2005b). This divides the population of people living with long-term conditions into three levels: the bottom level, composed of approximately 70–80% of the 'long-term condition' population, who are stable and able to self-manage; the middle level indicative of a population with more complex condi-

tions requiring disease-specific services; and the final small level identifying a population with highly complex physical and possibly social circumstances that require case management. It is thought that these people account for a disproportionate number of emergency admissions and bed days, being responsible for 42% of emergency admissions (Department of Health 2005b). Case study 22.1 illustrates the role of the community matron in a typical scenario involving a client with complex needs.

What is the role of the community matron?

The case manager role is complex and requires the practitioner to acquire new ways of working, collaborate with other agencies while working across organizational boundaries and challenge existing ways of working in order to provide seamless patient care in the community setting. As an advanced practitioner, matrons should be able to comprehensively assess, perform physical examinations, diagnose, refer for investigations, design, implement and evaluate care plans to improve the quality of life and disease management for patients on their caseload (NMC 2006). Specialist courses are being developed to equip nurses for such advanced roles (Board 2007) and a framework has recently been developed to ensure competence (Department of Health 2006b).

Challenges for community matrons

- Matrons do not generally provide a 24-hour service and are therefore developing innovative communication methods to ensure an accessible care plan is available to agencies that may be called upon 'after hours' in both health and social care.
- There is evidence citing the lack of social care available for patients in 'crisis' resulting in avoidable hospital admissions (Boaden et al 2006). Matrons are therefore challenging existing ways of working and collaborating with other health and social care providers in the development of services responsive to local need.
- There is still a need to develop relationships and communication with secondary care to

Case study 22.1

Lily is an 87-year-old widow who lives on her own in a ground floor flat. Her elderly sister lives next door. She has 15 children; most live within a 10-mile radius and visit regularly. Lily is elderly and frail, she has poor eyesight, hypertension and rheumatoid arthritis which limit her functional abilities and for which she has to take methotrexate.

I am a community matron and became involved when it was highlighted that she had had several hospital admissions over a 6-month period. These admissions were related to deterioration in mobility and she required a blood transfusion on one occasion.

Liaison from the hospital indicated that the family managed Lily's care at home. An assessment highlighted several issues:

- Although numerous family members were involved and visited Lily, there was no clarity about who did what for Lily, with very limited interaction between the caregivers.

- Lily was not taking her medication.

- Lily was bright and chatty, but on the second home visit her short-term memory problem was obvious. She could not recall the previous meeting, was happy to engage in small talk but had no depth of under-standing of the illness or tablets. She was unaware of

her functional deterioration or new symptoms since the previous visit. Memory testing score was 4/10. She appeared anaemic, was falling over frequently, her ankles were swollen and she appeared very breathless. She was admitted to hospital under the care of the Care of the Elderly team. I linked with the hospital to raise concerns. Lily required a transfusion and was diagnosed with dementia.

When planning for Lily's discharge I worked with the family on their understanding of her diagnosis of dementia and the disease pathway. I encouraged several open and frank discussions with the family resulting in an agreement on a home care package being provided. This package assists Lily with her day-to-day routine, monitoring her condition and prompting her medication. It has allowed her children to continue to provide support and care in their role as family members, not as care providers.

I continue to monitor Lily's physical and mental condition, respond to early symptoms of anaemia and other changes in condition and monitor blood results. I linked with the hospital team on the effectiveness of donepezil, which was not continued long term. Eighteen months on, Lily continues to live at home with her family support and the home care package; she has not been readmitted to hospital in that time.

---

ensure that when a patient is admitted the matron is informed immediately to assist in diagnosis, care planning and early discharge, thus avoiding unnecessary investigations and reducing length of stay.

- It is essential for the community matron to have the optimum effective caseload. If caseload numbers are too large then this proactive way of working is compromised. The success of meeting the targets of reduced emergency hospital admissions depends not only on matrons case managing the most at-risk patients but also on having the necessary health and social care available to prevent deterioration in health, and hospital admission, and to promote self-care in the general population.

Research on the effectiveness of the community matron role

The NHS improvement plan (Department of Health 2005b) set out priorities for the next 4 years that

highlight the importance of providing support for people with chronic diseases and complex needs.

One project aimed at addressing this was the high-profile pilot 'Evercare', the foundations of which originated from the United States where studies showed a 50% reduction in unplanned hospital admissions in nursing homes where patients were case managed (Kane et al 2003). The Department of Health enlisted the help of a US company 'United Healthcare' to run nine pilot sites within the UK over a period of 12 months. Unlike America, most of the patients in the studies were living in their own homes. Highly experienced nurses with various clinical backgrounds were recruited and provided with specialist training in clinical examination skills, diagnostics and management of long-term conditions. The main aim was to reduce unnecessary hospital admissions in elderly at-risk groups by having a community matron managing their care. Patients were referred to the service and considered to be 'at risk' if they were over 65 and had had two or more emergency hospital admissions in the preceding year.

Results collated after an 18-month period indicated an increase in satisfaction in the quality of care patients and carers received and a better understanding of how to manage their chronic diseases. Access to case management also added a frequency of contact, regular monitoring and a range of referral options that had not previously been provided by other health or social care professionals (Boaden et al 2006). The study, however, concluded that any reduction in admissions in this target group would have occurred spontaneously and so the effect of the intervention could not be measured. Interpretation and evaluation of the findings should be done with caution as the design of the trial had many limitations identified (Boaden et al 2006).

Developments following the research findings

Following the conclusions of the Evercare project, work is being done to develop and improve systems. Currently the number of admissions they have avoided within their caseload measures matrons' effectiveness. The results of the Evercare report highlighted the inadequacy of using two or more admissions as referral criteria. In response, the King's Fund (2005) developed a more stringent 'predictor of admission tool' to assist case finding. The 'Patients at Risk of Rehospitalisation' (PARR) tool uses 3 years of admissions data and other variables including extent of prior utilization, diagnosis and socio-demographic information. This tool can be combined with GP data, the 'Combined Predictive Tool', to provide more robust information and identify those patients whose condition has not reached a 'crisis point'. Croydon PCT has been using the Combined Predictive model in its award-winning 'virtual wards' project whereby people identified as having a very high risk of future hospitalization are provided with a proactive, educational approach to care by a team of professionals, led by a community matron.

The case management approach and use of community matrons is still in its infancy. There is no doubt that community matrons are in a prime position to coordinate and deliver optimum care within the community to patients with long-term conditions, thus improving standards of care and patient satisfaction. However, this role cannot be truly effective while working in isolation. It must be supported by changes in community services to provide safe, high-quality alternatives to hospital care that retain high rates of patient satisfaction.

Nurse-led walk-in centres

History of walk-in centres

Tony Blair first announced NHS walk-in centres (WICs) in 1999 as part of a programme of reforms that aimed to modernize and improve patient access to NHS services. The development of WICs as an alternative to conventional services, and the introduction of innovative new roles, were seen as being integral to achievement of the targets set out in *The NHS Plan* (Department of Health 2000).

The centres were proclaimed as a way of providing quicker and more convenient access to advice and treatment for minor ailments and injuries. Somewhat implicit within these stated aims was the recognition that existing primary care services were not offering the accessibility needed by patients; this was leading to increasing numbers of inappropriate attendances to A&E departments by patients with minor health problems. WICs also relieved demand on general practice by providing an alternative, situated in convenient locations with wider opening times and minimal waiting. The idea was to fully exploit the development of nursing skills and roles within the UK, while allowing GPs to fully utilize their extensive knowledge and skills by concentrating on those patients with more complex needs.

The British Medical Association, however, were unimpressed by the idea of nurse-led WICs (BBC Online 1999); while there were justifiable concerns raised over continuity of patient care, safety and effectiveness of the centres, other opposition voiced was perhaps more related to the perceived erosion of their status and traditional gate-keeping role within the NHS. Despite this dissent, 39 WICs had opened by September 2001. Today, the total number in England has risen to 77, with a further 18 sites in development. Scotland has opted for a different approach, and is promoting the role of its community pharmacists to provide a walk-in service for patients with minor illnesses. In Northern Ireland, just one centre based on the 'walk-in' concept has been developed. In Wales, while the Assembly supports the principle of nurse-led WICs, information is currently being gathered from the English experience of WICs to ascertain if their development would deliver better care for Welsh patients.

Research on effectiveness

A national evaluation of the first wave of centres was commissioned by the Department of Health (Salisbury et al 2002) to address the questions raised over the function of WICs within the NHS. It was designed to assess the quality, appropriateness and efficiency of WICs, their impact on other NHS providers and the extent to which they improved patient access to healthcare.

NHS WICs were found to improve access for certain groups of patients such as young and middle-aged men, who are known to be relatively low users of GP services. However, visitors also tended to be more affluent than attendees at GP surgeries, leading to concerns that WICs are not addressing existing inequalities for groups with the greatest health needs. Users of WICs appeared very satisfied with the care they received; respondents in the research were seen mainly by nurses, and had reduced waiting times and longer consultations compared with general practice. Quality of clinical care was also evaluated against that provided by GP services and NHS Direct using simulated patients presenting with one of five standardized scenarios. Results showed that nurses at WICs provided a quality of care at least as high as in general practice, within these specified areas.

Attendance at a WIC was felt to be entirely appropriate by both patients and the nurses they consulted. This finding is supported by the relatively low level of referral on to a GP (13%) or A&E department (6%) from the WICs evaluated. Nurses tended to justify all attendances as appropriate, even in instances where self-care would have been appropriate or where the patient needed to be directly referred to other health services for treatment. Nurses felt that the opportunity to provide advice or health promotion justified the visit as appropriate; however, the outcomes of such interventions are notoriously difficult to evaluate. Concerns over appropriateness have therefore tended to focus on the finding that WIC users have relatively low levels of health need.

At the time of evaluation, WICs had higher costs per consultation than any of the alternatives that patients stated they would otherwise have used. Clearly, improved accessibility (achieved through shorter waiting times), together with comparatively lengthy consultations will result in higher cost care for relatively minor illnesses. The escalating number of visitors to WICs will no doubt improve efficiency, in terms of cost per consultation, but will also have a knock-on effect upon accessibility as waiting times increase.

Most visitors to WICs (~75%) stated they would either have attended a GP practice or an A&E department if the centre had not existed. A subsequent reduction in the use of other local NHS services is therefore to be anticipated. However, past studies of WICs in North America have not shown this to be the case (Bell and Szafran 1992). While the UK evaluation showed a trend towards reduced utilization of GP services and A&E departments local to the WICs, this was not large enough to be statistically significant. However, the evaluation took place 12 months after the centres first opened, which is a relatively short time over which to demonstrate such impacts on other services – numbers of people attending centres have clearly increased since 2001. Additionally, WICs by nature see patients who are commuters, travellers and those unregistered with a GP practice, so it is difficult to evaluate any significant impact over such a large number of diverse NHS services.

Future challenges for nursing in WICs

The national evaluation showed that WICs had broadly met their aims of developing an accessible, nurse-led service, providing high-quality care – but at additional cost. Salisbury (2003) suggests several issues that need to be considered in order to achieve maximum benefits from WICs, including the following:

• *Increased accessibility has encouraged escalating numbers of visitors to the centres – is new demand being generated or are WICs providing a convenient alternative to existing services?* Salisbury et al (2002) found that most people attending WICs consulted very soon after their problem began, primarily with minor self-limiting illnesses. There is the suggestion that open-access services like WICs are undermining the confidence of patients to successfully manage their own conditions, in effect inhibiting 'watch and wait' approaches and medicalizing minor problems. However, most attendees are given advice and information rather than treatment or referral to another provider. Nurses need to explore if this intervention is helping patients to successfully self-manage future minor conditions in order to demonstrate the effective use of NHS resources.

- *How do nurses balance the conflict between professional autonomy and the use of computerized protocols when making clinical decisions?* WICs are staffed by a variety of nurses of differing experiences and backgrounds. To ensure consistent high-quality care, nurses are expected to use computerized clinical assessment software. However, Salisbury (2003) suggests that more highly trained nurses may experience a conflict between exercise of their professional autonomy and reliance on assessment software when making clinical decisions. Nurses at WICs have been allowed to supply and administer certain medications in identified clinical situations via patient group directions (PGDs). While PGDs allow more patients to be treated without referral to a medic, it could be argued that due to limitations in the number of conditions they cover and the restrictive patient inclusion criteria, professional autonomy is hindered. Since the development of WICs, independent nurse prescribing rights have been granted which could maximize the benefits of WICs. However, it has proved difficult for nurses working within WICs to find the medical mentors required to complete the prescribing course since doctors are not normally employed within WICs.

- *Could an integrated approach to urgent care be more beneficial to both patients and nurses?* Salisbury (2003) acknowledges that NHS WICs are currently isolated from other providers in the local healthcare economy, which can cause problems in terms of continuity of care, duplication of effort and inconsistent messages to patients. For nurses, while a role in a WIC is an attractive proposition, they may not necessarily be the best learning environment. The 'feedback' part of the experiential learning cycle is missing as there is no patient follow-up, and doctors are not usually on site to discuss uncertain cases with. This uncertainty surely leads nurses to practise more cautiously and refer more patients for medical review.

Salisbury (2003) recommends integration of WICs, out-of-hours GP providers and pharmacies and A&E departments, forming 'urgent-care centres' to maximize efficiency and improve continuity of care. Clearly, this would be an environment of benefit to nurses, in terms of providing the support needed to develop autonomous and prescribing practice.

Nurse prescribing

History of nurse prescribing

The concept of nurse prescribing began in 1986 with the Cumberlege Report (DHSS 1986). Nurses' roles were expanding and a government review of community nursing highlighted nurses' frustrations at having to get treatments sanctioned and prescribed by the GP even though they had assessed the patient and were highly skilled in areas such as palliative care. In 1992 new legislation enabled district nurses and health visitors to prescribe from a limited formulary, of mainly dressings, appliances and over-the-counter products. A Department of Health report published in 1999 suggested needs were still not being met due to restrictions in the nurse's formulary in relation to the expanding role of nurses, particularly in chronic disease management, and recommended increasing the range of nurses who could prescribe and standardizing formal training for new prescribers.

In 2001 the government announced that following consultation, non-medical prescribing would be extended to more nurses and also pharmacists, giving them access to a wider range of medicines. This would be on completion of a specific prescribing training programme approved by the NMC. This development supported initiatives in *The NHS Plan* (Department of Health 2000), which called for 'harnessing skills', and highlighted key roles for nurses.

In a bid to provide patients with quicker, more efficient access to medicines and to make better use of the skills of health professionals, the Department of Health announced the introduction of supplementary and independent nurse prescribing (Department of Health 2004). Supplementary prescribing is a prescribing partnership between the non-medical prescriber, independent prescriber and patient, using a patient-specific clinical management plan. This type of prescribing relies on a close working partnership between the doctor and supplementary prescriber and was seen to be useful in the management of patients with long-term conditions. Extended formulary nurse prescribers could prescribe from a formulary of all general sales list and pharmacy medicines and some prescription-only medicines relating to four main areas of treatment: minor ailments, minor injuries, health promotion and palliative care. However, prescribing within this formulary remained fairly restrictive (Latter et al 2005).

May 2006 heralded the most radical change in non-medical prescribing practice, with new legislation allowing nurses virtually the same prescribing rights as doctors (Department of Health 2006c). Although this legislation applied across the UK, England has led the four nations by discontinuing the *Nurse Prescribers' Extended Formulary*, allowing nurse independent prescribers to prescribe any licensed medicine, except controlled drugs, for any medical condition within their area of competence.

Challenges for nurse prescribers

This move was met with dismay from the medical profession who were not generally supportive of this new freedom nurses have been given (Young 2005). There are currently around 10 000 nurse independent prescribers on the NMC register, mainly working in primary care. Supplementary prescribing is less popular with nurses and has been problematic mainly in the restrictive use of the clinical management plan, which does not lend itself to acute episodes. Nurse prescribing rights are still in their infancy and there is little research to support the effectiveness of the role; however, the role has been evaluated to support future policy, education and practice (Latter et al 2005).

The medical perspective: are nurses qualified to diagnose and prescribe for patients?

Doctors have raised concerns that nurses lack the clinical skills that underpin prescribing, the training is inadequate and there is a risk to patient safety (Avery and Pringle 2005, Young 2005). Recent data suggest nurse prescribers generally have experience exceeding 10 years and have undertaken studies in advanced practice (Latter et al 2005, Young 2005).

The prescribing and pharmacology training nurses receive is extremely rigorous and nurses have to provide evidence that they have achieved 84 competencies laid down by the NMC in order to qualify. As well as completing the programme they must also have worked for 12 days under medical supervision. This is more prescribing training than medical students currently receive.

Unfortunately some doctors have withdrawn their support in mentoring trainee nurse prescribers and are seeking payment for this service. In the current financial climate of the NHS there is limited money for training and development and this action could seriously restrict the number of nurses accessing the module and deny essential clinical support.

The nurses' perspective: have we got the tools to do the job?

It is fundamental that prescribers work in an environment that allows them clinical support and encourages and facilitates joint decision-making and fosters ongoing development. (Latter et al 2005, Young 2005). A better working relationship complementing doctors' and nurses' roles supports safer prescribing practice promoting positive patient outcomes. It is a concern that in 2005 it was noted that only 5% of nurse prescribers were prescribing electronically (Latter et al 2005). The training still has an emphasis on handwritten prescriptions even though electronically generated prescriptions are safer, allowing the prescriber to review current medication and be alerted to drug interactions and allergies while creating an audit trail. This is a logistical and technical issue but system updates are available and employers should ensure nurses have the same access as doctors. This would also improve documentation and sharing of information.

The future development of nurse prescribing

Prescribing should not be seen as a stand-alone module and evidence supports the need for training in history taking and diagnosis, essential competencies in performing the role, and this is being addressed by education providers. While the prescribing role supports autonomy in advanced practice, nurse independent prescribers must continue to work in a supportive framework with other health professionals to promote positive patient outcomes and within the remit of the National Prescribing Centre (2007) competency framework and the NMC code of conduct.

In taking the service forward, there needs to be a more structured, standardized system of continued professional development which will ensure that nurses feel supported. This requires commitment by nurse employers, educators and the nurses themselves, through developing less formal networks such as prescribing forums, thereby ensuring that the nurse still achieves and maintains the prescribing competencies to stay on the NMC register. To meet the changing needs of healthcare and to support and enhance advanced nursing roles, prescribing rights for nurses have become essential. This more than any other expansion of role has allowed nurses to become autonomous and manage complete episodes of care.

Public health and older people

Community nurses for older people – is there value in a health visiting service for older people?

Over the last 5 years there has been a reduction in the numbers of health visitors working with older people as they increasingly concentrate on the health needs of the under-5s and their families. This change in role had been endorsed by recent government documents and policy, such as *Facing the Future: a Review of the Role of Health Visitors* (Department of Health 2006e).

There is little research into the effectiveness of a health visiting programme with older people although most indicate a positive effect. Rogers (2003) describes a diminishing work programme in this area despite evidence from a systematic review of studies of home visiting which found that this could reduce mortality and admission to long-term care. The role of secondary health promotion with individuals appears to be appreciated by older people and their carers in particular. Smoking cessation with the over-65 age group indicates greater successes than with younger groups (Wall 2005) and confirms that older people are often ready to accept health-promoting messages. The impact of more measurable performance management targets specifically centred on the prevention of admission to

hospital places staff with a primary prevention role in a difficult position. Despite emphasis on a shift towards preventative care and intervention based in the community (Department of Health 2006d), primary prevention and the promotion of independence remains difficult to quantify.

Box 22.1

Bristol CNOPs

In Bristol, Community Nurses for Older People (CNOPs), using the principles of health visiting, work closely with the community matrons to deliver a medical–social model of care. This service uses case finding to identify older people with a range of health and social needs and provides a range of services from case management for older people with complex needs to signposting to services to prevent ill health and maintain independence. CNOPs support the development of health-enhancing activities to support older people such as befriending services and exercise classes. This role has been part of the Bristol experience for over 30 years.

Conclusion

In this chapter we have described some of the alternative ways of working that are developing within nursing. Although the roles, settings and skills that we have described here are very different, there are some common key themes for nursing in general for the future. The chapter has highlighted the importance and difficulties of evaluation. Quantitative research is seen as a gold standard approach but randomized controlled trials are lengthy and expensive and may not answer the questions that arise in practice, i.e. which is the best model to use to provide care? Many of the new models are criticized for lack of evidence of effectiveness but there is little research into the traditional models of care. It is of fundamental importance that we continue to evaluate nursing roles but research methods are needed which are responsive to the practicalities of healthcare delivery. The developments and expansions of nursing practice have not been without difficulties as they have encroached on traditional medical practice, raising concerns about competencies and safety. It is still uncertain as to whether many of the approaches described save money or increase the ability of doctors to deal with more complex medical problems, but research has shown them to be safe, effective and popular with patients.

Regulation and professional recognition of advanced practice has been another theme from the chapter. There is evidence that we have learned from the early development of roles such as the nurse practitioner, which was introduced without recognized competencies or standards. This is illustrated by the work undertaken through the Department of Health and educational establishments to develop competency frameworks for community matrons at an early stage in the development of this role. The NMC is developing a register for advanced practitioners and this is welcome and urgently needed to support the recognition of advanced practice and to protect patients.

These problems are not insurmountable and should not discourage development. Nursing is in a key position to face the challenges of the future. All of the nursing roles in this chapter have achieved high rates of patient satisfaction, and partnership between professionals and patients will be key to achieving future developments. Nurses have stepped forward and shown that they are an essential part of the team ready to provide and develop innovative, high-quality services to meet the needs of the healthcare consumers of the future – the 'expert patients'.

SUMMARY

- Nursing is developing new and exciting roles to improve the care provided to patients.
- Many of the new roles increase the autonomy of nurses to work independently of the traditional medical model and to supplement and improve care that is already provided, e.g. community matrons, walk-in centres.
- Research and robust evaluation are needed to underpin the development of these roles, particularly acknowledging qualitative as well as quantitative research as valid tools.
- Relationships with patients remain at the heart of nursing practice with new models showing high levels of patient satisfaction and improved accessibility.

DISCUSSION POINTS

1. Do community nurses make the best use of health promotion models to deliver the key messages to promoting independence and health?
2. Does the changing emphasis on targets designed to improve performance, while laudable, disadvantage those professional groups who work in the areas of health promotion and promotion of independence? How could you overcome this?
3. Do we need clinical leadership in nursing and, if so, what is the purpose and who should provide it?
4. If you were setting up a research project to evaluate a nursing role, how would you go about it?
5. How can we measure and disseminate 'best practice' in nursing when practices vary so much?

References

Avery AJ, Pringle M 2005 Extended prescribing by UK nurses and pharmacists. BMJ 331: 1154–1155

BBC Online 1999 Walk-in centres could be a danger. BBC News: Health, 16 Jul. Online: http://news.bbc.co.uk/1/hi/health/395755.stm

Bell N, Szafran O 1992 Use of walk-in clinics by family-practice patients.

Canadian Family Physician 38: 507–513

Boaden R, Dusheiko M, Gravelle H, Parker S, Pickard S, Roland M 2006 Evaluation of Evercare: executive summary. National Primary Care Research and Development Centre, University of Manchester

Board M 2007 Education and support needs for the community matron role. Primary Health Care 17(4): 22–24

Booth J, Hutchison C, Beech C, Robertson K 2006 New nursing roles: the experience of Scotland's consultant nurses/midwives. Journal of Nursing Management 14: 83–89

Burke-Masters B 1986 The autonomous nurse practitioner: an answer to a chronic problem of primary care. Lancet 1(8492): 1266

Department of Health 1999 Review of prescribing, supply, and administration. Final report (Crown 11 Report). The Stationery Office, London

Department of Health 2000 The NHS plan: a plan for investment, a plan for reform. The Stationery Office, London

Department of Health 2004 Extending independent nurse prescribing within the NHS in England: a guide for implementation, 2nd edn. The Stationery Office, London

Department of Health 2005a Supporting people with long-term conditions: liberating the talents of nurses who care for people with long-term conditions. DH, London

Department of Health 2005b Supporting people with long-term conditions: an NHS and social care model to support local innovations and integration. DH, London

Department of Health 2006a Modernising nursing careers – setting the direction. DH, London

Department of Health 2006b Caring for people with long-term conditions: an education framework for community matrons and case managers. DH, London

Department of Health 2006c Nurse independent prescribing. Online: www.dh.gov.uk/en/ Policyandguidance/ Medicinespharmacyandindustry/ Prescriptions/theNonMedical PrescribingProgramme/ nurseprescribing/index.htm

Department of Health 2006d Our health, our care, our say: a new direction for community services. DH, London

Department of Health 2006e Facing the future: a review of the role of health visitors. DH, London

Department of Health and Social Security 1986 Neighbourhood nursing: a focus for care (Cumberlege Report). The Stationery Office, London

Guest D, Peccei R, Rosenthal P, et al 2001 Preliminary evaluation of the establishment of nurse, midwife and health visitor consultants. Report to the Department of Health. University of London, Kings College, London

Horrocks S, Anderson E, Salisbury C 2002 Systematic review of whether nurse practitioners working in primary care can provide equivalent care to doctors. British Medical Journal 324: 819–823

Jones D 1999 Nurse-led PMS pilots. In: Lewis R, Gillam S (eds) Transforming primary care: personal medical services in the new NHS. King's Fund Publishing, London: 41–50

Kane R, Keckhafer G, Flood S, Bershadsky B, Flood S, Siadaty M 2003 The effect of Evercare on hospital use. Journal of American Geriatrics Society 51: 1427–1434

King's Fund 2005 Patients at risk of rehospitalisation (PARR) case finding tool. Online: http://www.kingsfund. org.uk/health_topics/patients_at_ risk.html

Latter S, Maben J, Myall M, Courtenay M, Young A, Dunn N 2005 An evaluation of extended formulary independent nurse prescribing. University of Southampton, Southampton

Laurant M, Reeves D, Hermens R, Braspenning J, Grol R, Sibbald B 2007 Substitution of doctors by nurses in primary care. Cochrane Database of Systematic Reviews

Manley K 2000 Organisational culture and consultant nurse outcomes: part 2 nurse outcomes. Nursing Standard 14(37): 34–39

NHS Management Executive 1993 Nursing in primary health care: new world, new opportunities. HMSO, London

National Prescribing Centre 2007 A competency framework for shared decision-making with patients. Medicines Partnership Programme. NPC Plus, Staffordshire

Nursing and Midwifery Council 2006 Advanced nursing practice – update. Online: www.nmc.org/aArticle.aspx ?ArticleID=2068&keyword=advan ced%20and%20practice

Reveley S, Walsh M 2000 Preparation of advanced nursing roles. Nursing Standard 14(31): 42–45

Rogers E 2003 Health visitors and older people: 'thinking out of the box'. Community Practitioner 76(10): 381–385

Salisbury C 2003 Do NHS walk-in centres in England provide a model of integrated care? Journal of Integrated Care 3:1–7

Salisbury C, Chalder M, Manku-Scott T, et al 2002 The national evaluation of walk-in centres. Final report. University of Bristol

Scottish Executive 2001 Caring for Scotland – the strategy for nursing and midwifery in Scotland. The Stationery Office, Edinburgh

Stilwell B 1982 The nurse practitioner at work. Nursing Times 78(43): 1799–1803

Sturdy D 2004 Consultant nurses; changing the future. Age and Ageing 33: 327–328

Tomlinson B 1992 Report of the Inquiry into London's Health Service, Medical Education and Research. HMSO, London

Wall A 2005 Preparing the population for a healthier old age. Journal of Family Health Care 15(6): 163

Young G 2005 The nursing profession's coming of age. BMJ 331: 1415–1416

Recommended reading

Schober M, Affara F 2006 International Council of Nurses: Advanced nursing practice (Paperback). Blackwell Publishing, Oxford

This text explores key issues in advanced nursing practice, education, research and role development. An international flavour is evident throughout and readers will find this a useful resource when examining current and future developments in practice.

23

Advancing public health in nursing practice

Dianne Watkins and Judy Cousins

KEY ISSUES

- Contexts of practice and their influence on the nurses' contribution to public health
- A framework that outlines current public health practice within nursing
- Recognition of the challenges and opportunities for advancing public health in nursing practice

Introduction

The enduring contact that nurses have with all sections of society means that enormous potential exists for them to make positive and worthwhile contributions to existing and future societal health. Whether the focus of practice is on the management of chronic or acute conditions, supporting clients with complex needs and social issues, or preventive care, the core nursing values remain the same. That is, identifying and assessing need, planning and delivering evidence-based therapeutic interventions, coordinating care, referring to other agencies, reviewing and monitoring outcomes, and working in partnership with others. Through these core values all nurses promote and protect health and thereby contribute to the public health agenda in some way. This is in accordance with the *National Occupational Standards for the Practice of Public Health* (Skills for Health 2004: 6) which states the purpose of public health is to 'improve the health and well-being of the population, prevent disease and minimize its consequences, prolong valued life, and reduce inequalities in health'. Nurses working in a variety of settings will make a contribution to achiev-

ing this maxim through their everyday practice. This chapter will focus on contexts of practice and their influence on the nurses' involvement in public health. It will present a framework that represents nurses' current public health engagement, outline opportunities for nurses to further enhance their contribution to the public health agenda and discuss the limitations to them pursuing such work.

Contexts of nursing practice and their influence on public health

Government policy advocates that nurses working in all contexts should take an active role in public health. However, not all nurses recognize such opportunities. These perceptions should be reconsidered in light of the political value attributed to nurses' contribution in this area. Government documents such as *High Quality Care for All* (Department of Health 2008), *Designed for Life* (Welsh Assembly Government (WAG) 2005) and the *Designed to Realise our Potential* consultation paper (WAG 2007) outline the changing face of healthcare. The Welsh Assembly states that 'a predominant focus on health promotion, illness prevention, managing long-term chronic conditions, supporting self-care and providing services in a community environment' is the future nurse's role (WAG 2007: 4). The Department of Health (DH; 2004: 12) reiterates the need for public sector workers to 'increase their knowledge and understanding of health issues and this increased health awareness should permeate all areas of work so everyone understands how they can contribute to improving health'. Despite these political imperatives, some nurses may find it challenging to articulate how they address public health within the context of their work. This is understandable considering the diversity of settings in which nursing is delivered, which may either hinder or help opportunities for public health interventions.

Although it could be presumed that nursing practice delivered in a community setting provides a more conducive environment for public health practice, there are distinct differences in the opportunities afforded according to practice priorities, client groups and domain of specialism. Health visitors, occupational health nurses, school nurses and any other nurse recognized as having a predominant public health role and categorized under the specialist community public health nursing umbrella may make a larger contribution to the public health agenda, when compared to other community nurses. District nurses, practice nurses, community mental health nurses, community children's nurses and community learning disability nurses, whose domain of practice usually includes an acute/chronic care dimension as well as a preventative focus, may find their priorities centre on reactive rather than proactive interventions. Nurses based in secondary settings where they are involved in the provision of acute and chronic care may be presented with limited opportunities to participate in broader public health work, and their roles may focus on promoting lifestyle changes and disease management.

The literature pertaining to public health in nursing focuses on a range of activities. There is growing evidence to illustrate the contribution of specialist community public health nurses (SCPHNs) and other community nurses to the public health agenda. With regard to health visitors, qualitative findings from Bowes and Meehan Domokos (1998), Bowns et al (2000) and McIntosh and Shute (2006) all share a common theme: the value parents place on health visitor support. The most highly valued aspects of the service were the availability of health visitors as a source of information to reassure on common childcare issues and their role in facilitating opportunities to meet other parents through networking strategies. Quantitative evidence of the effectiveness of practice also exists – Elkan et al's (2000) systematic review and Bull et al's (2004) review of reviews concluded that the professional practice of health visiting enhances parenting abilities and parental management of common childhood dif-

ficulties; improves cognitive functioning in children of low birthweight; reduces incidence of childhood accidental injury; improves detection and management of postnatal depression; enables supportive environments for mothers; and improves breastfeeding rates. These beneficial outcomes may be due in part to health visitors' ability to discriminate their services positively to those clients with the greatest needs, as a means to ensure equity of service provision, while the availability of the service to all enables the profession to maintain a primary preventative approach to public health. Health visitors are recognized as the most likely group of nurses to engage in broader public health work (Whitehead 2003) and the principles they adhere to which include searching for health needs, stimulating an awareness of health needs, facilitation of health-enhancing behaviours and influencing policies affecting health place them in a unique position to undertake broad public health practice (Cowley and Frost 2006, United Kingdom Public Health Association).

Brooks et al (2007) identify how school nurses are ideally placed to deliver key public health interventions for children and adolescents. They are recognized to be effective links between education, health and social care and thereby make health services more accessible to pupils, parents, carers and staff (Department for Education and Skills, DH 2006). However, an evidence base to demonstrate the effectiveness of school nursing remains weak (Brooks et al 2007). Similarly, the Department for Work and Pensions et al (2005) recognize the potential for occupational health nursing to reduce health inequalities and improve the health of the working population but again evidence to support this is currently lacking. Both school nurses and occupational health nurses work with well populations and engage in primary preventive public health practice.

Community psychiatric nurses play a vital part in delivering behaviour modification programmes for people with problems associated with drug misuse and deliver early interventions for people with enduring mental health problems. With regard to community nursing, the Scottish Executive (2006) reported evidence of effectiveness in relation to community nurses reducing readmission rates through effective discharge planning and evidence of proactive risk assessment interventions conducted by community nurses reducing hospital admission in the over-75s. The Executive also revealed that there is some evidence that focused and prolonged community nursing interventions can improve the health of clients/patients or at least prevent them from getting worse.

The report (Scottish Executive 2006) highlighted that individuals and families value the relationships they are able to develop with nurses. This is an often overlooked yet significant aspect of public health working. For vulnerable individuals, in particular, their relationships with nurses may be the only contact available to them where they feel able to confide their concerns and seek support or assistance. In such circumstances individuals may disclose their deepest concerns; for example, women confide in health visitors their experiences of domestic violence, children disclose to school nurses their experiences of physical or sexual abuse, the learning disabled adult conveys inappropriate care to the learning disability nurse and it is the district nurse who is informed of the inadequate and abusive care experienced by the older, vulnerable adult. These are just some examples of how different nursing disciplines may act as key resources for different populations and make an important contribution to the public health agenda.

Hospital-based nurses working in a variety of roles in a secondary setting usually have less opportunity to encompass the total remit of public health within their work (Whitehead 2003), although it is recognized that there may be exceptions to this based on role and areas of practice. Early work undertaken by Watkins (1995) into factors which facilitate and inhibit health promotion in nursing practice found that implementation of health promotion initiatives were higher among nurses who worked in a community setting compared to hospital nurses. This may have been associated with the higher grade of staff, thus providing greater autonomy over practice, as well as the context of the patient's home providing a more conducive environment to discuss issues relating to the achievement of health. This view is supported by an early study by Caraher (1994: 544) who states that 'the institution of the hospital militates against the development of health promotion in a clinical setting as the organizational structure demands compliance and order'. The very acute nature of hospital work can be a constraint to promoting health, thus confounding the traditional role of the nurse in caring for the sick, although, as the patient moves to recuperation, opportunities to promote health may present. Political imperatives to move care into the community and care for only very acute conditions in a hospital environment may further inhibit opportunities for nurses to promote health in acute settings.

Public health in nursing practice – a framework of engagement

Public health in nursing practice is presented in this chapter as a 'framework of engagement' and divides nurses' work into biomedical public health practice and socio-political public health practice. Biomedical is defined as an individualistic approach that uses disease prevention or disease management as its focus. Its aim is to activate a behaviour change, or compliance, and in doing so utilizes a medical/preventative/behavioural approach to practice based on objective evidence. Education is usually the way in which interventions are delivered, and in the main there is limited consideration given to the determinants of health and how these influence decision-making (Blinkhorn 2002, Whitehead 2001, 2003). Behaviour change is seen as a simple process whereby the acquisition of knowledge will result in a change in lifestyle or adherence to prescribed outcomes. Socio-political includes consideration of the social and economic influences on health and aims to address these through using a more radical and empowering approach to public health practice. This includes empowerment of individuals and communities and is based on a philosophy of partnership working and collaboration. It aims to shape and influence healthy public health policy and to raise awareness through adopting a critical consciousness approach (Whitehead 2003).

There are advantages and disadvantages to basing public health practice on biomedical or socio-political perspectives and using approaches that mirror the underpinning philosophies (refer to Chapter 7 for further discussion of this). An evidence-based, pathogenic, biomedical approach to public health practice ignores social inequalities and as a result may marginalize those who are the most vulnerable (Ilett and Munro 2000). Adopting a socio-political perspective can provide insight into the impact of social circumstances on health and broaden thinking in public health practice. It can reveal differences in social groups, and discrimination and oppression; it can identify unmet needs and promote the establishment of services for the disadvantaged, thus making a contribution to reducing health inequalities. However, public health practice based on a biomedical perspective is the most common approach adopted by nurses and it is criticized for being individualistic and ignoring socio-economic, political and environmental issues (Whitehead 2001, 2003). While the importance of understanding these influences on health achievement cannot be ignored and should be considered in any public health work, it is often beyond the control of the nurse in a secondary setting to be able to directly influence these issues. This may be one reason why the nurse's contribution to public health is undervalued, although they play a very important part in promoting and supporting individuals through lifestyle changes and in managing chronic disease. These activities play a large part in helping to meet the public health agenda in the United Kingdom by minimizing the consequences of disease and prolonging valued life.

The framework presented in this chapter illustrates how hospital-based nurses engage in a greater proportion of biomedical public health compared to SCPHNs, who undertake more socio-political public health activity, although it is recognized that the practice of some SCPHNs retains a biomedical element. Community nurses are depicted as having slightly more socio-political public health within their practice than hospital-based nurses, but maintain a predominant focus on biomedical practice, the former being constrained by looking after clients/patients with acute and chronic health or social care needs.

To help identify public health in nursing practice, the framework takes guidance from the *National Occupational Standards for the Practice of Public Health* (Skills for Health 2004). This document outlines what is expected of someone whose work has a primary public health orientation (Box 23.1, Table 23.1) and this has been drawn upon to illustrate the degree of involvement in public health working of nurses who work within a hospital environment, community-based nurses and SCPHNs. The framework illustrates how nurses' current engagement in public health is largely dependent upon their practice foci, environment and mode of care delivery.

Public health in nursing practice – describing the framework of engagement

Domain 1

The first domain of practice includes all nurses who work within secondary care which is predominantly undertaken in a hospital setting. It is recognized that

---

Box 23.1

Public health practice

- Takes a population perspective
- Mobilizes the organized efforts of society and acts as an advocate for the public's health
- Enables people and communities to increase control over their own health and well-being
- Protects from and minimizes the impact of health risks to the population
- Ensures that preventative, treatment and care services are of high quality, based on evidence and are of best value

Adapted from the *National Occupational Standards for the Practice of Public Health* (Skills for Health 2004).

---

the public health practice of nurses in this section may be constrained by the environment and the provision of acute/chronic care. When matched against public health practice as defined by the *National Occupational Standards for the Practice of Public Health* (Skills for Health 2004), it is apparent that hospital-based nurses are able to undertake some of the fundamental public health activities described. For instance, acting on biological determinants of health and well-being is certainly within hospital nurses' remit and control. They are ideally positioned to offer information and support to patients on a range of conditions such as smoking cessation, diabetes management, and asthma control and prevention. Professional standards and regulations should ensure that any preventive treatment and care services provided by nurses are of high quality, based on evidence and of best value. Hospital-based nurses are in a prime position to advocate on behalf of those unable to advocate for themselves and are able to identify and refer those deemed vulnerable. The predominant health promotion approaches used are medical/behavioural/preventive. Many nurses may argue they use empowerment approaches. However, evidence from the literature suggests that the majority use persuasive, cajoling methods and that limited attention is paid to addressing the barriers or health determinants that may detrimentally affect health decisions (Whitehead 2001, 2002, 2003). West and Scott (2000) indicate that nurses are reluctant and lack the skills required to undertake socio-political activity.

Table 23.1 Public health in nursing practice: a framework for engagement

Domain 1 Hospital-based nurses	Domain 2 Community-based nurses	Domain 3 Specialist community public health nurses
	Socio-political public health practice	
Biomedical public health practice		
Emphasis – Biomedical with minimal socio-political public health practice	**Emphasis – Biomedical with limited socio-political public health practice**	**Emphasis – Biomedical and socio-political public health practice**
Acts on the biological determinants of health and well-being	Acts on the biological and social determinants of health and well-being	Acts on the biological, social, economic and environmental determinants of health and well-being
Ensures that preventive, treatment and care services are of high quality based on evidence	Ensures that preventive, treatment and care services are of high quality based on evidence	Ensures that preventive, treatment and care services are of high quality based on evidence
Utilizes a medical/preventive/behavioural approach to practice	Utilizes a medical/preventive/behavioural and an empowerment approach to practice	Utilizes a medical/preventive/behavioural and an empowerment approach to practice
Delivers education-based interventions	Enables individuals, families and groups to increase control over their health and well-being	Enables individuals, families, groups and communities to increase control over their health and well-being
Advocates for the health of individuals	Advocates for the public's health	Advocates for the public's health
	Protects and minimizes the impact of health risks to the population	Protects and minimizes the impact of health risks to the population
		Takes a community/population perspective
		Mobilizes the organized efforts of society
		Adopts a primary preventative approach

Adapted from the *National Occupational Standards for the Practice of Public Health* (Skills for Health 2004).

There are also other differences evident in the working practices between nurses positioned in domain 1 when compared against the second and third domains of the framework. For instance, it is extremely rare for hospital-based nurses to be involved in surveillance and assessment of the population's health and well-being, or to develop health programmes and services to reduce inequalities. As Whitehead (2003, 2004, 2006) points out, the majority of nurses may well carry out 'health education' in their work and their contribution to public health is usually work undertaken on an individual level with patients, promoting lifestyle and behaviour change.

It is recognized that not all hospital-based nurses will be confined to public health practice in the first domain; some may cover all three areas. Specialist and consultant nurses in cardiac rehabilitation, TB or oncology, for instance, have opportunities to practise across all three domains, as they engage with clients in primary and secondary settings.

Domain 2

The second domain of the framework illustrates the degree of involvement of a range of nurses who are usually community based, although outreach nurses, those who work across primary and secondary care settings and midwives also fall into this sphere. A large number of nurses from many different specialisms, including district nursing, practice nursing, community mental health nursing, community learning disability nursing, community children's nursing and midwifery, fit into this domain. Their work in socio-political public health is limited as these roles generally include a proportion of acute care, chronic care, social care, etc., although it is acknowledged this is dependent upon the position and role performed.

Similar to domain 1, when matched against public health practice as described in the *National Occupational Standards for the Practice of Public Health* (Skills for Health 2004), nurses in this second domain are capable of undertaking all the activities identified in that of domain 1. The majority of nurses categorized into this second domain undertake individualized public health work that focuses on disease prevention and disease management. They may work in promoting population health through involvement in immunization, screening and surveillance and in so doing protect and minimize risks to health (for more examples see Chapters 13 and 14). There are occasions when the practice of nurses placed within the second domain adopts a socio-political philosophy. For example, district nurses who work with homeless populations have opportunities to engage with the commissioning process to develop homeless healthcare services and in so doing advocate on behalf of a vulnerable, marginalized population (Queen's Nursing Institute 2007). Community psychiatric nurses may work in a general practice setting undertaking a primary preventive role in working to reduce mental health illness in the community.

The approaches used by nurses in this domain encompass medical/preventive/behavioural/educational and empowerment. Work at an individual level includes behaviour change programmes, dietary advice and support to the diabetic patient, etc. Community mental health nurses provide cognitive behavioural interventions for those with drug or alcohol problems or enduring mental health problems (for more illustrative examples see Chapter 18). Community learning disability nurses advocate on behalf of the disabled and community children's nurses are pivotal in assisting individuals in self-management of chronic conditions, which enables people to gain greater control over their health management (for further examples see Chapters 19 and 20). The context of practice, i.e. the home environment, affords more opportunity for nurses to observe the social, environmental and economic influences on health, and in so doing, it is likely to engender the use of more empowering approaches that take cognizance of these determinants. Working on a community level may also facilitate socio-political working based on community needs identified.

Domain 3

SCPHNs, including health visitors, school nurses, occupational health nurses or others who hold a recognized specialist public health nursing position, comprise those nursing disciplines in the third domain of the framework. In matching the work of the SCPHN with the areas of public health work outlined by Skills for Health (2004), it is evident that they incorporate much of this into their everyday practice. Nurses working in this domain utilize both biomedical and socio-political approaches to their practice. It is proposed that the latter dominates SCPHN working, although there is limited evidence to support this thinking (Whitehead 2003). The principles of practice previously alluded to within this chapter would indicate that the practice foci place SCPHNs in a unique position to be able to utilize socio-political type working and there is a close affiliation with the public health principles outlined by Skills for Health. However, SCPHNs form a small proportion of the nursing workforce in the United Kingdom and hence their potential to play a large part in advancing the public health agenda is constrained by both numbers and other dimensions of their role, which maintain an individual reactive focus.

The socio-political dimension of SCPHN practice is enhanced by the fact that they usually take a community/population perspective as well as an individual caseload. Health needs assessment of a population, workplace, community or school, and initiating and leading programmes to address needs identified, are a major part of their role. Such programmes can seek to address social and environmental factors that impact upon health, thus utilization of a socio-political perspective can be more easily adopted. Community development initiatives that focus on the social inclusion of the most marginalized in society are undertaken by health visitors, and individual empowerment strategies in schools that help children develop the skills of assertion and decision-making are examples of school nurses' involvement in public health (see Chapters 15 and 16 for further information). The occupational health nurse is ideally placed to undertake a health needs assessment in the workplace and to initiate programmes of prevention to avoid accidents and promote safety at work (see Chapter 17 for further information). Integral to the practice of SCPHNs is primary prevention, which includes working on an individual, family, group, community and a population level. They are sometimes involved in working with communities and groups in society in 'critical consciousness raising', and utilization of an empowering approach, which facilitates working to address a range of social/environmental/political factors influencing health and well-being. Through using a community development approach they mobilize organized efforts in society and advocate for health enhancement. It is these dimensions that distinguish SCPHNs from other nurses within the framework of public health engagement and place them in the third domain.

Challenges and opportunities – advancing public health in nursing practice

Opportunities exist for nurses to expand their public health work, although the challenges they face and further education they may require need to be recognized and addressed to enable practice to progress. Public health is an important part of every nurse's role in whatever setting, clinical specialty or environment that nursing takes place. The Nursing and Midwifery Council (NMC) code of conduct states that 'as a registered nurse, midwife or specialist community public health nurse, you must work with others to protect and promote the health and well-being of those in your care, their families and carers, and the wider community'. This is further confirmed by the Royal College of Nursing (RCN; 2007), who suggest that the contribution of nursing to public health is to:

- increase life expectancy through influencing healthy behaviours
- reduce health inequalities, e.g. targeting vulnerable populations to improve health outcomes and access to services
- improve population health, e.g. reducing obesity, alcohol abuse, improving sexual health behaviour
- increase the awareness of positive healthy behaviours in communities
- promote and develop social capital
- engage with individuals, families and communities to influence the design and development of services.

Modernising Nursing Careers (Department of Health et al 2006: 7) also discusses a need for nursing to change to meet the needs of society and to 'lay a greater emphasis on prevention, health promotion and supporting self-care'. In an effort to meet the objectives set by the government, the regulatory and professional body, a change in nurses' perception of their role in public health is required. It must no longer be seen as an 'add-on' activity that nurses cannot find time to include in their daily practice, but as a core component of *all* nursing practice embedded in all activities. In order to move towards effective and competent health promotion interventions in nursing practice, it is essential that:

1. There is a greater emphasis on the development of nurses' socio-political awareness and of the determinants of health and how they impact on health achievement.
2. There is a greater emphasis on development of 'empowering strategies' and their utilization in all nursing practice.
3. Attention is given to the further development of nurse leadership in public health practice.
4. Nurses are prepared and engage in further evaluation of public health work to demonstrate effectiveness and the contribution they make to the public health agenda in the United Kingdom.

Developing nurses' socio-political awareness and understanding of the determinants of health

It is recognized that not all nurses will be in a position to utilize socio-political and radical approaches to public health, as the very nature of their work and the environment in which they practise may inhibit socio-political action. However, adopting a 'socio-political perspective' is necessary for nurses working in *all settings* so that they understand the wider influences on health and acknowledge this in their public health practice, when working with individuals, families, groups, communities and populations. Even when using a predominantly biomedical approach where practice is disease orientated, there is a necessity to acknowledge health determinants and the important role they play in shaping people's behaviour and decisions relating to their health.

It is crucial that nurses understand the impact of factors such as unemployment, social exclusion, poverty, gender, stress, violence, inadequate housing, etc. on health and to consider how their roles can contribute to reducing inequalities in health experiences. Kendall and Lissauer (2003) describe the skills necessary to undertake roles in public health practice as the ability to appreciate how a range of determinants affect health; to access appropriate knowledge and use it to guide practice; to make links between individual patients' and clients' needs and those of the wider community; and to promote social capital. Adopting socio-political awareness to biomedical approaches will enable nurses to address the social, environmental and emotional needs of individuals, families, groups and populations as well as their physical ones.

Development of the skills required to practise public health work effectively and competently requires a radical rethink of how nurses are prepared for their roles. Although current pre-registration educational programmes that prepare nurses of the future include a focus on public health, perhaps the emphasis remains on the provision of acute care and students may find this more attractive and exciting then learning about empowering people to give up smoking. It is acknowledged that at a post-registration level public health working in its many guises forms the majority of the curriculum for SCPHNs and a strong public health emphasis is present in programmes to prepare the community nurses outlined in previous chapters within this book. However, there remains potential to develop this further and to debate in greater depth the value of socio-political action, particularly as literature determining the effectiveness of these nurses in public health is largely centred on individualistic practice (Blinkhorn 2002, West and Scott 2000, Whitehead 2003).

Role modelling has an important effect on learning and what is currently missing in hospital and community nursing environments is a proliferation of role models who adopt socio-political approaches to their practice. Investment is required if we are to change nurses' and others' perceptions of the role nursing can play in taking forward the public health agenda.

Developing empowerment strategies and their use in nursing

Approaches used in nursing to promote the health of the public should focus on the principles of empowerment as outlined in Chapter 7, which acknowledge and respect the patient's involvement in decision-making (Rafael 1999, Smith et al 1999, Whitehead 2001, 2003). These principles should be adopted regardless of clinical specialism or context of care, and to enable nurses to undertake such activities, adequate preparation is required. For some nurses this way of working is not new;

however, others may require further development of their knowledge and skills to facilitate working in an empowering way with confidence and competence.

An opportunity exists for nurses to lead on, and make explicit, therapeutic ways to increase user involvement through partnership working initiatives. Nurses need to appreciate that promoting user involvement is not necessarily about relinquishing control to users but on changing the nature of care, where practitioners make more transparent their decision-making processes and the resources available to support those decisions, thus enabling users to become part of that process (Andrews et al 2004). For clients or groups to be actively involved in the design and evaluation of healthcare services, nurses will be required to develop new relationships that not only value user involvement but that more accurately reflect their civil and human rights.

Kendall and Lissauer (2003) discuss how practitioners, as well as engaging service users in healthcare decisions, also need to enable users to take greater responsibility for their own healthcare management. Such a philosophical shift will undoubtedly prove challenging to both practitioners and patients/clients alike, as arguably there has long existed a culture of 'expert knows best' in the NHS. Nurses will need confidence in their professional knowledge and skills 'so that they do not hide behind professional veneers but instead, find ways to engage and involve their patients/clients in better balanced relationships' (Welsh Assembly Government 2007: 5). Similarly, patients/clients, who in the past have so easily slipped into passive, dependent roles, will have to adjust to the responsibility of becoming more involved in decisions concerning their health and well-being. Ultimately, both professionals and service users will need support and guidance in order to rise to the challenge of what may be a small yet significant revolution in healthcare delivery.

Developing nurse leadership in public health practice

Areas where nurses have already demonstrated abilities to lead on public health include management of minor illness via NHS Direct and walk-in centres. Nurse prescribing is now well established and consultant nurses, community matrons, specialist nurse practitioners and advanced nurse practitioners operate in primary care environments, contributing to public health across the social strata and age range of the population. Future areas for developing public health practice include leading within and across professional boundaries, ensuring seamless client-centred care, and supporting clients to develop a greater sense of responsibility for their health and care, including self-management of chronic, long-term illnesses (Kendall and Lissauer 2003). Such outcomes may be accomplished through advocating for and involving users through partnership working, and through demonstrating effective and responsive interventions.

As well as comprehensive knowledge and understanding of public health principles and approaches, nurses who lead public health will require advanced leadership abilities that allow them to work autonomously and in partnerships with confidence and competence in order to provide safe and responsive care. There is an emphasis and particular importance attributed to partnership and collaboration in public health working. This will require nurses to possess knowledge of factors that promote or hinder joint working relationships to better enable them to develop effective partnership opportunities. Understanding the roles and responsibilities of others and negotiating tensions in power-based relationships are just some of the skills required by nurses when working in interprofessional or multidisciplinary teams, or across agencies to address socio-political factors (see Chapter 21 for further information on partnership working in health and social care). Lissauer and Kendall (2002) state that public health advanced practice also requires an ability to span medical and social dimensions of health, and to work with practitioners who practise according to different health models and paradigms. Interprofessional collaboration with such practitioners will be crucial and will require nurses in the future to work across professional boundaries and share leadership with others. The NHS Institute for Innovation and Improvement (2003), in their 'Leadership Qualities Framework', propose that sophisticated communication skills will be needed to facilitate such practice as practitioners will be required to articulate overviews of community health needs and priorities and raise awareness of the needs of the most marginalized and vulnerable, such as parents with learning disabilities, looked after children, asylum seekers, travellers, or disadvantaged ethnic minority groups. Advocating for the most marginalized in society

should be a central feature of public health and community nursing.

Demonstrating effectiveness and the contribution of nursing to public health

In the present fiscally challenged and competitive NHS, it is essential that nurses are capable of evaluating their public health practice effectively and demonstrating whether the services they provide are valued by service users and meet their needs. Beresford and Branfield (2006) remind that measures to assess effectiveness often fall short of considerations of service users, despite the political rhetoric behind the need for services to be developed according to and around service user requirements. Even when this does occur, it is not always according to quality indicators as perceived by service users, but instead, according to professional considerations of what constitutes quality.

This means that professionals may define outcomes of service interventions positively when they are delivered in, for example, a timely fashion, according to specific criteria and result in predetermined demonstrable outcomes. Indeed, professionals are encouraged to adopt such approaches to practice evaluation (for example, see the 2008 Queen's Nursing Institute briefing paper no. 9 on evaluating outcomes) and from a professional perspective, little is wrong with this. However, outcome measures such as *involvement and confidence in decision-making, treated with respect and raised self-esteem and confidence* gained through empowerment strategies are not types of information routinely collected, even though they are in fact some of the most important issues to service users. Beresford and Branfield (2006) consider how these broader civil and human rights orientated measures should underpin any strategy aiming to evaluate the effectiveness of services. Information on improved choice of and accessibility to services, improvements in health status, well-being, or social inclusion of marginalized populations will better enable nurses to demonstrate their wider contribution to public health and such an approach will also work to place service users squarely in the centre of service planning. A challenge exists for nurses to develop robust means to capture such information alongside more traditional forms of evaluation.

Regardless of where on a continuum of public health practice hospital, public health or community nurses work, what is evident is a need for all to make transparent the value of their public health interventions. Familiarization with public health language is a useful first step. The discourse associated with public health working is characterized by terminology such as enabling, empowering, advocating, involving, supporting, informing, including, etc., and these help to describe interventions which aim to promote equality and equity of healthcare experience, promote user involvement and collaborative working, promote inclusion of marginalized individuals, groups or populations, and describe non-judgemental and anti-discriminatory practice. Use of discourse associated with public health working when describing care and health-enhancing interventions enables practitioners to illustrate how public health principles and approaches form part of day-to-day practice and enable nurses to articulate their contribution to the public health agenda.

All nurses must demonstrate their contribution to the public health agenda through raising awareness of the range and diversity of public health working activities that they are able to undertake. Such action would enable nurses to market themselves as leading participants in the multiprofessional world of public health, thereby raising their professional profile.

Conclusion

This chapter aimed to provide an overview of nurses' current practice in public health and to identify how context may influence the contribution they can make. It has attempted to illuminate the differences between nurses working in an institutional setting and community-based nurses. This differentiation is not always easy, as it is dependent on role and practice foci; thus delineation between these groups is arbitrary. The authors present a framework of engagement which is matched with the National *Occupational Standards for the Practice of Public Health* (Skills for Health 2004) principles of public health working. Tentative conclusions are arrived at and recommendations made as to how public health in nursing practice may be developed further. The issue of biomedical and socio-political philosophies is debated and the authors present a view that centres on nurses incorporating a 'socio-political perspective' into their public health work that includes empowerment strategies. These are considered integral to the success of nurses in their quest to become effective in public health practice. What is presented is a limited view that aims to promote further debate and discussion among academics and practitioners who are actively engaged in the world of public health.

SUMMARY

- All nurses possess qualities and abilities which enable them to contribute to public health.
- For those practitioners unable to adopt socio-political approaches to practice, gaining a greater appreciation of this philosophy will help broaden understanding of factors which impact upon an individual's ability to react to health promotion advice.
- Nurses should assume greater leadership in public health and work across boundaries.

DISCUSSION

1. What opportunities to develop socio-political working exist in your work?
2. What barriers would prevent this?
3. How would you adopt a greater emphasis on using empowerment strategies in your practice?

References

Andrews J, Manthorpe J, Watson R 2004 Involving older people in intermediate care. Journal of Advanced Nursing 46(3): 303–310

Beresford P, Branfield F 2006 Developing inclusive partnerships: user-defined outcomes, networking and knowledge – a case study. Health and Social Care in the Community 14(5): 436–444

Blinkhorn AS 2002 Editorial. Health Education Journal 61: 195

Bowes AM, Meehan Domokos T 1998 Health visitors work in a multiethnic society: a qualitative study of social exclusion. Journal of Social Policy 27(4): 489–506

Bowns IR, Crofts DJ, Williams TS, Rigby AS, Hall DMB, Haining RP 2000 Levels of satisfaction of 'low-risk' mothers with their current health visiting service. Journal of Advanced Nursing 31(4): 805–811

Brooks F, Kendall S, Bunn F, Bindler R, Bruya M 2007 The school nurse as navigator of the school health journey: developing the theory and evidence for policy. Primary Health Care Research & Development 8: 226–234

Bull J, McCormick G, Swann C, Mulvihill C 2004 Ante- and post-natal home-visiting programmes: a review of reviews. Health Development Agency, London

Caraher M 1994 A sociological approach to health promotion for nurses in an institutional setting. Journal of Advanced Nursing 20(3): 544–551

Cowley S, Frost M 2006 The principles of health visiting: opening the door to public health practice. CPHVA/ UKSC, London

Department for Education and Skills, Department of Health 2006 Looking for a school nurse. The Stationery Office, London

Department of Health 2004 Choosing health. The Stationery Office, London

Department of Health 2008 High quality care for all: NHS next stage review final report. The Stationery Office, London

Department of Health, Social Services and Public Safety; Scottish Executive; Welsh Assembly Government; Department of Health 2006 Modernising nursing careers. The Stationery Office, London

Department for Work and Pensions, Department of Health, Health and Safety Executive, Scottish Office, Welsh Assembly 2005 Working for health. Online: http://www. workingforhealth.gov.uk

Elkan R, Robinson JJA, Blair M, Williams D, Brummell K 2000 The effectiveness of health services: the case of health visiting. Health and Social Care in the Community 8(1): 74–79

Ilett R, Munro E 2000 Introducing the social model of health. In: Craig PM, Lindsey GM (eds) Nursing for public health. Churchill Livingstone, Edinburgh

Kendall L, Lissauer R 2003 The future health worker. Institute for Public Policy Research, London

Lissauer R, Kendall L 2002 New practitioners in the future health service: exploring new roles for practitioners in primary and intermediate care. Institute for Public Policy Research, London

McIntosh JB, Shute L 2006 The process of health visiting and its contribution to parental support in the Starting Well demonstration project. Health and Social Care in the Community 15(1): 77–85

NHS Institute for Innovation and Improvement 2003 NHS leadership qualities framework. Online: http:// www.nhsleadershipqualities.nhs.uk/ portals/0/the_framework.pdf

Queen's Nursing Institute 2007 Briefing: evaluating outcomes (No. 8). QNI, London

Queen's Nursing Institute 2008 Briefing: evaluating outcomes (No. 9). QNI, London

Rafael F 1999 The politics of health promotion: influences on public health promoting nursing practice in Ontario, Canada from Nightingale to the nineties. Advances in Nursing Sciences 22(1): 23–39

Royal College of Nursing 2007 Nurses as partners in delivering public health: a paper to support the contribution to public health, developed by an alliance of organisations. RCN, London

Scottish Executive 2006 Improving health by providing visible, accessible, consistent care: the review of nursing in the community in Scotland. TSO, SE, Edinburgh

Skills for Health 2004 National occupational standards for the practice of public health. The Stationery Office, London

Smith P, Masterson A, Lloyd-Smith S 1999 Health promotion versus disease and care: failure to establish 'blissful charity' in British nurse education and practice. Social Science and Medicine 48: 227–239

United Kingdom Public Health Association 2007 Health visiting and public health: a paper by the UK Public Health Association's Special Interest Group on Health Visiting and Public Health. Online: http:// www.ukpha.org.uk/media/HV%20 SIG%20docs/hv&phpaper.doc

Watkins D 1995 Factors facilitating and inhibiting health promotion in nursing practice. Unpublished Masters Dissertation, UWCM, Cardiff

Welsh Assembly Government 2005 Designed for life: creating world class health and social care for Wales in the 21st century. Wales Assembly Government, Cardiff

Welsh Assembly Government 2007 'Designed to Realise Our Potential': a 'beliefs and action' statement for nurses, midwives and specialist community public health nurses in Wales for 2007 and beyond: a consultation paper. HMSO, Cardiff

West E, Scott C 2000 Nursing in the public sphere: breaching the boundary between research and policy. Journal of Advanced Nursing 32: 817–824

Whitehead D 2001 Health education, behavioural change and social psychology: nursing's contribution to health promotion? Journal of Advanced Nursing 34: 822–832

Whitehead D 2002 The 'health promotional' role of a pre-registration student cohort in the UK: a grounded theory study. Nurse Education in Practice 2: 197–207

Whitehead D 2003 Incorporating socio-political health promotion activities in clinical practice. Journal of Clinical Nursing 12: 668–677

Whitehead D 2004 Health promotion and health education: advancing the concepts. Journal of Advanced Nursing 47: 311–320

Whitehead D 2006 Health promotion in the practice setting: findings from a review of clinical issues. Worldviews on Evidence-Based Nursing 3(4): 165–184

Index

Note: page numbers in *italic* refer to figures, tables, boxes or case studies